Viral Vectors for Vaccine Delivery

Scrivener Publishing
100 Cummings Center, Suite 541J
Beverly, MA 01915-6106

Publishers at Scrivener
Martin Scrivener (martin@scrivenerpublishing.com)
Phillip Carmical (pcarmical@scrivenerpublishing.com)

Viral Vectors for Vaccine Delivery

Edited by

Vivek P. Chavda
Dept. of Pharmaceutics and Pharmaceutical Technology, L. M. College of Pharmacy, Ahmedabad, Gujarat, India

and

Vasso Apostolopoulos
School of Health and Biomedical Sciences, RMIT University, Melbourne, Victoria, Australia

Scrivener Publishing

WILEY

This edition first published 2025 by John Wiley & Sons, Inc., 111 River Street, Hoboken, NJ 07030, USA and Scrivener Publishing LLC, 100 Cummings Center, Suite 541J, Beverly, MA 01915, USA

For more information about Scrivener publications please visit www.scrivenerpublishing.com.

Wiley Global Headquarters
111 River Street, Hoboken, NJ 07030, USA

For details of our global editorial offices, customer services, and more information about Wiley products visit us at www.wiley.com.

Library of Congress Cataloging-in-Publication Data

ISBN 978-1-394-27153-5

Front cover image courtesy of Adobe Firefly
Cover design by Russell Richardson

Set in size of 11pt and Minion Pro by Manila Typesetting Company, Makati, Philippines

Printed in the USA

10 9 8 7 6 5 4 3 2 1

Contents

Preface

The development of vaccines has been a cornerstone of public health, preventing countless diseases and saving millions of lives. However, traditional vaccine approaches often face limitations, such as the need for multiple doses, the potential for adverse reactions, and the inability to induce long-lasting immunity against complex pathogens. In recent decades, viral vectors have emerged as a promising alternative, revolutionizing the field of vaccine development.

This book provides a comprehensive overview of viral vectors and their applications in vaccine delivery. Its chapters explore various aspects of viral vector technology, from the basic principles of viral vector construction to the latest advancements in gene editing and manufacturing.

To begin, the book introduces the concept of viral vectors and their advantages over traditional vaccine platforms. Subsequent chapters delve into the intricacies of viral vector construction, including the selection of appropriate viral backbones, the insertion of foreign genes, and the optimization of vector design for maximum immunogenicity. The role of adjuvants in enhancing the efficacy of viral vector vaccines is also discussed, highlighting their importance in boosting immune responses and improving vaccine potency.

The next section explores the different types of viral vectors used for vaccine delivery, including replication-competent and non-replicating vectors. Replication-competent vectors mimic natural infections, inducing a robust immune response, while non-replicating vectors are safer but may require multiple doses. Genetically modified viral vectors, such as those engineered for targeted delivery or enhanced antigen presentation, are also covered.

The book further delves into the specific applications of viral vectors in vaccine development, including their use in veterinary medicine and the development of vaccines against emerging infectious diseases. The advantages and challenges associated with viral vector vaccines are discussed, along with the commercially available viral vector vaccines and the future potential of this technology.

This book serves as a valuable resource for researchers, scientists, and healthcare professionals working in the field of vaccine development. It provides a comprehensive understanding of viral vector technology and its potential to address the challenges of vaccine design and delivery. By exploring the latest advancements and future prospects, this book aims to contribute to the development of safer, more effective, and more accessible vaccines for a healthier global population. The editors are grateful to everyone who has supported their work and also wish to thank Martin Scrivener and Scrivener Publishing for their support and publication.

Editors
Vivek P. Chavda
Vasso Apostolopoulos

1

Introduction to Viral Vectors

Anjali P. Bedse[1]*, Suchita P. Dhamane[2], Shilpa S. Raut[1], Komal P. Mahajan[3] and Kajal P. Baviskar[4]

[1]Department of Pharmaceutics, K K Wagh College of Pharmacy, Nashik, Maharashtra, India
[2]Department of Pharmaceutics, JSPM's Jayawantrao Sawant College of Pharmacy & Research, Hadapsar, Pune, Maharashtra, India
[3]Department of Pharmacology, K K Wagh College of Pharmacy, Nashik, Maharashtra, India
[4]Department of Pharmaceutical Chemistry, K K Wagh College of Pharmacy, Nashik, Maharashtra, India

Abstract

Viral vector manipulation is the most effective way to transfer genes to modify a specific cell type or tissue. Therapeutic genes can also be expressed through this technique. Many virus species are currently being studied for their ability to introduce genes into cells for transgenic expression, which can be either temporary or permanent. These comprise herpes simplex viruses, baculoviruses, adeno-associated viruses, poxviruses, γ-retroviruses, lentiviruses, and adenoviruses (Ads). The selection of a virus for regular clinical usage depends upon several factors, including transgenic expression effectiveness, production ease, safety, toxicity, and stability. An introduction to the general properties of viral vectors frequently used in gene transfer, as well as their benefits and drawbacks for gene therapy applications, is given in this chapter.

***Keywords*:** Viral vectors, gene transfer, transgene expression, adenoviruses, gene therapy

**Corresponding author*: dranjalibedse@gmail.com

Vivek P. Chavda and Vasso Apostolopoulos (eds.) Viral Vectors for Vaccine Delivery, (1–24) © 2025 Scrivener Publishing LLC

1.1 Introduction

For decades, traditional vaccination platforms such as live-attenuated or killed viral vaccines have been utilized effectively in inducing long-term immunity to various kinds of pathogenic human diseases. However, for many human infections, such vaccination platforms, especially live-attenuated vaccines, are unsuitable for human usage due to safety issues, low efficacy, or basic impracticality [1].

In a phase 1 clinical trial of a live-attenuated dengue virus vaccine, side effects produced by the vaccine virus strain's under-attenuation were observed [2].

Certain infections, including the Ebola and Marburg viruses belonging to the Filoviridae family, are so deadly that live-attenuated vaccines are not even considered because the risk of the vaccine strain becoming under-attenuated or reverting to a pathogenic state would be too great. The persistent need for developing novel, safer, and more effective vaccine platforms has led researchers to explore alternate approaches for vaccine production, including DNA vaccines, viral-vectored immunizations, and recombinant protein subunit vaccines. One of the most promising platforms for recombinant vaccine research is the viral vector. A viral vector is comparable to a small delivery device that can transport genetic material to the cell nucleus. The viral vector has the genetic material loaded and packaged into it. The purpose of using viral vectors for vaccination is to introduce the target pathogen's naturally existing antigens to the immune system without the infectious pathogen [1].

Viral vectors can be categorized into two main groups based on their genomic behavior within host cells: those that integrate into the host cellular chromatin, such as oncoretroviruses and lentiviruses, and those that primarily exist as extrachromosomal episomes within the cell nucleus, including adeno-associated viruses (AAV), adenoviruses (Ads), and herpesviruses. This classification is crucial for understanding their mechanisms of action and potential applications in gene therapy and vaccination. The selection of viral vectors for clinical use is influenced by several critical factors, including stability, toxicity, safety, ease of manufacturing, and the efficiency of transgene expression. These considerations ensure that the chosen vector is suitable for the intended therapeutic application while minimizing risks to the patient. Viral vectors encompass both RNA and DNA viruses, which can be further divided based on their genomic structure into single-stranded (ss) and double-stranded (ds) genomes. For instance, retroviruses typically possess an ssRNA genome that must be reverse-transcribed into dsDNA before integration into the host genome. In contrast, Ads are characterized by their dsDNA genomes and are known for their ability to transiently express genes without integrating into the host genome.

The distinct properties of each viral vector type contribute to their effectiveness in various therapeutic contexts. For example, retroviral vectors are particularly effective for stable gene integration in dividing cells, while AAVs are favored for their low immunogenicity and ability to transduce both dividing and nondividing cells. Ads offer high transduction efficiency and large packaging capacity, making them suitable for delivering larger genetic payloads [3, 4].

1.2 Baculovirus Vectors

A safe, nontoxic, non-integrative vector with a high replication capability is the baculovirus. Since baculoviruses may infect both latent and growing cells, they are also a highly versatile, inexpensive vector with a wide tissue and host tropism. Additionally, they are more biosafe since they only reproduce in insect cells—not in mammalian cells. Baculoviruses are a desirable choice for gene transfer due to their advantageous characteristics. Regenerative medicine, anticancer treatments, and vaccine development have all benefited greatly from the substantial advancements made in using baculoviruses in gene therapy. Nowadays, the main applications of baculoviruses are in the manufacture of vaccines and recombinant proteins. New avenues for the production of vaccines of the next generation have been made possible by the stimulation of mucosal and systemic immune responses by baculoviruses through oral or intranasal delivery. This human-friendly virus will undoubtedly be promoted as a viable vector for clinical applications if further knowledge about the biology of baculoviruses and their interactions with non-native hosts is obtained [5, 6].

The term "baculovirus" refers to the unique rod-shaped viral particles produced in infected insect cells, known as occlusion bodies. Baculoviruses are frequently employed in insect cell culture systems as expression vectors. The baculovirus can be modified to include foreign genes in its genome, which allows the virus to infect insect cells. This makes it possible to produce significant quantities of recombinant proteins for scientific or commercial uses.

Baculoviruses have been assessed as potential carriers of antigens to elicit immunological responses, making them attractive candidates for the production of vaccines [5].

1.3 Adenovirus Vectors

Adenoviral vectors (AdVs) have emerged as the most widely used vehicle for gene therapy in cancer treatment. These vectors are also employed in vaccination strategies to deliver foreign antigens and in various gene therapy applications. In many cases, AdVs are engineered to be replication-defective; this involves the deletion of essential viral genes, which are then replaced with a genetic cassette that expresses a therapeutic gene. Such modifications allow for targeted gene delivery while minimizing the risk of viral replication in healthy tissues. In the context of cancer therapy, replication-competent AdVs, known as oncolytic vectors, have been developed. These vectors are specifically designed to replicate within cancer cells, utilizing the natural lytic cycle of the virus to induce cell death selectively. By exploiting the unique vulnerabilities of tumor cells, oncolytic Ads can effectively target and destroy malignant tissues while sparing normal cells.

Numerous clinical trials have demonstrated the safety and therapeutic efficacy of both replication-defective and replication-competent AdVs. For instance, studies have shown that these vectors can elicit robust immune responses against tumors, enhancing their potential as therapeutic agents. The ability of AdVs to infect a broad range of cell types and their capacity to induce strong cellular and humoral immune responses further support their utility in cancer treatment. Moreover, AdVs can be engineered to express immune-modulatory molecules or tumor-specific antigens, which can enhance antitumor immunity. This versatility makes them suitable not only for direct cancer therapies but also for combination strategies with existing treatments such as immune checkpoint inhibitors [7].

Although Ads have been used as gene delivery vehicles since the invention of gene therapy, Ad vaccines, like mRNA vaccines, are a more recent approach [8, 9]. The viral replication genes E1 and/or E3 are removed and substituted for the desired transgene, like an antigen, to form a vector. This prevents the virus from expressing the desired antigen and stops it from replicating its genome after infection. In comparison to mRNA vaccines, Ads have a number of advantages, such as the previously mentioned low cost and thermostability [10].

Ad vector vaccinations generally elicit robust transgenic antigen-specific cellular (specifically, $CD8^+$ T cells) and/or humoral immune responses, making them immunogenic vaccines [11].

The potential of AdVs to elicit a potent and well-balanced immune response makes them ideal for use in the COVID-19 pandemic. These vectors have been studied as vaccine agents for a variety of infectious diseases

[12, 13]. Early AdV systems faced biological challenges, but the distinct molecular characteristics of these vectors facilitated the rapid development of vaccines with complex designs [10, 14].

AdVs have the benefit of high infection effectiveness and a significant cargo limit. AdVs have a significant disadvantage in that they are highly cytotoxic; nevertheless, this characteristic can be useful when the vectors are employed as oncolytic viruses. Although there are drawbacks of transient gene expression, safety benefits outweigh them as gene expression on unintentional targets would be transient [14].

AdVs are categorized into first, second, and third generations based on their genetic makeup. First-generation AdVs can only be produced using a packaging cell line that expresses the E1 protein; they are not capable of self-replication. The most widely utilized packaging cells are human embryonic kidney 293 cells.

Most human cells produce E1A-like proteins; therefore, even first-generation AdVs with deleted E1 sections can cause robust host immune responses and persistent cytotoxicity in transduced host cells. Another strategy was to develop a second-generation Ad without E2 and E4 deletions in order to lessen the host cell's immune response to the vector. The E2 section encodes genes related to Ad replication, while the E4 region encodes regulatory proteins related to DNA transcription.

Second-generation Ads continue to elicit host immune responses and reduce transgenic expression in target cells by expressing adenoviral proteins through the remaining genes. The production of third-generation AdVs, often referred to as "helper-dependent vectors," involves co-introducing a "helper adenovirus"—a virus that carries the genes required for replication—into the packed cells. Third-generation Ads can be contaminated by helper Ads, and self-propagating Ads can result from homologous recombination between helper viruses and packing cells [15].

Gendicine, a recombinant human p53 adenovirus, was approved by the China Food and Drug Administration (CFDA) in 2003 as a first-in-class gene therapy product for head and neck cancer treatment. Gendicine is a biological medication that can be given in three different ways: intravascular infusion, intracavity, or minimally invasive intratumoral injection. The wild-type (wt) p53 protein produced by Gendicine-transduced cells has a tumor-suppressive role in response to cellular stress. It induces apoptosis, senescence, and/or autophagy, depending on the conditions of the cellular stress. It also promotes cell-cycle arrest and DNA repair. Gentacine has demonstrated notably higher response rates when combined with radiation and chemotherapy than when used with traditional therapies alone. Additionally, its safety record is really good. Apart from head and neck cancer, other cancer types and illness stages have also been effectively treated with metronidazole. No major side effects have been noted, with the exception of 50 to 60% of patients experiencing vector-associated transient fever, which persisted for a few hours [16].

1.4 Poxvirus Vectors

Poxviruses are a large, complex virus belonging to the Poxviridae family that can affect both vertebrates and invertebrates. Poxviruses are comparatively large and oval-shaped viruses. Poxviridae is subdivided into two subfamilies: Chordopoxvirinae (vertebrate poxviruses) and Entomopoxvirinae (insect poxviruses). The subfamily Chordopoxvirinae has been further divided into nine genera, four of which contain viruses that cause diseases in humans (Orthopoxvirus, Parapoxvirus, Molluscipoxvirus, and Yatapoxvirus). Smallpox and molluscum contagiosum are diseases that affect humans, whereas the other two are zoonotic infections. The virion is enclosed, and the genome is protected in a protein sheath. Among all DNA viruses, poxviruses are distinct in that they can only reproduce outside of the nucleus, in the cytoplasm of the host cell. To encode the various enzymes and proteins involved in viral DNA replication and gene transcription, a large genome is therefore required [17].

Poxvirus infections can cause lesions, skin nodules, or a severe rash. Variola virus, the causative agent of smallpox, caused enormous morbidity and mortality in human communities before its effective eradication. The smallpox vaccine, which was essential in the eradication of smallpox, is based on the vaccinia virus (VV), a poxvirus closely related to the variola virus. The vaccination protected against smallpox without developing it. Though smallpox is no longer around, other poxviruses can infect humans. Monkeypox and VVs are two examples. Monkeypox is related to smallpox but produces a less severe sickness in humans. The smallpox vaccine is based on the VV.

Poxviruses have been utilized as vectors for foreign gene expression in mammalian cells. Modified poxviruses, such as modified vaccinia Ankara (MVA), are used as vaccine vectors in the treatment of a variety of infectious diseases. Poxviruses are open to genetic modification because of their enormous genomes. This has been used for various applications, including gene delivery vector application in research and the development of recombinant vaccines [18].

The ability of poxviruses to produce cellular and humoral immunity, their huge genome size with several immunomodulatory genes, and their tolerance for significant heterologous gene insertions are the major characteristics that make them good antigen delivery platforms and vaccine vectors. Initially, the VV was designed to express heterologous genes. Later, with promising results, the potential of using swinepox, parapoxvirus, and avipoxvirus as vectors was additionally examined. In order to mitigate the safety risks associated with wt poxviruses, a variety of severely attenuated strains with replication defects have been created, primarily by repetitive cycles in cell culture [19].

The thymidine kinase (TK) gene has been specifically targeted for insertional inactivation in the majority of recombinant poxviruses produced too far. This involves introducing a heterologous gene into the TK locus within the poxvirus genome. Poxviridae family recombinant VV vectors proliferate and transcribe their genome in infected cells' cytosol. Thus, it is important that viral DNA is incorporated into the host's genome. VV is the preferred vector for transient gene expression since it infects almost all types of mammalian cells. Its massive, adaptable genome makes it possible to insert large DNA segments up to 25 kb in size. This virus has three distinct stages in its infectious cycle. Genes in the early phase code for enzyme proteins, while genes in the intermediate phase control the expression of genes in the late phase, which codes for structural proteins. Promoting the expression of the inserted gene of interest is possible by means of the 7.5-kDa protein that encodes the promoter gene, which is active during both the early and late phases of infection. The wt VV is cytolytic, while less virulent poxvirus vectors like MVA or fowl pox virus are commonly used for cell transduction.

To create safer and more versatile poxvirus-vectored vaccine candidates, other immunomodulatory genes have also been used recently. In heterologous prime-boost vaccination regimens, in which poxvirus vectors are combined with other killed or DNA vaccine formulations, it has been demonstrated that poxvirus vectors are highly effective. The number of vaccinations based on the poxvirus has been approved for use against various animal infections, such as the canine distemper virus (CDV), rabies virus (RabV), avian influenza virus (AIV), and West Nile virus (WNV) [19].

VV is a member of the poxvirus family. An icosahedral papovavirus is called Simian virus-40(SV40). Recently, alterations have been implemented in Simian virus-40 (SV40) to enable it to serve as a vector for gene delivery. Gene transfer vectors that exhibit certain distinctive characteristics include recombinant SV40 (rSV40) vectors: SV40 is a widely recognized virus, and it is simple to create nonreplicative vectors at titers of 1012 IU/ml. Additionally, these successfully transduce both dormant and proliferating cells, are nonimmunogenic, and provide a broad variety of cell types with sustained transgene expression. The limited ability to clone viruses and the potential risks associated with the random integration of the viral genome into the host genome are currently the drawbacks of using rSV40 vectors for gene therapy [20].

1.5 Herpes Virus Vectors

Herpesviruses are well known for being able to cause latent infections. Some cells may experience the virus going dormant after an initial active infection, and subsequent reactivations can result in recurring infections. Many individuals carry herpes viruses without showing any symptoms, and these kinds of viruses are very widespread. Some people, particularly those with compromised immune systems, may experience more severe herpesvirus infections and consequent complications [21].

Alphaherpesvirinae, Betaherpesvirinae, and Gammaherpesvirinae are the three subfamilies of the nine herpes viruses that are known to infect humans (Figure 1.1).

Herpesviruses with reduced virulence are engineered to carry heterologous immunogens that specifically target a number of hazardous and important infections. These compounds are remarkable for their ability to elicit humoral and cell-mediated immune responses, as well as to accept large amounts of foreign DNA.

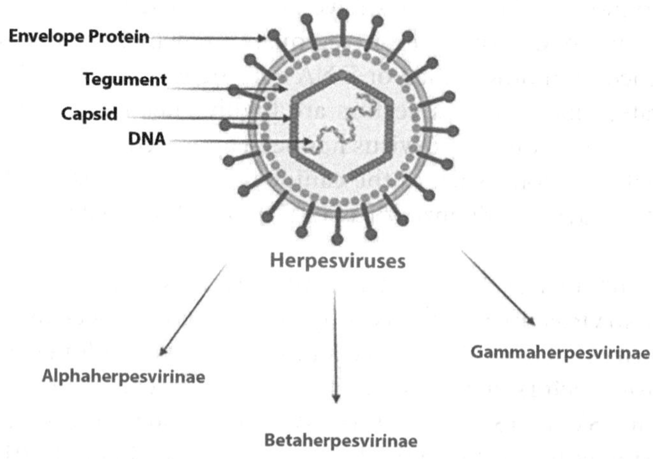

Figure 1.1 Structure and types of herpesviruses.

A strong basis for the advancement of herpesvirus-based vectors is established by a better understanding of the interaction between the vector and the host. Currently, a variety of molecular techniques, including codon optimization, homologous and two-step en passant mutagenesis, BAC technology, and the CRISPR/Cas9 system, are used to facilitate the generation of herpesvirus-based recombinant vaccine vectors [22].

Herpes simplex virus (HSV) vectors are appropriate for transferring and expressing several large therapeutic genes in brain neurons over an extended period of time, even in the total absence of viral gene expression. The advanced vector technologies are safe, long-lasting, and non-inflammatory within the nucleus of nerve cells. HSV may eventually be utilized to treat a number of neurodegenerative disorders with an identified inherited cause [21].

1.6 Epstein-Barr Virus Vectors

The Epstein-Barr virus (EBV) vector is characterized by its ability to persist in the host cell nucleus as an episome, rather than integrating into the host genome. This property renders it a highly accessible and efficient vector for use in human cell lines. The EBV vector comprises two key DNA components: the nuclear antigen-1 (EBNA1) gene, which is expressed by the virus, and the OriP sequence, which serves as the origin of plasmid replication. The EBNA1 protein plays a crucial role in maintaining the stability of the episome by binding to the OriP sequence. This interaction facilitates the anchoring of OriP-containing plasmids to nuclear proteins within the host cell, allowing them to remain stable episomes during cell division. As a result, these plasmids can replicate alongside the host's cellular machinery without disrupting genomic integrity. The unique characteristics of EBV vectors make them particularly suitable for various applications in gene therapy and vaccine development. Their episomal nature allows for sustained expression of therapeutic genes without the risks associated with genomic integration, such as insertional mutagenesis. This aspect is especially important in therapeutic contexts where long-term gene expression is desired. Furthermore, EBV vectors can be engineered to enhance their functionality. For instance, modifications can be made to improve their replication efficiency or to include additional regulatory elements that enhance transgene expression. This adaptability makes EBV vectors a valuable tool in both research and clinical settings [23].

Research on alpha herpes virus has significantly improved several genetic techniques, and EBV replication is comparable to that of other herpes viruses. However, EBV is distinct from alpha herpes viruses in that it induces latency in human B cells and modifies their growth [24].

EBV vectors with OriP-containing plasmid replicate once throughout the cell cycle in parallel with the host chromosomes. The high-affinity matrix attachment area containing oriP is responsible for anchoring EBV vectors, which have a chromatin-like structure, to the nuclear matrix in latently infected cells.

The two noncontiguous portions that make up OriP are the dyad symmetry (DS) element and the family of repetitions (FR). A 30-bp repeat sequence is present in 20 tandem flawed copies in the FR and four similar copies in the DS, the other region. The majority of sequences for EBNA1 binding are present in these 30-bp repeats.

With the use of EBV-based vectors, deficient human cell lines can be effectively corrected by cDNA or genomic DNA transfections leading to complementation and cloning of the correcting gene. It is possible to target tumor cells that express EBNA-1 specifically with vectors containing only oriP in EBV-associated neoplasms such as nasopharyngeal carcinoma and Burkitt's lymphoma [25].

1.7 Retrovirus Vectors

Gene therapy commonly uses viruses, specifically retroviruses, as vectors. The genetic material found in retroviruses is RNA. Reverse transcription is the process by which the retrovirus converts RNA into DNA once it enters the host cell. The provirus, which is the viral DNA that has been created, is integrated into the host cell's DNA. Proviruses often provide no risk to users. There is a significant risk, though, as some retroviruses have the ability to turn healthy cells malignant.

Retroviruses must render them harmless prior to using them as a vector. For instance, by deliberately deleting a gene that codes for the viral envelope, the retrovirus can be made inert. A retrovirus cannot enter the host cell if it does not have the envelope. A single envelope-defective retrovirus can multiply into many viral particles with the help of helper viruses. Helper viruses possess the usual genes that produce envelopes. Because the vector virus has a malfunctioning envelope gene, it can multiply together with the helper virus when it infects host cells (Figure 1.2). The vector and helper viruses multiply billions of times by repeatedly replicating in the host cells. It is possible to isolate and purify the vector viruses from the helper viruses. It is crucial to isolate vector viruses and ensure they are

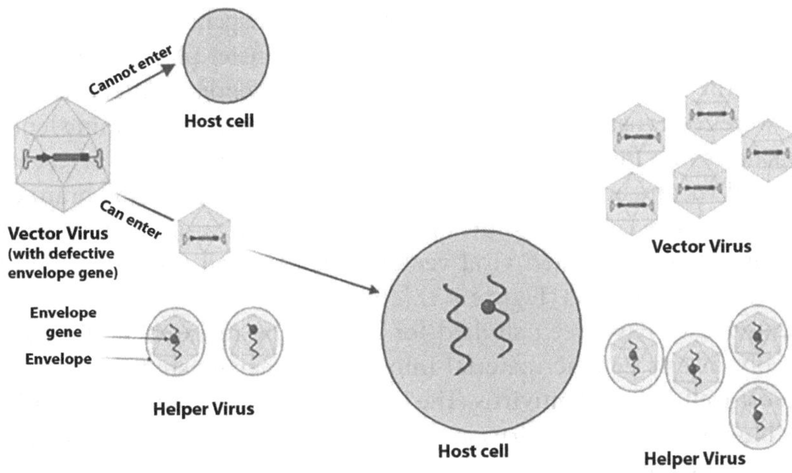

Figure 1.2 Large-scale production of vector viruses using helper viruses.

completely free of helper viruses. The health of patients receiving gene therapy is seriously threatened by helper virus contamination.

A retroviral vector carrying a maximum 8-kb size therapeutic DNA is useful for transforming the cells. However, the integration and delivery efficiency of therapeutic DNA is poor. To achieve high efficiency of integration, packaged retroviral RNA particles are used.

1.8 Lentivirus Vectors

Lentiviruses are among the most popular and useful viral vectors in the laboratory. Lentiviruses have two advantages: they have a large genetic capacity and can transduce both proliferating and nondividing cells. At the beginning of the 1990s, investigators developed viral vector systems based on retroviruses, such as the Moloney murine leukemia virus (MMLV).

Only actively dividing cells were susceptible to infection by the vectors, but they also had the ability to integrate into the genome and support transgenic expression for a long time. While nondividing cells might be infected by a different type of adenovirus-based vector, transgenic expression would not be produced over time. The packaging, envelope, and transfer plasmids constituted the original lentiviral vector system. The HIV-1 provirus mutant included in the packaging plasmid was unable to package itself because it lacked a few necessary proteins. The cell types that the vector could infect were determined by the viral envelope present on the envelope plasmid. Finally, the necessary transgene and HIV-1 long-terminal repeats (LTRs) were included in the transfer plasmid, helping to facilitate the integration of the virus into the host genome. After these plasmids were co-transfected, 293T cells released transgene-containing lentiviral particles into the medium, which could be collected for use in research. Lentiviral vectors are still widely used for tracing and targeting brain cells because they can carry a significantly larger genetic cargo (8 kb versus 4.5 kb) than adeno-associated viral vectors, even though the latter can also target nondividing cells (Figure 1.3) [26, 27].

Lentiviruses have been studied for decades by researchers. Because it naturally inserts genetic material into cells, especially stem cells, HIV is the most well-known lentivirus. The lentiviral vector is built using an HIV virus blueprint. The HIV virus is made up of nine genes. Researchers take three or four different genes from the HIV virus's blueprint to create the lentiviral vector, which increases the vector's ability to transfer genetic material. Now, more genes will be added in order to produce the desired therapeutic effect. Since only a small portion of the nine genes from the original viral blueprint are used, HIV infection is impossible due to incomplete genomes.

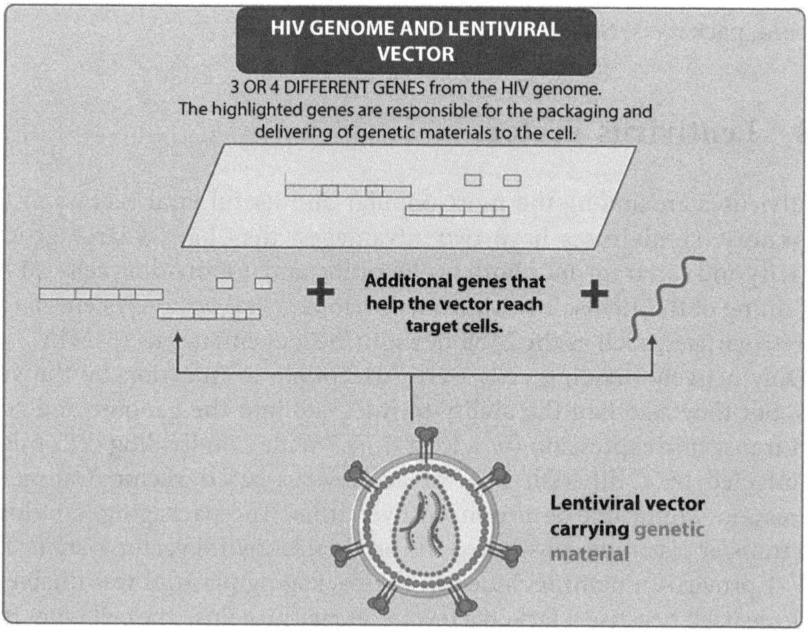

Figure 1.3 HIV genome and lentiviral vector.

Lentiviral vectors, which are derived from the human immunodeficiency virus, have been extensively researched and improved during the past 20 years. To treat hemoglobinopathies and primary immunodeficiencies, third-generation, self-inactivating lentiviral vectors have been used in several clinical trials recently to transfer genes into hematopoietic stem cells (Figure 1.4). Furthermore, in order to create immunity against cancer, these vectors have been utilized to clone T cell receptors or introduce chimeric antigen receptors (CARs) into mature T cells. After CAR T cell therapies developed with lentiviral vectors demonstrated substantial clinical effectiveness in patients with B cell malignancies, regulators approved the first genetically modified cellular therapy [28].

1.9 Adeno-Associated Virus (AAV)

AAV is one of the gene therapy vehicles that is currently undergoing the most research. It was first discovered to be a contamination of viral preparations, which is where its name originates. A protein shell encloses and protects the 4.8-kb ssDNA genome that composes up AAV. AAV is a member of the parvovirus family [29].

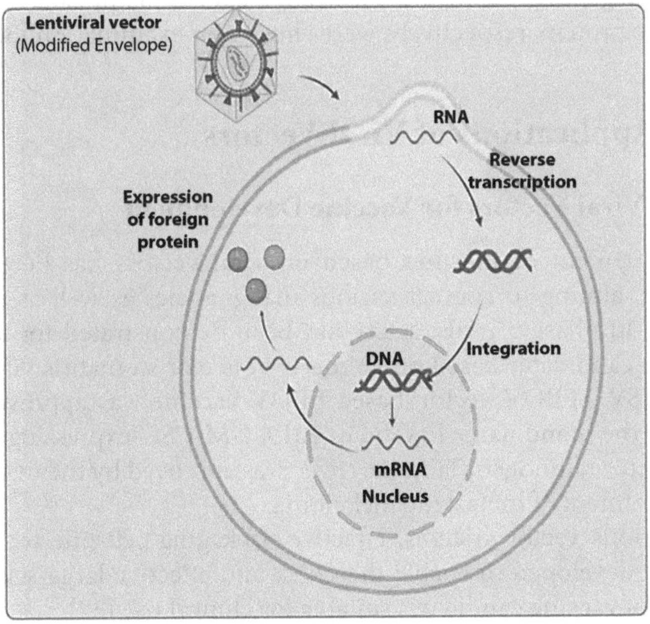

Figure 1.4 Lentiviral vector in gene therapy.

Its ss genome has three genes: aap (Assembly), Rep (Replication), and Cap (Capsid). The most important consideration when creating a decent rAAV vector is the packing size of the expression cassette that will be placed in between the two ITRs (inverted terminal repeats). It is widely accepted that, even for viral ITRs, anything under 5 kb works as a good point of origin. The rate of transgene recombination (truncations) or viral production yields is considerably reduced when rAAV vectors larger than packaging cassettes (5 kb) are attempted to be generated. AAV vectors are not designed to efficiently package long coding sequences. Using dual overlapping vector techniques can aid in changing the packing. In order to achieve transgene expression, the ss AAV-delivered transgene must be transformed into a ds transgene upon delivery to the nucleus, according to its biology. Self-complementary AAV is beneficial because it bypasses that process by using its ss packed genome to complement itself and generate a ds genome in the nucleus. In contrast to the vector's decreased packaging capacity, transgene expression occurs more quickly.

AAV is a highly effective vector for effecting gene integration into the host cell chromosome and transporting the gene into both dividing and nondividing cells. Furthermore, the genes delivered through the AAV vector may exhibit persistent expression. Using the AAV vector as a mediator, the prospect of introducing a gene into EBV-transformed B cells is investigated. The genes 6A8 and 5D4, which code for α-mannosidase and a cell membrane protein, respectively, were chosen for examination [30, 31].

1.10 Applications of Viral Vectors

1.10.1 Viral Vectors for Vaccine Development

The development of vaccines based on viral vectors has been steadily advancing, aiming to combat various malignancies as well as infectious disorders. In phase 3 trials, safety has been demonstrated for a number of vaccine candidates based on chimeric vesicular stomatitis virus (VSV) vectors. VSV-ZEBOV vector–based EBOV vaccine was approved by the FDA with the brand name Ervebo in 2019. GM-CSF–expressing oncolytic HSV-1 vector talimogene laherparepvec was approved by the FDA in 2015 for the treatment of metastatic melanoma.

For various vector systems, effective packaging cell line technologies have been developed to enable the quick and effective large-scale manufacturing of vaccine candidates suitable for clinical use [32].

1.10.2 Gene Therapy: The Performance of Viral Vectors

Promising in treating a wide range of diseases, gene therapies are presently among the most researched therapeutic approaches in both the clinical and preclinical phases. Gene therapies are a promising means of treating diseases that were previously thought to be incurable by traditional methods. It works by inserting a gene into target cells. A vector is frequently needed to transfer gene therapies into target cells; viral vectors are among the most researched vectors because of their unique benefits, including exceptional transduction efficiency. After decades of research and development, viral vector–based gene treatments have shown promise in the clinic, with multiple drugs now approved for the treatment of various infectious diseases, cancer, and monogenic disorders [33, 34].

In gene therapy, a vector is used to deliver genetic material to the cells. The molecules that make up genetic material, known as DNA or RNA, are responsible for storing information and sending instructions to the cells on what to do. It might include directions on how to make a certain protein, for instance.

Viral vectors are devices that are used in genetic engineering and molecular biology to introduce genetic material into cells. These viruses have been modified such that they can be utilized to transfer particular genes into the target cells. As a part of their normal life cycle, viruses have acquired the capacity to effectively transfer their genetic information into host cells.

Genome editing techniques have rapidly evolved, with CRISPR-Cas9 emerging as a leading method due to its precision, efficacy, and efficiency. This system relies on the collaboration of clustered regularly interspaced short palindromic repeats (CRISPR) and their associated protein, Cas9. The CRISPR/Cas9 system comprises two essential components: a Cas9 protein and a guide RNA (gRNA). A significant hurdle in therapeutic CRISPR/Cas9 applications has been the development of safe and efficient delivery methods. Viral vectors, renowned for their *in vivo* delivery capabilities, have emerged as promising candidates. Lentivirus vectors (LVs), AAVs, and AdVs are commonly employed due to their superior delivery efficiency compared to other methods [35].

1.10.3 Clinical Trials

Many therapeutic investigations utilizing viral vectors have been undertaken and are currently ongoing [32]. For instance, following three decades of development, pivotal-stage clinical studies for gene therapy for hemophilia are currently underway, which mainly focus on AAV-based vectors. There have been eleven clinical trials for hemophilia gene therapy, while with some degree of effectiveness, liver-directed AAV expressing either FVIII or FIX has been used in six ongoing phase 1/2 clinical trials [36, 37].

As reported by Carbonero *et al.*, intravenous administration of enadenotucirev in patients with different cancers including colorectal cancer, urothelial cell cancer, non–small cell lung cancer, and renal cell cancer was studied. Enadenotucirev is a chimeric adenovirus that selectively targets tumors and has exhibited preclinical activity. This virus delivery was accompanied by significant local $CD8^+$ cell infiltration in 80% of examined tumor samples, suggesting an enadenotucirev-driven immune response. In the majority of tumor samples, tumor-specific delivery was found, and there were no treatment-related significant side effects [38]. A phase 1 clinical trial with oncolytic VVs was also conducted in 11 patients with resistant advanced colorectal or other solid tumors [39]. Viral vectors under clinical trial are given in Table 1.1.

1.11 Safety Issues of Viral Vector/Biosafety Challenges

Although the introduction of viral vector gene delivery methods has resulted in a promising new chapter in gene therapy recently, not all cell types can be treated by a single delivery method, either *in vitro* or *in vivo.*

Table 1.1 Viral vectors under clinical trial.

Viral vector	Disease	Outcome	Reference
Oncolytic HSV HF10	Different cancers	Antitumor activity, low adverse effects	[40]
Oncolytic HSV M032	Glioblastoma	Significant antitumor activity	[41]
NDV expressing multiple tumor-associated antigens (TAAs)	Ovarian, stomach, and pancreatic cancer	Long-term survival in phase 2 trials	[42]
CAV21	Melanoma	Antitumor activity	[43, 44]
Lenti-FVIII	Hemophilia	Potential cure	[38]

Additionally, there are unique occupational health and safety issues associated with the use of viral vector systems. The safe use of viral vector systems in human gene therapy research is a concern shared by the majority of IBCs in research and clinical settings, as there is currently no single document outlining best practices for using them. Institutional biosafety committees (IBCs) and healthcare providers have limited resources when it comes to risk assessment and developing protocols to minimize risk and exposure in a research/clinical context [4].

➢ **AAV**

Clinical investigations and preclinical animal research have shown that AAV vectors are extremely safe. Eighty percent of people have positive antibodies against AAV strains. Frequent doses, however, may be a limiting factor since it may trigger an immune response. Furthermore, a number of gene clinical studies have shown that AAV vectors do not induce an enhanced immune response. The incorporation of recombinant AAV enhanced the incidence of tumor formation in various animal models, although this connection has not been found in humans [4].

➢ **Adenovirus Vectors**

Adenoviral genes are currently challenging to produce, even though their genomes have a carrying capacity of over 30 kb. Another problem with AdVs in general is that, unlike the relatively harmless AAV virions, the particles themselves cause cellular inflammatory responses [45, 46].

➢ **Retrovirus Vectors**

Retroviral vectors have been widely employed to deliver therapeutic genes in the field of gene therapy and clinical applications for monogenic disorders, cancer, and infectious diseases, providing patients with steady and efficient transgene expression [4]. However, the greatest safety risk associated with the use of RV stems from their potential to integrate into the host cell genome, which elevates the chance of insertional mutagenesis and oncogene activation [47].

➢ **Lentivirus Vectors**

Since lentiviral vectors are more effective at transducing non-proliferating or slowly proliferating cells—like CD34 stem cells—they have become more and more popular for use in therapeutic settings. However, there are still hazards associated with using LVVs in research, and evaluations are being done regarding the clinical procedures' long-term safety. The limitations of using LVVs in clinical trials today result mostly from inadequate techniques for the production of high-titer virus stocks and safety concerns regarding their origin from HI, despite the engineering of packing cell lines and the removal of genes required for viral replication [4].

Some Other Challenges are as Follows:

- Immunogenicity: The immune system may recognize and mount a response against the viral vectors, potentially limiting their effectiveness.
- Insertional Mutagenesis: Some viral vectors may integrate into the host cell's genome, which can lead to unintended consequences, such as activating or disrupting other genes.
- Overexpression of target gene
- Immune response to native protein or viral capsid
- Hepatotoxicity

1.12 Conclusion

Gene therapy is a promising field that aims to introduce, replace, or alter genetic material within a person's cells in order to treat or prevent disease. It is noteworthy that the selection of the viral vector is dependent upon a number of parameters, such as the intended duration of gene expression, the target tissue, and safety considerations. Therapeutic genes are delivered to target cells primarily by viral vectors. Many viral vectors exist, but retroviral and AdVs in particular, have shown great efficacy in transferring therapeutic genes to target cells. Viral vectors can either remain episomal (adenoviruses) or integrate into the host genome (retroviruses) in order to sustain gene expression. Despite their efficacy and safety, viral vectors can trigger immune responses in the host, leading to inflammation or the destruction of transduced cells. Insertional mutagenesis poses a concern since the integration of the viral genome into the host DNA can interfere with normal gene activity, particularly when using retroviral vectors. In gene therapy, viral vectors are useful tools, but more investigation and development are required to address safety issues, increase targeting specificity, and boost overall efficacy. In order to conduct competent research and apply gene therapy using viral vectors in the future, it will be necessary to balance potential benefits with ethical considerations.

References

1. Barrett, A.D.T. and Stanberry, L.R., *Vaccines for biodefense and emerging and neglected diseases*, 1st ed., Academic Press/Elsevier, Amsterdam Boston, 2009.
2. Blaney, J.E., Matro, J.M., Murphy, B.R., Whitehead, S.S., Recombinant, Live-Attenuated Tetravalent Dengue Virus Vaccine Formulations Induce a Balanced, Broad, and Protective Neutralizing Antibody Response against Each of the Four Serotypes in Rhesus Monkeys. *J. Virol.* [Internet], 79, 9, 5516–5528, 2005, Available from: https://journals.asm.org/doi/10.1128/JVI.79.9.5516-5528.2005.
3. Chen, Y.H., Keiser, M.S., Davidson, B.L., Viral Vectors for Gene Transfer. *CP Mouse Biol.* [Internet], 8, 4, e58, 2018, Available from: https://currentprotocols.onlinelibrary.wiley.com/doi/10.1002/cpmo.58.
4. Ghosh, S., Brown, A.M., Jenkins, C., Campbell, K., Viral Vector Systems for Gene Therapy: A Comprehensive Literature Review of Progress and Biosafety Challenges. *Appl. Biosaf.* [Internet], 25, 1, 7–18, 2020, Available from: https://www.liebertpub.com/doi/10.1177/1535676019899502.
5. Madhan, S., Prabakaran, M., Kwang, J., Baculovirus as Vaccine Vectors. *CGT* [Internet], 10, 3, 201–213, 2010, Available from: http://www.eurekaselect.com/openurl/content.php?genre=article&issn=1566-5232&volume=10&issue=3&spage=201.
6. Schaly, S., Ghebretatios, M., Prakash, S., Baculoviruses in Gene Therapy and Personalized Medicine. *BTT* [Internet], 15, 115–132, 2021, Available from: https://www.dovepress.com/baculoviruses-in-gene-therapy-and-personalized-medicine-peer-reviewed-fulltext-article-BTT.
7. Wold, W. and Toth, K., Adenovirus Vectors for Gene Therapy, Vaccination and Cancer Gene Therapy. *CGT* [Internet], 13, 6, 421–433, 2014, Available from: http://www.eurekaselect.com/openurl/content.php?genre=article&issn=1566-5232&volume=13&issue=6&spage=421.
8. Chavda, V.P., Ghali, E.N.H.K., Balar, P.C., *et al.*, Protein subunit vaccines: Promising frontiers against COVID-19. *J. Control. Release*, 366, 761–782, 2024.
9. El-Maradny, Y.A., Ramadan, A.A., Chavda, V.P., Balar, P.C., Redwan, E.M., The fast-track development of COVID-19 vaccines [Internet], in: *Advanced Vaccination Technologies for Infectious and Chronic Diseases*, pp. 415–440, Elsevier, Amsterdam, Netherlands, 2024, [cited 2024 May 31], Available from: https://linkinghub.elsevier.com/retrieve/pii/B9780443185649000278.
10. Mendonça, S.A., Lorincz, R., Boucher, P., Curiel, D.T., Adenoviral vector vaccine platforms in the SARS-CoV-2 pandemic. *npj Vaccines* [Internet], 6, 1, 97, 2021, Available from: https://www.nature.com/articles/s41541-021-00356-x.
11. Coughlan, L., Factors Which Contribute to the Immunogenicity of Non-replicating Adenoviral Vectored Vaccines. *Front. Immunol.* [Internet], 11, 909, 2020, Available from: https://www.frontiersin.org/article/10.3389/fimmu.2020.00909/full.

12. Chavda, V.P., Teli, D., Balar, P.C., *et al.*, Potential Anti-SARS-CoV-2 Prodrugs Activated by Phosphorylation and Their Role in the Aged Population. *Molecules*, 28, 5, 2332, 2023.
13. Chavda, V.P., Vuppu, S., Mishra, T., Balar, P., The Emergence of Hybrid Variants of SARS-CoV-2: Towards Hybrid Immunity. *Vaccines*, 11, 4, 764, 2023.
14. Sayedahmed, E.E., Kumari, R., Mittal, S.K., Current Use of Adenovirus Vectors and Their Production Methods [Internet], in: *Viral Vectors for Gene Therapy*, F.P. Manfredsson and M.J. Benskey (Eds.), pp. 155–175, Springer New York, New York, NY, 2019, [cited 2023 Dec 11]. Available from: http://link.springer.com/10.1007/978-1-4939-9065-8_9.
15. Matsunaga, W. and Gotoh, A., Adenovirus as a Vector and Oncolytic Virus. *CIMB* [Internet], 45, 6, 4826–4840, 2023, Available from: https://www.mdpi.com/1467-3045/45/6/307.
16. Zhang, W.-W., Li, L., Li, D., *et al.*, The First Approved Gene Therapy Product for Cancer Ad- *p53* (Gendicine): 12 Years in the Clinic. *Hum. Gene Ther.* [Internet], 29, 2, 160–179, 2018, Available from: http://www.liebertpub.com/doi/10.1089/hum.2017.218.
17. Krauzewicz, N. and Griffin, B.E., Polyoma and Papilloma Virus Vectors For Cancer Gene Therapy [Internet], in: *Cancer Gene Therapy*, N.A. Habib (Ed.), pp. 73–82, Springer US, New York, NY, 2002, [cited 2023 Dec 11]. Available from: http://link.springer.com/10.1007/0-306-46817-4_8.
18. Poxvirus, Description, Types, Features, & Disease, Britannica [Internet], Available from: https://www.britannica.com/science/poxvirus.
19. Carroll, M.W. and Moss, B., Poxviruses as expression vectors. *Curr. Opin. Biotechnol.* [Internet], 8, 5, 573–577, 1997, Available from: https://linkinghub.elsevier.com/retrieve/pii/S0958166997800316.
20. Vera, M. and Fortes, P., Simian Virus-40 as a Gene Therapy Vector. *DNA Cell Biol.* [Internet], 23, 5, 271–282, 2004, Available from: http://www.liebertpub.com/doi/10.1089/104454904323090903.
21. Artusi, S., Miyagawa, Y., Goins, W., Cohen, J., Glorioso, J., Herpes Simplex Virus Vectors for Gene Transfer to the Central Nervous System. *Diseases* [Internet], 6, 3, 74, 2018, Available from: http://www.mdpi.com/2079-9721/6/3/74.
22. Kamel, M. and El-Sayed, A., Utilization of herpesviridae as recombinant viral vectors in vaccine development against animal pathogens. *Virus Res.* [Internet], 270, 197648, 2019, Available from: https://linkinghub.elsevier.com/retrieve/pii/S016817021930005X.
23. Kiyosue, K. and Miwa, Y., Epstein-Barr virus-derived vector suitable for long-term expression in neurons. *Heliyon* [Internet], 6, 3, e03504, 2020, Available from: https://linkinghub.elsevier.com/retrieve/pii/S2405844020303492.
24. (NAS Colloquium), *Genetic Engineering of Viruses and Viral Vectors* [Internet], National Academies Press, Washington, D.C., 1996, Available from: http://www.nap.edu/catalog/5708.

25. Van Craenenbroeck, K., Vanhoenacker, P., Haegeman, G., Episomal vectors for gene expression in mammalian cells. *Eur. J. Biochem.* [Internet], 267, 18, 5665–5678, 2000, Available from: https://febs.onlinelibrary.wiley.com/doi/10.1046/j.1432-1327.2000.01645.x.
26. Dong, W. and Kantor, B., Lentiviral Vectors for Delivery of Gene-Editing Systems Based on CRISPR/Cas: Current State and Perspectives. *Viruses* [Internet], 13, 7, 1288, 2021, Available from: https://www.mdpi.com/1999-4915/13/7/1288.
27. Zufferey, R., Dull, T., Mandel, R.J., *et al.*, Self-Inactivating Lentivirus Vector for Safe and Efficient *In Vivo* Gene Delivery. *J. Virol.* [Internet], 72, 12, 9873–9880, 1998, Available from: https://journals.asm.org/doi/10.1128/JVI.72.12.9873-9880.1998.
28. Milone, M.C. and O'Doherty, U., Clinical use of lentiviral vectors. *Leukemia* [Internet], 32, 7, 1529–1541, 2018, Available from: https://www.nature.com/articles/s41375-018-0106-0.
29. Kaplitt, M.G. and Loewy, A.D., *Viral Vectors: Gene Therapy and Neuroscience Applications*, Academic Press, San Diego, California, USA, 1995.
30. Shi, G.X., Wang, Y., Liu, Y., Cui, W., Zhao, F.T., Zhu, L.P., Long-Term Expression of a Transferred Gene in Epstein–Barr Virus Transformed Human B Cells. *Scand. J. Immunol.* [Internet], 54, 3, 265–272, 2001, Available from: https://onlinelibrary.wiley.com/doi/10.1046/j.1365-3083.2001.00924.x.
31. Grieger, J.C., Choi, V.W., Samulski, R.J., Production and characterization of adeno-associated viral vectors. *Nat. Protoc.* [Internet], 1, 3, 1412–1428, 2006, Available from: https://www.nature.com/articles/nprot.2006.207.
32. Lundstrom, K., Application of Viral Vectors for Vaccine Development with a Special Emphasis on COVID-19. *Viruses* [Internet], 12, 11, 1324, 2020, Available from: https://www.mdpi.com/1999-4915/12/11/1324.
33. Li, X., Le, Y., Zhang, Z., Nian, X., Liu, B., Yang, X., Viral Vector-Based Gene Therapy. *IJMS* [Internet], 24, 9, 7736, 2023, Available from: https://www.mdpi.com/1422-0067/24/9/7736.
34. Zhao, Z., Anselmo, A.C., Mitragotri, S., Viral vector-based gene therapies in the clinic. *Bioeng. Transl. Med.* [Internet], 7, 1, e10258, 2022, Available from: https://aiche.onlinelibrary.wiley.com/doi/10.1002/btm2.10258.
35. Asmamaw Mengstie, M., Viral Vectors for the *in Vivo* Delivery of CRISPR Components: Advances and Challenges. *Front. Bioeng. Biotechnol.* [Internet], 10, 895713, 2022, Available from: https://www.frontiersin.org/articles/10.3389/fbioe.2022.895713/full.
36. Spencer, H.T., Riley, B.E., Doering, C.B., State of the art: gene therapy of haemophilia. *Haemophilia* [Internet], 22, S5, 66–71, 2016, Available from: https://onlinelibrary.wiley.com/doi/10.1111/hae.13011.
37. Mingozzi, F. and High, K.A., Immune responses to AAV vectors: Overcoming barriers to successful gene therapy. *Blood* [Internet], 122, 1, 23–36, 2013, Available from: https://ashpublications.org/blood/article/122/1/23/31570/Immune-responses-to-AAV-vectors-overcoming.

38. Garcia-Carbonero, R., Salazar, R., Duran, I., *et al.*, Phase 1 study of intravenous administration of the chimeric adenovirus enadenotucirev in patients undergoing primary tumor resection. *J. Immunother. Cancer* [Internet], 5, 1, 71, 2017, Available from: https://jitc.bmj.com/lookup/doi/10.1186/s40425-017-0277-7.
39. Downs-Canner, S., Guo, Z.S., Ravindranathan, R., *et al.*, Phase 1 Study of Intravenous Oncolytic Poxvirus (vvDD) in Patients With Advanced Solid Cancers. *Mol. Ther.* [Internet], 24, 8, 1492–1501, 2016, Available from: https://linkinghub.elsevier.com/retrieve/pii/S1525001616336012.
40. Eissa, I.R., Naoe, Y., Bustos-Villalobos, I., *et al.*, Genomic Signature of the Natural Oncolytic Herpes Simplex Virus HF10 and Its Therapeutic Role in Preclinical and Clinical Trials. *Front. Oncol.* [Internet], 7, 149, 2017, Available from: http://journal.frontiersin.org/article/10.3389/fonc.2017.00149/full.
41. Markert, J.M., Razdan, S.N., Kuo, H.-C., *et al.*, A Phase 1 Trial of Oncolytic HSV-1, G207, Given in Combination With Radiation for Recurrent GBM Demonstrates Safety and Radiographic Responses. *Mol. Ther.* [Internet], 22, 5, 1048–1055, 2014, Available from: https://linkinghub.elsevier.com/retrieve/pii/S1525001616312369.
42. Schirrmacher, V., Clinical trials of antitumor vaccination with an autologous tumor cell vaccine modified by virus infection: Improvement of patient survival based on improved antitumor immune memory. *Cancer Immunol. Immunother.* [Internet], 54, 6, 587–598, 2005, Available from: http://link.springer.com/10.1007/s00262-004-0602-0.
43. Pandha, H., Harrington, K., Ralph, C., Melcher, A., Grose, M., Shafren, D., Phase I/II storm study: Intravenous delivery of a novel oncolytic immunotherapy agent, Coxsackievirus A21, in advanced cancer patients. *J. Immunother. Cancer* [Internet], 3, Suppl 2, P341, 2015, Available from: https://jitc.bmj.com/lookup/doi/10.1186/2051-1426-3-S2-P341.
44. Andtbacka, R.H., Curti, B.D., Hallmeyer, S., *et al.*, Phase II calm extension study: Coxsackievirus A21 delivered intratumorally to patients with advanced melanoma induces immune-cell infiltration in the tumor microenvironment. *J. Immunother. Cancer* [Internet], 3, Suppl 2, P343, 2015, Available from: https://jitc.bmj.com/lookup/doi/10.1186/2051-1426-3-S2-P343.
45. Lowenstein, P., Mandel, R., Xiong, W., Kroeger, K., Castro, M., Immune Responses to Adenovirus and Adeno-Associated Vectors Used for Gene Therapy of Brain Diseases: The Role of Immunological Synapses in Understanding the Cell Biology of Neuroimmune Interactions. *CGT* [Internet], 7, 5, 347–360, 2007, Available from: http://www.eurekaselect.com/openurl/content.php?genre=article&issn=1566-5232&volume=7&issue=5&spage=347.
46. Morsy, M.A. and Caskey, C.T., Expanded-capacity adenoviral vectors—the helper-dependent vectors. *Mol. Med. Today* [Internet], 5, 1, 18–24, 1999, Available from: https://linkinghub.elsevier.com/retrieve/pii/S1357431098013768.

47. Romano, G., Development of Safer Gene Delivery Systems to Minimize the Risk of Insertional Mutagenesis-Related Malignancies: A Critical Issue for the Field of Gene Therapy. *ISRN Oncol.* [Internet], 2012, 1–14, 2012, Available from: https://www.hindawi.com/journals/isrn/2012/616310/.

2

Viral Vector Construction

Suneetha Vuppu*, Toshika Mishra, Shatakshi Mishra, Stany B. and Anushka Das

Department of Biotechnology, Science, Innovation, and Society Research Lab 115, Hexagon (SMV), Vellore Institute of Technology, Vellore, Tamil Nadu, India

Abstract

Viral vectors comprise a class of efficient vectors that are utilized in gene delivery to the target site in a patient's body attributed to its mechanism of entering the cell and transduction of dividing as well as nondividing cells. These are further categorized into DNA- and RNA-based vectors based on the molecular composition. In addition to gene therapy, viral vectors find application in the domains of molecular biology and vaccine development. During the construction of viral vectors, the viral genomes are manipulated to utilize their ability to infect the host cells while significantly reducing the pathogenicity. Usually, the genes responsible for replication are deleted, and the transgene cassette comprising therapeutic genes is incorporated into the viral genome. Although there are several restrictions associated with the construction of viral vectors like immune response, specificity of transgene delivery, and insertional mutagenesis, these challenges can be overcome with the development of improved techniques. The advancements in the construction of viral vectors provide an opportunity to develop effective and safe therapeutic interventions for a wide array of genetic and acquired diseases. This chapter provides insight into the properties of viral vectors and their important applications in therapeutics and research. In this chapter, we also investigate various viruses utilized for the development of viral vectors, the construction process, obstacles, and advancements in the construction of viral vectors. Furthermore, the future prospects of viral vectors are also discussed.

***Keywords*:** Viral vectors, gene therapy, vaccine development, adenovirus, lentivirus, poxvirus, immune response, transgene

**Corresponding author*: vsuneetha@vit.ac.in

Vivek P. Chavda and Vasso Apostolopoulos (eds.) Viral Vectors for Vaccine Delivery, (25–64) © 2025 Scrivener Publishing LLC

2.1 Introduction

The fundamental concept of *in vivo* gene transfer involves the introduction of a gene into an organism using a vector that delivers the gene of interest only to particular target cells. While the transfer of genes serves as a crucial tool for investigating molecular mechanisms *in vitro* or animal models, the ultimate objective is "gene therapy," wherein genes are employed as therapeutic agents in humans. The goal of gene therapy is to transfer genetic information to target cells to either establish a new function for treating (like cancer) or preventing diseases (like vaccinations) or to replace a faulty function (like in monogenic diseases) [1]. There are two primary approaches for achieving gene transfer: *ex vivo* and *in vivo*.

The fundamental barrier to *in vivo* gene therapy is the lack of an efficient, nontoxic gene delivery mechanism, not a scarcity of therapeutic genes. Viruses, which are capable of transducing genetic information into host cells for self-replication, provide a natural solution. Recombinant viral vectors, which are generated by replacing nonessential viral genes with therapeutic foreign genes, can efficiently transduce the cell types that they infect. Despite the potential immune response triggered by viruses, their evolution has equipped them with effective countermeasures, allowing the viruses to be delivered and replicated in target cells. Using viral vectors as "Trojan horses" to get access to specific cells takes advantage of millions of years of evolutionary development. This strategy was first investigated in 1973 when Rogers *et al.* used the Shope papilloma virus, in an unsuccessful attempt to stimulate arginase activity in tissue culture cells of hyperargininemic patients. Despite these initial challenges, there is still a lot of research being done on the direct use of replication-competent viruses as therapeutic agents, especially when it comes to oncolytic viruses and cancer treatment.

After the promising prospects of gene therapy in the 1990s, a significant setback occurred with the use of adenovirus (Ad) vectors in treating ornithine transcarbamylase, leading to the unfortunate death of a patient [2]. Leukemia then developed as a result of therapies for severe combined immunodeficiency (SCID) integrating therapeutic genes provided by retroviruses into the LMO2 proto-oncogene area [3, 4]. These challenges were attributed to clinical trial design inexperience and an overly optimistic approach to viral vector safety in gene therapy. Consequently, skepticism arose, impacting funding, clinical trials, and industry support. However, dedicated gene therapists persisted in addressing delivery and safety concerns through vector engineering, contributing to the resurgence of gene therapy. In the current scenario, viral and nonviral vectors are experiencing renewed interest in innovative modifications and applications. Some of the key properties of the viral vectors include with respect to their host ranges, toxicity, and immunogenicity. Some of these properties could be justified with certain viral vectors such as Ad which shows a broad host range with a transient expression and a strong immunogenicity [5, 6]. AAV, another viral vector that consists of a single-stranded DNA genome has a much broader host range and a slow expression onset [7–10]. Herpes simplex virus (HSV) has a broad host range with long-term expression along with low toxicity [11, 12]. Lentiviruses and alphaviruses too show a broad host range accompanied by a long-term expression [13–15].

2.2 Applications of Viral Vector

The utilization of viral vectors in gene therapy has emerged as a transformative approach, capitalizing on the evolutionary adaptability of viruses over millions of years. Viruses, having evolved to survive and replicate within host cells, serve as carriers and vectors for gene delivery in gene therapy research. This method has shown promise, with the ability of viral vectors to safeguard transgenes from degradation and efficiently traverse cellular barriers. The inaugural success in 1999, treating SCID disorder using viral vectors, marked a pivotal moment. The subsequent years witnessed over 68% of gene therapy clinical trials employing viruses as vectors, demonstrating the significant role they play in this field [16]. Despite their potential, the safety concerns surrounding the inherent harmful nature of viruses necessitate strategic engineering approaches. These include preventing viral replication, promoting inactivation, and mitigating natural toxicity [17]. Viruses offer a diverse range of types and species, characterized by variations in size, morphology, genetic material, and tropism, providing flexibility for tailored gene therapy applications. Criteria such as the presence of an envelope, capsid symmetry, genetic material nature, replication site, and virion size are instrumental in classifying viruses for gene therapy selection [18]. The choice of a specific viral vector is guided by these criteria, considering both advantages and disadvantages to ensure efficient gene delivery. Various viral vectors, such as adenoviral vectors [19], retroviruses [20], adeno-associated viruses (AAVs) [21], and poxviruses [22], are explored for gene therapy applications. Adenoviral vectors, studied for two decades, are categorized into three generations based on gene deletion levels. Although they possess a large coding capacity, their immunogenicity and potential for severe immune responses limit their use. Retroviruses, especially lentiviruses, offer the unique capability to integrate their genetic material into host cells, allowing for stable gene expression.

Viral vectors play a crucial role in advancing neuroscience research by serving as powerful tools for *in vivo* gene delivery. Recombinant viruses are frequently used by researchers to introduce a range of components, including recombinases, sensors, tracers, reporters, and gene regulatory elements to neural cells. These vectors facilitate the manipulation and delivery of essential research tools, contributing to a robust platform for experimentation. To comprehend its architecture and assess neural activity, the mammalian brain—which is divided into neural circuits that control cognitive processing and the formulation of actions—uses fluorescent markers, sensors, and neural circuit tracers [23]. Viruses, including AAVs [24], retro/lentiviruses [25], and glycoprotein-deleted rabies viruses (rabies dG), emerge as effective vectors for the *in vivo* transportation of such tools. AAVs are preferred for gene delivery in both research and clinical trials because of their selectivity in transduction, low immunological reaction, and long-lasting gene expression in neurons and glia [26]. However, their small packaging capacity is a limitation. Lentiviruses, which can transduce both proliferating and nondividing cells, transcend this barrier by having a greater packing capacity of up to 9 kb [27]. Despite concerns about insertional mutations, lentiviral (LV) vectors remain robust for gene delivery in neurobiology research. Rabies dG viruses, particularly strains SADB19 and CVS-N2c, are employed for understanding brain architecture by delivering fluorescent neural tracers [27]. Recombinant technologies have enabled the modification of rabies dG to create safer alternatives for mapping neural circuits through trans-synaptic retrograde infection.

Since the first viral vector carrying a foreign gene from the SV40 virus was created in 1972, viral vectors have been essential to the development of vaccines for more than 40 years [28]. These vectors offer advantages such as eliciting both potent antibody and cellular responses, high immunogenicity without adjuvants, and the potential for long-lasting immunity, sometimes achieved after a single dose. Vaccine studies against diseases, such as HIV, malaria, Ebola, and, more recently, SARS-CoV-2, have made considerable use of viral vectors in preclinical and clinical settings [29].

Viral vectors have undergone distinct generational developments for protein expression in plants. First-generation vectors involve functional viruses expressing both wild-type viral genes and the coding sequence of a target protein. Second-generation vectors, such as deconstructed vectors and magnifection, address the limitations of first-generation ones [30].

Biodefense is a problem because biological agents have historically been used in terrorism and conflict. Countries that produced biological weapons violated the Biological and Toxin Weapons Convention (BWC), including Russia and Iraq [31]. Events such as the anthrax attacks in the United States in 2001 and the attempts by tiny organizations demonstrate the accessibility of biological agents Centers for Disease Control and Prevention [32]. The development of vaccines is the main goal of countermeasures; live-attenuated viruses, bacterial vectors, and viral vectors all show promise. TC-83 for VEEV and live vaccine strain for tularemia are examples of live-attenuated vaccinations that elicit protective immune responses [33]. Replication-competent and replication-defective viral vectors carry genes related to vaccines and have the potential to be used in state-sponsored projects and biodefense initiatives against bioterrorism.

Table 2.1 presents applications of viral vectors in biological domains.

2.3 Viral Vectors

2.3.1 Adenoviruses

The Ad capsid, 70 to 100 nm in diameter, consists of 12 trimeric hexon proteins and pentameric penton base proteins, with trimeric fiber proteins extending from them. The linear, double-stranded DNA genome (26 to 40 kb) is organized within the capsid into a nucleosome-like structure with inverted terminal repeat sequences. The early region (E1, E2, E3, and E4 units) and the late area are the two main transcription regions found in the genome [46]. Certain viral vectors, such as oncolytic Ads, have demonstrated promise in the treatment of cancer using gene therapy. For instance, scientists created an oncolytic Ad that targets pancreatic cancer cells specifically. This virus effectively infected and replicated within cancer cells, leading to the destruction of pancreatic tumors. Another approach involved creating chimeric Ad vectors that selectively replicate in cancer cells. These vectors were designed to express therapeutic genes, causing targeted death of tumor cells when injected into the tumors. To improve treatment efficacy, a strategy involved encapsulating the chimeric Ad in microbubbles for "stealth delivery" and using ultrasound to release and activate the virus within tumors. Ad-based gene therapy has a limited duration of therapeutic activity; thus, researchers looked into hybrid Ad vectors that incorporate CRISPR technology or the Sleeping Beauty transposon system for permanent gene editing and chromosomal integration [17, 47]. Additionally, oncolytic Ad vectors were combined with the expression of immunomodulatory proteins to change the tumor microenvironment, making it more responsive to the immune system. One specific oncolytic Ad,

Table 2.1 Applications of viral vectors in various biological fields.

Applications	Viral vectors	Advantages	Disadvantages	Comments	References
Gene therapy	AAV	Long-term gene expression - Low immunogenicity - Efficient transduction of dividing and nondividing cells	Limited cargo capacity - Immune response in some cases - Integration risks with lentiviruses	AAV vectors have demonstrated success in delivering therapeutic genes with minimal adverse effects.	[21]
Vaccine development	Adenovirus	Induces strong immune response - Allows antigen expression for presentation to the immune system	Potential preexisting immunity - Limited cargo capacity - Safety concerns in some cases	Adenoviral vectors are widely used in vaccine development, leveraging their immunogenic properties	[34]
Cancer gene therapy	Oncolytic viruses	Selective targeting of cancer cells - Enhanced tumor cell killing - Potential for combination therapies	Potential for off-target effects - Immune response against the vector - Safety concerns in clinical applications	Oncolytic viruses hold promise as a targeted approach for cancer gene therapy, with ongoing clinical trials.	[35]

(*Continued*)

Table 2.1 Applications of viral vectors in various biological fields. (*Continued*)

Applications	Viral vectors	Advantages	Disadvantages	Comments	References
Stem cell research	Lentivirus	Stable and heritable gene expression - Efficient transduction of stem cells - Integration into the host genome	Risk of insertional mutagenesis - Potential immune response - Limited cargo capacity	Lentiviral vectors are valuable tools in stem cell research, enabling stable genetic modifications	[25]
Neuroscience research	AAV	Neuronal cell targeting - Long-lasting gene expression - Tropism for specific brain regions	- Limited cargo capacity - Potential immune response - Variable transduction efficiency	AAV vectors are widely employed in neuroscience research for targeted gene expression in neuronal populations.	[36]
Functional genomics	AAV	Efficient gene delivery - Long-term gene expression - Cell type–specific targeting	Potential immunogenicity - Limited cargo capacity -Variable transduction efficiency	AAV vectors play a crucial role in functional genomics, allowing large-scale manipulation of gene expression	[37]

(*Continued*)

Table 2.1 Applications of viral vectors in various biological fields. (*Continued*)

Applications	Viral vectors	Advantages	Disadvantages	Comments	References
In vivo gene editing	AAV	Efficient delivery to target tissues - Persistent expression of editing components	Limited cargo capacity - Potential immunogenicity - Off-target effects	AAV-based delivery of CRISPR/Cas9 components shows promise for *in vivo* gene editing applications.	[38]
Cardiovascular gene therapy	AAV	Efficient transduction of cardiac cells - Persistent gene expression - Potential for treating heart diseases	Limited cargo capacity - Immune response in some cases - Safety concerns in clinical applications	AAV vectors are explored for delivering therapeutic genes to the heart, aiming to address cardiovascular diseases.	[24]
Immunotherapy	Lentivirus	Efficient modification of immune cells - Long-lasting expression of therapeutic genes - Potential for targeted cancer immunotherapy	Risk of insertional mutagenesis - Potential immune response - Limited cargo capacity	Lentiviral vectors are crucial for modifying immune cells in adoptive cell transfer therapies for cancer.	[39]

(*Continued*)

Table 2.1 Applications of viral vectors in various biological fields. (*Continued*)

Applications	Viral vectors	Advantages	Disadvantages	Comments	References
Metabolic disorders gene therapy	AAV	Efficient transduction of liver cells - Persistent and regulated gene expression - Potential for treating metabolic disorders	Limited cargo capacity - Preexisting immunity in some cases - Immune response against the vector	AAV vectors show promise in gene therapy for metabolic disorders, targeting the liver for sustained therapeutic effects.	[40]
Respiratory gene therapy	Adenovirus	Efficient transduction of respiratory epithelial cells - Potential for treating lung diseases - Induction of strong immune responses	Limited duration of gene expression - Potential immunogenicity - Safety concerns in clinical applications	Adenoviral vectors are explored for delivering therapeutic genes to the respiratory system, addressing lung diseases.	[41]
Ophthalmic gene therapy	AAV	Tropism for retinal cells - Long-lasting gene expression - Potential for treating inherited retinal disorders	Limited cargo capacity - Preexisting immunity in some cases - Potential for immune response against the vector	AAV vectors are utilized for delivering therapeutic genes to the eyes, showing promise in treating inherited retinal disorders.	[42]

(*Continued*)

Table 2.1 Applications of viral vectors in various biological fields. (*Continued*)

Applications	**Viral vectors**	**Advantages**	**Disadvantages**	**Comments**	**References**
Muscle gene therapy	Lentivirus	Efficient transduction of muscle cells - Long-lasting gene expression - Potential for treating muscular dystrophies	Risk of insertional mutagenesis - Potential immune response - Limited cargo capacity	Lentiviral vectors hold potential for gene therapy in muscle-related disorders, aiming to correct genetic defects.	[43]
Dendritic cell targeting for immunotherapy	Lentivirus	Efficient modification of dendritic cells - Induction of robust immune responses - Potential for cancer immunotherapy	Risk of insertional mutagenesis - Potential immune response - Limited cargo capacity	Lentiviral vectors play a role in modifying dendritic cells for enhanced cancer immunotherapy.	[44]
Antibody gene delivery for passive immunization	AAV	Long-lasting expression of therapeutic antibodies - Potential for treating infectious diseases - Low immunogenicity	Limited cargo capacity - Preexisting immunity in some cases - Potential for immune response against the vector	AAV vectors are explored for delivering genes encoding therapeutic antibodies, providing passive immunization against infections.	[45]

enadenotucirev, demonstrated selective propagation and killing of tumor cells [48]. It was tested for its resistance to inactivation by human blood components, implying that it may be administered intravenously.

2.3.2 Retroviruses

The retroviral capsid enveloped with a diameter measuring 80 to 100 nm, encloses the genome of the virus within a lipid bilayer derived from the host cell. Retroviruses, including HIV-1, share a basic structure. Three major coding segments (gag, pol, and env) for integration, replication, and encapsulation make up their linear, nonsegmental, single-stranded RNA genome (7–12 kb), which also includes one small coding domain including the pro gene, which codes for the viral protease [46]. Researchers have explored the utilization of AAV vectors (adeno-associated virus) for the treatment of various genetic disorders in animal models. For Rett Syndrome (RTT), a neurodevelopmental disorder linked to the X chromosome, AAV vectors carrying the MeCP2 gene were directly delivered to the cerebrospinal fluid in a mouse model. While there were some side effects, the treatment enhanced the survival rate of mice with RTT. In Huntington's disease (HD), a neurodegenerative disorder, AAV-based therapy was tested in a mouse model [49]. Delivering microRNA that targets the disease-causing gene using AAV vectors led to a decrease in the amount of the toxic protein and showed promise for secure and efficient gene silencing. AAV vectors encoding the cystic fibrosis transmembrane conductance regulator (CFTR) were used to target cystic fibrosis in animal models; however, there was unclear evidence of any clinical benefit [50]. In another study, different AAV serotypes were tested in Rhesus macaques for lung delivery, with AAV1 showing a higher vector genome number, although both serotypes demonstrated safe administration. AAV vectors were used to express therapeutic genes for muscular dystrophies such as Duchenne and limb-girdle muscular dystrophies. This resulted in improved muscle size distribution, decreased muscle degeneration, and extensive gene expression in animal models. AAV vectors bearing an altered human coagulation factor VIII (hFVIII) gene were created for hemophilia A, a bleeding condition. Different AAV vectors were evaluated in a mouse model, and some generated antibodies against hFVIII. The results suggest potential for AAV-based gene therapy for hemophilia A, with considerations for immune responses in future clinical trials [51].

2.3.3 Lentiviruses

The LV capsid mirrors that of simple retroviruses, containing a single-stranded RNA genome consisting of a 7- to 12-kb RNA genome with essential genes (gag, pol, and env). In addition, lentiviruses possess six other genes encoding regulatory and accessory proteins crucial for replication, binding, infection, and release. Commonly derived from HIV-1, LV vectors eliminate original genes and incorporate foreign genes. Transfecting HEK293 or 293T cells yields LV vectors, which, in contrast to common retroviruses, involve helper plasmids with specific gene components (gag, pol, rev, and env) and a separate plasmid for the recombinant LV vector sequence [46]. Pyruvate kinase deficiency (PKD) is a metabolic condition that has been addressed by researchers using LV vectors containing the PKLR gene and the human PKD (hPKD) promoter [52]. Hematopoietic stem cells (HSCs) transduced with the lentivirus were used to restore organ pathology, normalize the erythroid compartment, and improve the hematological phenotype in PKD animals without generating genotoxicity. Lentivirus vectors have also been used in central nervous system (CNS) gene therapy to silence RNA [53]. In Parkinson's disease (PD), lentivirus-based RNA interference (RNAi) was used to counteract the dysregulation and overexpression of α-synuclein, a protein associated with PD, in human dopaminergic cells and neurons in a rat model [54]. To reduce neurodegeneration and behavioral abnormalities in a mouse model of Alzheimer's disease, lentivirus vectors were utilized for RNA silencing to knock down BACE1, a protein implicated in amyloid precursor protein breakdown [55]. Furthermore, in a different Alzheimer's disease animal model, lentivirus-based small interfering RNA (siRNA) expression decreased tau phosphorylation and neurofibrillary tangles. Lentivirus vectors were used to deliver short hairpin RNAs (shRNAs) directed against the HIV-1 long terminal repeat (LTR) regulatory region and the HIV-1 co-receptor CCR5. This approach effectively reduced HIV infection in humanized bone marrow/thymus (hu-BLT) mice, pointing to a possible HIV treatment. Pigtailed macaques were used to assess Cal-1, another lentivirus vector, which showed preclinical and safe integration in the setting of anti-HIV treatment [17].

2.3.4 Poxviruses

The poxvirus capsid is generated in the cytoplasm of the host cell during DNA replication, with some viral genome replication products contributing to capsid production. Mature virions are encased by trans-Golgi structures and develop into intracellular enveloped viruses. These viruses eventually fuse with the inner cell membrane, are liberated from the Golgi envelope, and are redeveloped by the host cell membrane upon departure. Poxviruses such as MVA and NYVAC have large dsDNA genomes (178 and 192 kb), with roughly 100 conserved genes and extra genes that distinguish different viral strains. Most viral strands lack introns [46]. Poxviruses, particularly vaccinia viruses, have shown promise in gene therapy applications for various types of cancer. PANVAC, a system made up of recombinant vaccinia and fowlpox viruses that contain specific tumor-associated antigens, was utilized to treat pancreatic cancer. When administered sequentially in preclinical animal models, these vectors induced immune responses and showed potential for pancreatic cancer treatment. For hepatocellular carcinoma (HCC), a modified recombinant GLV-2b372 vaccinia virus was injected into HCC xenografts in mice [17]. The medication caused a considerable decrease in tumor sizes when compared to control mice, indicating potential efficacy against HCC. In prostate cancer, a GLV-1h153 vaccinia virus expressing the NIS gene, combined with radiotherapy, showed superior results in inhibiting tumor growth and improving survival rates in both xenograft and immunocompetent mouse models. Another modified vaccinia virus with a defective F4L gene displayed selective replication and cell death in bladder cancer models, resulting in significant tumor reduction or full ablation without affecting normal cells [17]. Additionally, this approach established antitumor immunity in animal models. When delivered systemically, a new cowpox virus (CPXV) vector containing a thymidine kinase gene deletion and the suicide gene FCU1 insertion showed preferential accumulation in tumor cells. Intratumorally administration in glioblastoma and colon cancer models resulted in significant inhibition of tumor growth [17].

2.3.5 Adeno-Associated Viruses

The AAV capsid is an icosahedral, nonenveloped protein shell with a diameter of 22 nm, exhibiting distinct serotypes with specific affinities for host cell receptors, facilitating targeted delivery to various tissues. AAV's genome comprises linear, single-stranded DNA flanked by 145-bp ITR sequences, featuring two open reading frames. The 5¢ frame encodes crucial replication proteins (Rep 78, Rep 68, Rep 52, and Rep 40), while the 3¢ frame codes for capsid proteins (VP1, VP2, and VP3) [46]. Researchers have been using AAV vectors (adeno-associated virus) in various genetic disorder treatments. For Rett syndrome (RTT), an AAV vector delivering the MeCP2 gene to the cerebrospinal fluid extended the survival of RTT mice, despite some dose-dependent side effects [56]. In HD, AAV-based therapy reduced the levels of the disease-causing HTT gene in transgenic HD sheep, indicating effective gene silencing in the striatum [17]. In cystic fibrosis, AAV vectors expressing the CFTR gene showed good safety in animal models, although clear clinical benefits were not evident. Tests with different AAV serotypes in Rhesus macaques showed that AAV1 had a higher vector genome number in the lungs compared to AAV5, but the AAV1-based activity was significantly low [57]. Further clinical trials, particularly with the more lung-tropic AAV1 serotype, are supported by the safety of AAV injection despite an increase in serum-neutralizing antibodies for both serotypes. For muscular dystrophies like Duchenne and limb-girdle muscular dystrophies, AAV vectors were used for the expression of the dystrophin gene, leading to widespread expression and improved muscle health in animal models. AAV vectors for hemophilia A were developed with a promoter and enhancer specific to the liver to contain the hFVIII gene. Evaluation in a mouse model showed varying levels of anti-hFVIII antibodies based on the AAV serotype used, suggesting considerations for potential immune responses in future treatments [19].

2.3.6 Herpes Simplex Viruses

The HSV features an icosahedral protein shell enveloped by a viral envelope containing glycoproteins crucial for host cellular attachment. The layer in between the capsid core and the envelope is known as the tegument, which is made up of virally encoded proteins and enzymes. Roughly 90 proteins are encoded in the 152-kb dsDNA that makes up the HSV genome and are necessary for the virus to adhere and replicate. The genome is divided into distinct long and short segments, each of which has an inverted repeat sequence to cap it [46]. HSV vectors have shown long-lasting effects and have been used in various medical applications. In treating painful diabetic neuropathy, HSV vectors were used to express pro-inflammatory cytokines. In mice with type I diabetes, constant injection of HSV-IL-10 into the nerve fibers inhibited pain responses, pointing to a possible treatment option for excruciating diabetic neuropathy [58]. Mice were injected with nonreplicating HSV vectors releasing growth factors to treat sensory neuropathy. With no adverse effects, this method effectively transduced dorsal root ganglions (DRGs) and stopped the advancement of sensory neuropathy. Preclinical research has investigated oncolytic HSV vectors in the setting of cancer [59]. An HSV-1 vector, called HF10, was engineered with specific deletions and mutations in its genome, allowing it to efficiently replicate in tumor cells and cause significant damage. This led to the activation of immune cells and a reduction in tumor growth, improving survival in animal models. Oncolytic HSV-2 vectors were also investigated for colon cancer cells and cancer stem-like cells in animal experiments. These vectors significantly inhibited the growth of the tumors, suggesting that they may be used to reduce cancer and stop it from spreading and reoccurring [17].

2.3.7 Alphaviruses

Alphaviruses have mostly been employed in preclinical research on gene therapy for the treatment of cancer [60]. The ability to transmit alphavirus vectors as naked RNA, multilayer plasmid DNA vectors, or recombinant particles with modified replication capabilities is one of their distinctive features. In one study, mice with A549 lung cancer xenografts had longer survival times when they received local delivery of a replication-proficient Semliki Forest virus (SFV) vector expressing enhanced green fluorescent protein (EGFP) [61]. In a different study, SFV-IL-12–based therapy was applied to a rat glioma model, leading to a notable decrease in tumor volume and an increase in survival time [62]. Researchers incorporated six microRNAs (miRNAs) into the SFV genome to inhibit tumor cell multiplication. When these modified SFV4-miRT124 particles were delivered to mice, they precisely targeted gliomas, restricted dissemination in the CNS, and greatly boosted survival rates [63]. Furthermore, M1, a naturally occurring oncolytic alphavirus, has been demonstrated to specifically target cancer cells that lack zinc finger antiviral protein (ZAP). In a liver tumor model, M1 displayed strong tumor tropism and potent oncolytic action [64].

2.3.8 Flaviviruses

In the setting of flaviviruses, gene therapy was carried out using a Kunjin viral vector encoding the granulocyte-macrophage colony-stimulating factor (GM-CSF). This vector was injected directly into tumors in mice with subcutaneous CT26 colon carcinoma [65]. More than half of the animals were cured after receiving Kunjin–GM-CSF treatment, with tumors becoming undetectable 18 days later. In the same way, while treating B16-OVA melanoma tumors, there was considerable tumor shrinkage after 5 days, and the cure rate reached 67% [65]. In addition, subcutaneous Kunjin–GM-CSF injections in mice resulted in the regression of CT26 lung metastases. In simpler terms, this gene therapy approach using the Kunjin virus vector expressing GM-CSF showed promising results in treating various types of tumors in mice, leading to tumor regression and a significant cure rate.

2.3.9 Rhabdoviruses

In the field of gene therapy, vesicular stomatitis virus (VSV) has been employed in preclinical trials. VSV is attractive because it has low prevalence in humans and is effective in expressing genes from other organisms. One application is in vaccine development, where VSV vectors expressing HIV-1 proteins triggered strong immune responses in nonhuman primates, protecting them from challenges with a pathogenic SIV/HIV recombinant [66]. However, concerns about VSV's potential to cause neurovirulence have led to efforts to create safer versions. In one technique, a chimeric VSV vector swapped its original envelope with one from another virus, causing no harm to normal brain cells while effectively eradicating brain tumor cells in diverse types. This vector can be safely delivered systemically, allowing for several injections. To prepare for clinical trials, an oncolytic VSV-IFNβ-NIS vector encoding interferon and sodium iodide transporter was investigated in preclinical mouse models [67]. The vector showed dose-dependent tumor regression in animals with plasmacytoma tumors, as well as regression in SCID mouse xenografts. In a dosage escalation trial using purpose-bred dogs with naturally occurring tumors, the maximum tolerable dose was identified with mild to moderate side effects, and the virus was swiftly eliminated from the bloodstream without generating infectious viruses in other bodily fluids. Another study showed that VSV-based expression of human mucin 1 (MUC1) dramatically reduced tumor growth in mice with pancreatic cancer xenografts [68]. When combined with the chemotherapy drug gemcitabine, the VSV-MUC1 treatment showed superior therapeutic efficacy.

2.3.10 Newcastle Disease Virus

Newcastle disease virus (NDV) is extensively studied for its potential in cancer treatment due to its oncolytic activity [69]. In one study, NDV vectors expressing different immune-stimulating proteins, IL-2 and IL-15, were injected directly into melanoma tumors in mice. Both treatments suppressed tumor growth, but NDV-IL15 showed higher survival rates compared to NDV-IL2 [69]. Another study produced recombinant NDVs with the GFP gene through genetic engineering; these NDVs selectively multiplied within tumors and caused mouse lung tumors to undergo apoptosis. Researchers have explored the use of NDV to express immune-stimulating proteins like IL-2 and TRAIL (tumor necrosis factor–related apoptosis-inducing ligand). When compared to NDV-IL2 alone, the modified NDV containing both TRAIL and IL-2 exhibited better apoptotic effects. This treatment induced the proliferation of immune cells ($CD4^+$ and $CD8^+$) and the expression of antitumor cytokines. In mice with liver cancer (HCC) and melanoma, the NDV carrying both IL-2 and TRAIL demonstrated prolonged survival. Additionally, a different NDV strain (Anhinga) was used to express soluble TRAIL, resulting in efficient suppression of liver cancer without significant toxicity [70, 71].

2.3.11 Coxsackieviruses

Scientists have explored the use of coxsackieviruses, specifically coxsackievirus B3 (CVB3) and coxsackievirus A21 (CAV21), for potential gene therapy applications. In one study, mice with ischemic hind limbs were given injections of CVB3, which expresses human fibroblast growth factor 2 (FGF2), to prevent ischemic necrosis [72]. For over 3 weeks, this treatment increased blood flow in limbs that were ischemia, and the changed CVB3 exhibited less pathogenicity than the wild form. In melanoma xenograft mice, CAV21 expressing decay-accelerating factor (DAF) and intercellular adhesion molecule-1 (ICAM-1) showed a decrease in tumor burden [73]. A single dose of CAV21 effectively lysed tumors, and the virus propagated systemically, producing regression in tumors distant from the injection site. The same CAV21 vector proved efficient for treating mice with breast tumor xenografts, causing considerable tumor shrinkage and eliminating metastases. Furthermore, when coupled with the chemotherapeutic medication doxorubicin hydrochloride, CVA21 expressing ICAM-1 and DAF demonstrated greater tumor regression than either the virus or the medicine alone. In the context of prostate cancer, low pathogenic enteroviruses such as CVA21, CVA21-DAFv, and Echovirus 1 (EV1) were studied in mice [74]. Systemic delivery caused tumor xenograft reduction, and increasing dosages of EV1 produced a therapeutic response in the LNCaP animal model.

2.3.12 Measles Virus

Measles viruses have been explored for gene therapy in various preclinical animal studies. In one method, an oncolytic measles virus (MV-Edm) was engineered to express NIS, a gene deficient in invasive and radioiodine-resistant anaplastic thyroid carcinoma (ATC) [75]. Treatment with this modified virus confirmed NIS expression and improved the killing of tumors.

In another approach, the measles virus was modified to produce a yeast-based bifunctional suicide gene named super-cytosine deaminase (SCD) [76]. This gene can transform a nontoxic prodrug (5-fluorocytosine) into an extremely cytotoxic chemical (5-fluorouracil), which addresses resistance difficulties in cancer treatment. The modified virus (MV-SCD) successfully lysed human ovarian cancer and primary tumor cells, indicating high oncolytic activity. It has also shown efficacy in a mouse model of human HCC, generating long-term virus replication in tumor tissue and cell death [77]. In several investigations, MV-SCD was delivered intratumorally coupled with systemic 5-FU in mice models of TFK-1 and HuCCT1 xenografts, leading to substantial tumor reduction and increased survival advantages [78].

2.4 Construction of Viral Vectors

Transient transfection and stable producer cell lines are the two basic methods in the field of viral vector manufacture; each is covered in the sections that follow, utilizing data from previous studies. Transient transfection serves as a laboratory method facilitating the short-term introduction of external genetic material, such as plasmid DNA or RNA, into cells to achieve temporary gene expression. Differing from stable transfection, where foreign DNA integrates into the host cell genome for sustained expression, transient transfection allows for the transient synthesis of introduced genes. The procedure involves preparing genetic material, transfecting cultured cells through various methods, facilitating gene expression temporarily, and subsequent analysis. Predominantly utilized in research, transient transfection provides a rapid and adaptable approach for studying gene function, assessing expression constructs, and conducting brief experiments, although it has inherent limitations, including variability and transient expression [79]. On the other hand, stable producer cell lines involve genetically modified cells designed to consistently generate a specific product, such as proteins, antibodies, or viral vectors, over an extended duration. In contrast to transient transfection, which yields short-lived gene expression, stable producer cell lines deliver a continuous and stable supply of the desired product. The process encompasses integrating the desired gene into the genetic material of host cells, typically using approaches like plasmid or viral vector delivery. Once established, these cell lines can be cultured over multiple generations, ensuring reliable and prolonged production of the targeted substance. Widely employed in biopharmaceutical manufacturing and gene therapy, stable producer cell lines offer a dependable and reproducible platform for large-scale production. To address the adverse events related to insertional mutagenesis and trans-activation of cellular proto-oncogenes that were seen in recent clinical trials for X-linked SCID, a scalable and dependable production method for high-titer ecotropic self-inactivating (SIN) gamma-retroviral (gRV) vectors that are compliant with current good manufacturing practice (cGMP) standards has been developed [80]. Safety-enhanced SIN gRV vectors and LV vectors have been produced to reduce the dangers associated with insertional mutagenesis. The SIN design has proven effective in this regard, rendering both LTRs transcriptionally silent upon vector integration into the genome. However, establishing stable producer cell lines for SIN gRV vectors is a challenge, necessitating the use of alternative methods for large-scale vector production. Among these strategies is the use of transfection-based techniques, which offer advantages over the traditional method of producing stable producer cell lines and master cell banks (MCBs) in terms of flexibility, cost savings, and time efficiency [79]. This approach has several advantages, such as the ability to edit vector plasmids without having to regenerate producer cell lines and the elimination of the need to verify stable producer lines for each vector, but it also has significant drawbacks. High amounts of plasmid DNA or cellular debris in the vector product pose challenges; however, inventive approaches have been suggested to overcome these limits, such as preloading gRV vector particles on fibronectin or treating LV vectors with Benzonase [81]. Additionally, the research explores the assessment of three transfection techniques: polycation use, cationic lipids (Fecturin and Lipofectamine), and DNA coprecipitation with calcium phosphate. The 38-year-old calcium phosphate technique is the focus of this study because of its low toxicity, good transduction efficiencies, and cost-effectiveness [82]. The effectiveness of transduction for adherent and nonadherent cells is evaluated with and without serum. Beyond transfection, the researchers investigate bioreactors for the synthesis of gRV vectors, emphasizing the advantages of fixed-bed reactor culture systems, especially those that make use of the Wave Bioreactor platform's Fibra-Cel cell carrier [83]. This cell carrier serves as a fully disposable, single-use closed-system bioreactor solution. It was previously employed in the production of the first gene therapy product to be licensed in China. A case study comprehensively describes the optimization process, including a comparison of adherent 293T and suspension-based 293F cells, optimal transfection temperatures and procedures, cell seeding density optimization, when to switch media, and plasmid concentration [79]. The 3′ untranslated region (UTR) of the virus receives the addition of the woodchuck hepatitis virus post-transcriptional regulatory element (wPRE). Notable alterations to the enhanced viral backbones made by the researchers include vectors with a modified primer binding site to avoid epigenetic repressors. These changes aim to improve RNA processing and increase the titer of non-concentrated vector stocks. The production and certification of five high-titer ecotropic SIN gRV vectors that are cGMP-grade and facilitate preclinical animal safety studies are the goals of the study. All things considered, this massive research project integrates the most recent advances in transfection methods, bioreactor systems, and vector design to produce a scalable and efficient production system for clinical-grade gRV vectors, paving the way for upcoming clinical trials and breakthroughs in gene therapy (Figure 2.1). In a study, plasmids encoding gRV and LV vectors were used to construct viral vectors intended for gene therapy applications. The gRV vectors utilized in genotoxicity tests were SERS11.EGFP.pre*, SRS11.EFS.EGFP.pre*, SERS11.SF.EGFP.pre*, RSF91.EGFP.pre*, and RSF91.uORF.EGFP.pre*; Jens Bohne donated the uORF element. Plasmid SRS11.EFS.IL2Rg.pre* was utilized in the production of the IL2Rg vector. For development, several vectors were used, including SRS11.SF.GFP.pre*SE, SRS11.SF.eGFP.pre*, and SRS11.SF.GFP.pre*. The MIEG3 gRV vector was created in the laboratory of D. Williams. For each gRV vector, the plasmid pCDNA3.MLVg/p encoded the necessary gag and pol sequences, while the LV vector used pCDNA3.g/p.4CTE. The pHCMV-RD114, pHCMV-VSV-G, pHCMV-GALVenv, and K73-Eco envelope plasmids were all included [79]. The Plasmid Factory in Bielefeld, Germany, provided Ccc-grade plasmids that were appropriate for the current good manufacturing practice (cGMP). Using 293T cells derived from HEK293 cells cultured in Dulbecco's modified Eagle's medium (DMEM) supplemented with 10% fetal bovine serum (FBS) and cryopreserved in a suitable freezing solution allowed adherent conditions to be maintained in cell culture. Serum-free FreeStyle293 media were used to cultivate 293F cells from HEK293 cells, which were then cryopreserved in a nonadherent environment. Glucose levels were monitored during the cell culture procedure. Adherent 293T cells were transfected using Ca-phosphate, Lipofectamine 2000, or Fecturin methods, while nonadherent 293F cells were transfected in a range of medium conditions. For transfection, Fibra-Cel disks or tissue culture flasks were used. After being filtered, the captured vectors were kept at −70°C or below. For large-scale production in the bioreactor, certified 293T cells were used, and following transfection, the growth medium was changed regularly. A closed-system fluid channel was used to process and store the harvested vectors. Titration of vectors involved calculating titers based on EGFP expression, which was used to determine expression in certain cell lines. After transfection, Trypan blue staining on Fibra-Cel disks was used under a microscope to evaluate the morphology of the cells. Overall, this thorough methodological approach demonstrates the painstaking procedures needed in the creation and titration of high-titer viral vectors for gene therapy applications. It does this by integrating a range of vectors, plasmids, and cell culture techniques [79].

The facts are briefly covered, another study focuses on developing a LentiPro 26 using the stable producer cell lines technique. The text that follows describes the experimental procedures that were used in a scientific study that focused on the culture of HEK293T cells and the creation of plasmids for the generation of LV vectors [84]. The core of the work is the use of HEK293T cells, a well-known cell line that is frequently used for a variety of molecular and cellular biology applications. The cells were cultured in 10% FBS-enhanced DMEM. The culture was kept under controlled conditions, with 7% CO_2 in the air and a temperature of 37°C. Plasmid creation was a crucial aspect of the research, involving the utilization of multiple essential plasmids. Among these, pMDLg/pRRE, pRSV-REV, pMD2.G, and pRRLIN.cPPT.PGK-GFP.WPRE were noteworthy since they each had a distinct role to play in the creation of LVs. These plasmids were either altered to meet the needs of the experiment or taken from the Addgene plasmid library. To accomplish the necessary changes, cloning techniques, primers, and templates were used during creation. To modify the LV vectors' characteristics, for example, a point mutation in the pGP(T26S)P plasmid was introduced, changing the viral protease sequence. Both transient and stable methods were used to produce the LV vectors. Using linear polyethyleneimine, cells were transfected with the appropriate plasmids for the temporary manufacturing procedure. To guarantee uniformity across several productions, the transfection settings were meticulously regulated, utilizing precise amounts of the vector genome, Gag-Pro-Pol, Rev, envelope glycoprotein, and a stuffer plasmid. After being collected, the supernatant containing the LVs was clarified and kept at −80°C for storage. Similar seeding procedures were used in stable viral productions, and supernatants were extracted at predetermined intervals. This helped to provide a more complex picture of the temporal dynamics of LV vector creation. An essential component of the research was identifying functional LV titers, which was done by using flow cytometric analysis to check for GFP expression in HEK293T cells that had been transduced. This process aided in the computation of transducing units per volume (TU/ml), a quantitative indicator of the vector's functionality, and gave information on how well the LV vectors transduced target cells [84]. Additionally, clones were screened and isolated using fluorescence-activated cell sorting

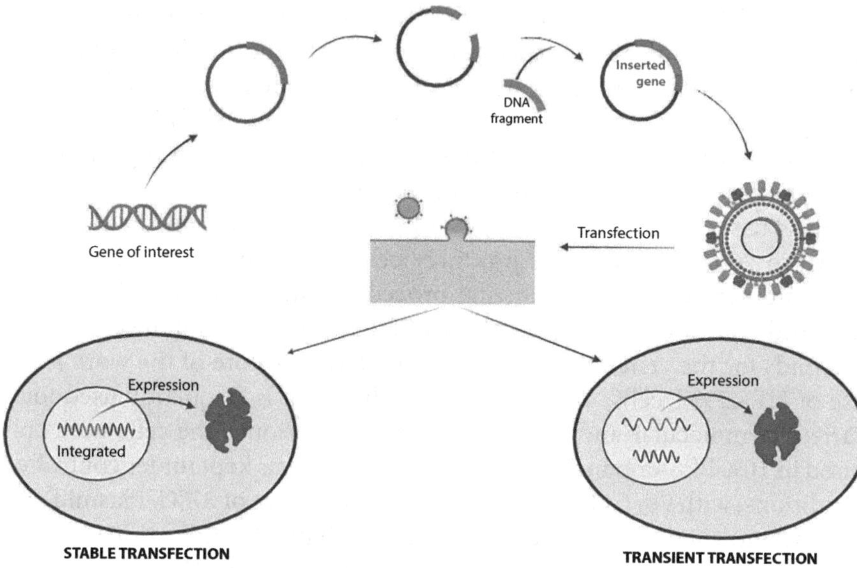

Figure 2.1 Transfection by viral vectors (created by Vuppu *et al.* using Biorender.com).

(FACS), a sophisticated method that allowed for the separation and investigation of cell populations based on fluorescent properties.

2.5 Challenges

The production of the viral vector is a critical component in the field of gene therapy and molecular biology, as it largely involves the development of vectors and aids in the efficient delivery of genetic material to target cells. Viral vectors have a prospective function in a variety of applications, but their creation can present several obstacles.

Some of the challenges are as follows:

2.5.1 Immune Response

One of the biggest obstacles that gene therapy using viral vectors encounters is the activation of the immune system. Among all the viral vectors, Ad vectors are particularly immunogenic, triggering multiple immune responses. The Ad capsid triggers humoral and inflammatory reactions, but cytotoxic T lymphocyte (CTL) [85] has been developed in an attempt to suppress T cell responses. Ad vectors that are "gutted" or "helper-dependent" (HD) [86, 87] have been developed in an attempt to suppress T cell responses. Although progress has improved prospects for long-term gene transfer, caution is necessary as HD Ads may still induce capsid-mediated inflammatory responses. The dose plays an important role in inducing harmful immune and inflammatory responses. Studies in immune-privileged rodent brains show a linear relationship between Ad vector dose and inflammatory responses, with a narrow range causing cellular toxicity [88]. Predicting vector-related side effects is complicated by individual variability in immune responses, as observed in the heterogeneous reactions to the Ad vector during the OTC trial [88, 89]. To mitigate risks, monitoring immune status, cytokine profiles, and underlying conditions in gene-transfer clinical trials is recommended. While T cell responses against transgenic products are taken into account, other viral vector systems, such as lentivirus or AAV vectors, cause less inflammation. Preexisting humoral immunity to wild-type viruses also poses challenges, necessitating strategies like switching capsid serotypes to address neutralizing antibodies [90, 91]. In summary, while gene therapy shows promise, addressing immunogenicity, inflammatory responses, and individual variability in immune reactions is crucial for ensuring the safety and efficacy of viral vectors in clinical applications.

2.5.2 Specificity of the Transgene Delivery

Wild-type viruses naturally infect tissues accessible via transmission routes, but recombinant vectors, such as Ads and AAVs, can bypass these limitations. For example, Ads and AAVs can effectively infect neurons when injected into the brain, despite the fact that they do not naturally infect the CNS. However, this broad infectivity can be detrimental, resulting in unexpected vector absorption by numerous cell types in multiple organs, even when delivered locally. While transgene expression can be controlled using tissue-specific promoters, vector dissemination remains a concern [92, 93]. The lack of specificity in Ad vectors was implicated in a fatal systemic immune response in 1999. Vector dose is closely linked to the severity of immunogenic reactions and other toxic effects. Improving the effectiveness of viral vectors in infecting specific cell groups is critical for gene therapy safety because it allows lower viral loads to be employed. One focus of vector development is achieving transductional targeting. Pseudotyping is a straightforward method, where the vector's outer protein coat is exchanged to alter its specificity [94–96]. Another method involves adding molecular adaptors, such as bispecific antibodies, to the vector's capsid to improve targeting. However, the practicality of this technique for clinical studies remains dubious. A third strategy involves genetically changing the capsid genes to alter receptor binding characteristics, hence redirecting vector tropism. This has been successful in cell culture but requires further evaluation *in vivo*. Ad vectors are more amenable to genetic retargeting than other vectors. Herpes and retrovirus internalization is complex, making genetic retargeting challenging. AAV engineering is also challenging, although recent advances in the AAV2 capsid structure might aid this process. Novel genetic targeting approaches involve DNA shuffling and randomized peptide insertions to create vector libraries with altered tropism. While vectors can be targeted to new cell types, limiting nonspecific uptake by other cells is difficult. Nonetheless, increasing transduction efficiency with focused techniques and optimum promoters can lessen the danger of hazardous side effects by allowing for lower viral dosages.

2.5.3 Insertional Mutagenesis

For over a decade, integrated viral vectors, primarily derived from retroviruses, have been used in clinical trials to enable sustained gene transfer in proliferative cells such as hematopoietic cells. The prevailing wisdom was that retroviral vector genomes were incorporated randomly into host DNA, with the presumed risk of altering a cellular sequence linked to cancer estimated to be around 1 in every 10 million insertions. Despite treating hundreds of patients in various gene therapy trials, no vector-induced cancers were observed, reinforcing the view that the risk was negligible due to the requirement for multiple genetic lesions for oncogenesis [97]. Recent research has challenged these beliefs, with one study indicating that retrovirally transduced bone marrow cells caused leukemia in mice. This prompted worries regarding the transgenic product's cooperation with the disruption of a leukemia-linked gene. In the SCID-XI trial [98], two patients developed a leukemia-like disorder due to retroviral vector integration near the oncogene LMO2 [99]. Another study found that retroviral insertion is not as random as previously thought, with a bias for incorporation into transcriptionally active genes. This selection could lead to the clonal growth of transformed cells and the onset of cancer. The concern is whether similar hazards exist for other therapeutic applications involving integrating vectors. Clonal expansion in *ex vivo* hematopoietic gene therapy appears to be a danger factor, but nondividing tissues in people with functioning immune systems are less likely to be affected. Efforts may be directed toward making existing integrating vectors safer, maybe by inserting suicide genes to enable self-destruct mechanisms in the event of oncogenesis. New vector systems, such as the bacteriophage ΦC31 integrase system, are being investigated to facilitate integration into certain predefined sites. Even recombinant AAV (rAAV) vectors, initially considered safe, are under scrutiny. Despite the low incidence of rAAV integration and the fact that most applications target nonproliferating cells, chromosomal rearrangements and deletions are linked to integrated rAAV genomes. Nonhomologous end joining (NHEJ) of rAAV-free ends with damaged chromosomes is the mechanism. Research indicates that rAAV integration is elevated by genotoxic drugs that cause double-strand breaks and that the number of integrated genomes in mice does not increase when the rAAV vector dose is exceeded [100].

2.6 Advancements in Technology of Viral Vector Construction

There are numerous strategies for producing viral vectors, the most common of which is the use of mammalian cells in adherent or suspension cell systems. Traditional laboratory-scale systems with adherent cells struggle to scale due to the need for multiple flasks, roller bottles, or cell factories. This lengthens the duration of processing and amplifies the danger resulting from aseptic processing. Larger disposable culture systems and bioreactors are becoming more common in the industry to address these issues and improve safety in clinical manufacturing. Different systems, such as the Corning HYPERFlask and HYPERStack, have been used depending on the kind of vector and cells [101]. By allowing cell proliferation on a gas-permeable surface, these approaches eliminate the need for headspace and allow for an increased number of cells to be cultivated in the same incubator footprint. For instance, the HYPERStack provides a much bigger area for cell growth than conventional techniques, leading to a notable increase in productivity for the creation of vectors [101]. Higher cell culture densities are possible using fixed-bed culture systems, such as the CellCube, iCELLIS™ bioreactor, and Celligen bioreactor [102–104], all of which provide adequate gas exchange and nutrition supply. The Celligen bioreactor, using a FibraCel cell carrier, manufactured China's first approved gene therapy product [105]. Unlike conventional stirred tank reactors, these systems can achieve superior vector producer cell development and are engineered to prevent the accumulation of byproducts. Techniques like chemical lysis or microfluidization could be investigated to release intracellular viruses. Lab-to-industrial-scale scalability is provided by suspension-based cell cultures, such as those made with the Wave Bioreactor and Sartorius stirred tank reactor. Serum-free suspension cultures are not suitable for all cell lines, and the cell densities per volume are typically lower than in fixed-bed reactors, even though they make it simple to collect both cells and culture fluid. The type of cells, the harvesting technique, and the type of vector all influence the manufacturing system selection. For example, the iCELLis™ fixed-bed bioreactor is a feasible choice for transfection-based technologies, indicating its potential for producing clinical-grade viral vectors in a scalable manner [102]. Transfection-based and stable producer cell lines are the two basic categories into which manufacturing techniques can be divided. Transient transfection of cells with vector, helper, or packing plasmids is a popular method for producing viral vectors. Due to differences in efficiency, it is seen as a bottleneck in clinical manufacturing. There are several transfection reagents available, each with pros and cons, including calcium phosphate, polyethyleneimine (PEI), and cationic lipids [106]. Clinical manufacturing is a field where scalability, consistency, and strict control are critical considerations. On the other hand, stable producer cell lines generate vectors over long times, making purification and scaling simpler. However, several genetic products required for vector manufacturing are toxic, making it difficult to establish producer cell lines. Each vector-specific producer cell line must be certified by a master cell bank before clinical manufacturing. Conventional transfection techniques have been replaced by the creation of scalable transfection systems like the MaxCyte and inducible cell lines [107]. Clinical-grade viral vector production on a wide scale requires substantial time and financial commitment. For every system to meet regulatory requirements—like the FDA's current good manufacturing practices—careful optimization and validation are needed (cGMP). The decision between stable producer cell line techniques and transfection-based approaches is influenced by various parameters, including downstream purification requirements, consistency, and scalability. Alternative transfection reagents are available, each having pros and cons, including calcium phosphate, PEI, and cationic lipids. Scalability and purification benefits are offered by stable producer cell lines; nevertheless, they need to be certified and may present issues with cell toxicity and the durability of high-titer vector production. Viral vectors with genome count between 10^{15} and 10^{16} are currently manufactured to a level that is considered adequate for low-dose gene therapy programs and orphan disease indications. The expanding needs in the field of gene therapy, however, are predicted to necessitate a large increase in manufacturing capacity as successful clinical programs progress to later stages and for diseases requiring higher per-patient vector dosages. The baculovirus system, which is used by uniQure to produce Glybera, is one method of attaining increased yields [108]. This technique, developed by Kotin and associates, produces AAV using SF9 suspension insect cells [109]. SF9 cells are infected with recombinant baculoviruses carrying the vector genome, capsid, and helper genes rather than transfected with the vector-generating genes. Recent system developments have integrated the AAV rep and cap genes into a single baculovirus, resulting in high outputs of roughly 10^{14} viral genomes per liter (vg/L) from 100- to 200-L bioreactors. The system's scalability has been demonstrated from 20 ml to 200 L, and projections for 500-L scale productions indicate a large increase in manufacturing capacity. HSV type 1 (HSV-1) recombinant replication-defective and wild-type Ad type 5 (Ad5) are two more technologies designed for large-scale AAV manufacturing. A 250-L production-scale producer cell line manufacturing procedure based on Ad5 was developed. Furthermore, the Wave Bioreactor was employed to manufacture AAV using the recombinant HSV-1 expression system with suspension baby hamster kidney (BHK-21) cells [110]. The system has demonstrated great productivity, reaching up to 10^{14} vg/L at a 10-L scale. Comparing this approach to a vector made by plasmid transfection, better virus survivability and higher expression per virion were shown. Ensuring the safety and efficacy of recombinant viral vectors for clinical trials, especially with expected manufacturing capacity increases, requires specialized quality control (QC) testing. The intricate nature of viral vectors demands unique analytical techniques for each gene therapy product. Two types of QC testing exist: vector-specific tests and approved protein or vaccine product tests. Potency assays, which are vital for proving drug stability and lot consistency, measure functional activity resulting from vector transgene expression. Limitations include persistent DNA contamination, particularly plasmids or bacmids, which are challenging to remove due to their similarity to the vector. Mitigation involves optimizing vector production and employing purifying techniques, ensuring stringent requirements and product consistency as gene therapy advances.

2.7 Conclusion and Future Prospects

Thus, the dynamic and ever-changing area of viral vector building contributes to creative advances in the creation of treatments such as gene therapy for a variety of diseases. Many scientists want to enhance procedures for creating more effective and secure viral vectors. The future of viral vector construction in gene therapy is marked by transformative progress and significant opportunities. Emphasis lies on enhancing precision and specificity, with a focus on minimizing off-target effects through advanced transductional targeting strategies. The engineering of viral capsids to achieve greater selectivity in terms of cell type or tissue is a key goal, enhancing therapeutic efficacy while minimizing unintended consequences. The future also involves refining safer integration strategies, particularly for retroviruses, by exploring alternative mechanisms such as the bacteriophage ΦC31 integrase to address concerns about insertional mutagenesis.

A notable trend is the pursuit of non-integrating vectors, particularly certain AAV variants optimized to persist in episomal form, mitigating the genotoxicity risks associated with integration. Synthetic biology and genome editing technologies play a crucial role, enabling precise customization of viral vectors with specific functionalities, regulatory elements, and payload capacities. Technologies like CRISPR/Cas systems empower researchers to design vectors with unparalleled precision for diverse therapeutic applications [17].

Efforts are directed toward optimizing vector production processes for scalability and consistency in large-scale manufacturing. Overcoming the immunogenicity of viral vectors remains a challenge, prompting the exploration of strategies like surface modifications and stealth technologies to attenuate immune responses and enhance therapeutic potential. Diversification of vector platforms involves exploring novel viruses or viral-like particles with unique advantages, such as increased payload capacity or the ability to infect specific cell types, broadening therapeutic options.

The integration of gene-editing technologies, specifically CRISPR/Cas systems, with viral vectors opens new frontiers in precision medicine, allowing targeted modifications of the host genome for potential cures of genetic disorders. *In vivo*, delivery strategies are undergoing refinement, including innovations in vector administration techniques and systemic distribution optimization for enhancement of efficiency and safety of gene delivery. Navigating the future of viral vector construction requires a multidisciplinary approach, converging insights from molecular biology, virology, immunology, and bioengineering [111]. This collaborative effort signifies a new era in precision medicine with transformative implications for patient care and treatment outcomes.

Acknowledgments

The authors want to express their sincere gratitude to Dr. G. Viswanathan, honorable Chancellor, VIT University, Vellore, for his constant encouragement. We would also like to acknowledge ICMR for awarding the JRF position to Toshika Mishra.

References

1. Chavda, V.P., Baviskar, K.P., Vaghela, D.A., Raut, S.S., Bedse, A.P., Nasal Sprays for Treating COVID-19: A Scientific Note. *Pharmacol. Rep.*, 75, 2, 249–265, **2023**, doi: 10.1007/s43440-023-00463-7.
2. Raper, S.E., Chirmule, N., Lee, F.S., Wivel, N.A., Bagg, A., Gao, G., Wilson, J.M., Batshaw, M.L., Fatal Systemic Inflammatory Response Syndrome in a Ornithine Transcarbamylase Deficient Patient Following Adenoviral Gene Transfer. *Mol. Genet. Metab.*, *80*, 148–158, **2003**, doi: 10.1016/j.ymgme.2003.08.016.
3. Hacein-Bey-Abina, S., Garrigue, A., Wang, G.P., Soulier, J., Lim, A., Morillon, E., Clappier, E., Caccavelli, L., Delabesse, E., Beldjord, K., *et al.*, Insertional Oncogenesis in 4 Patients after Retrovirus-Mediated Gene Therapy of SCID-X1. *J. Clin. Invest.*, *118*, 3132–3142, **2008**, doi: 10.1172/JCI35700.
4. McCormack, M.P. and Rabbitts, T.H., Activation of the T-Cell Oncogene *LMO2* after Gene Therapy for X-Linked Severe Combined Immunodeficiency. *N. Engl. J. Med.*, *350*, 913–922, **2004**, doi: 10.1056/NEJMra032207.
5. Wang, F., Wang, Z., Tian, H., Qi, M., Zhai, Z., Li, S., Li, R., Zhang, H., Wang, W., Fu, S., *et al.*, Biodistribution and Safety Assessment of Bladder Cancer Specific Recombinant Oncolytic Adenovirus in Subcutaneous Xenografts Tumor Model in Nude Mice. *Curr. Gene Ther.*, *12*, 67–76, **2012**, doi: 10.2174/156652312800099599.
6. Wei, Q., Fan, J., Liao, J., Zou, Y., Song, D., Liu, J., Cui, J., Liu, F., Ma, C., Hu, X., *et al.*, Engineering the Rapid Adenovirus Production and Amplification (RAPA) Cell Line to Expedite the Generation of Recombinant Adenoviruses. *Cell. Physiol. Biochem.*, *41*, 2383–2398, **2017**, doi: 10.1159/000475909.
7. Grieger, J.C. and Samulski, R.J., Packaging Capacity of Adeno-Associated Virus Serotypes: Impact of Larger Genomes on Infectivity and Postentry Steps. *J. Virol.*, *79*, 9933–9944, **2005**, doi: 10.1128/JVI.79.15.9933-9944.2005.
8. Mingozzi, F. and High, K.A., Immune Responses to AAV Vectors: Overcoming Barriers to Successful Gene Therapy. *Blood*, *122*, 23–36, **2013**, doi: 10.1182/blood-2013-01-306647.
9. Samulski, R.J. and Muzyczka, N., AAV-Mediated Gene Therapy for Research and Therapeutic Purposes. *Annu. Rev. Virol.*, *1*, 427–451, **2014**, doi: 10.1146/annurev-virology-031413-085355.

10. Santiago-Ortiz, J.L. and Schaffer, D.V., Adeno-Associated Virus (AAV) Vectors in Cancer Gene Therapy. *J. Control. Release*, *240*, 287–301, **2016**, doi: 10.1016/j.jconrel.2016.01.001.
11. Epstein, A., Marconi, P., Argnani, R., Manservigi, R., HSV-1-Derived Recombinant and Amplicon Vectors for Gene Transfer and Gene Therapy. *Curr. Gene Ther.*, *5*, 445–457, **2005**, doi: 10.2174/156652305774329285.
12. Holmes, K.D., Cassam, A.K., Chan, B., Peters, A.A., Weaver, L.C., Dekaban, G.A., A Multi-Mutant Herpes Simplex Virus Vector Has Minimal Cytotoxic Effects on the Distribution of Filamentous Actin, α-Actinin 2 and a Glutamate Receptor in Differentiated PC12 Cells. *J. Neurovirol.*, *6*, 33–45, 2000, doi: 10.3109/13550280009006380.
13. Kay, M.A., Glorioso, J.C., Naldini, L., Viral Vectors for Gene Therapy: The Art of Turning Infectious Agents into Vehicles of Therapeutics. *Nat. Med.*, *7*, 33–40, **2001**, doi: 10.1038/83324.
14. Piedrahita, D., Hernández, I., López-Tobón, A., Fedorov, D., Obara, B., Manjunath, B.S., Boudreau, R.L., Davidson, B., LaFerla, F., Gallego-Gómez, J.C., *et al.*, Silencing of CDK5 Reduces Neurofibrillary Tangles in Transgenic Alzheimer's Mice. *J. Neurosci.*, *30*, 13966–13976, **2010**, doi: 10.1523/JNEUROSCI.3637-10.2010.
15. Vigna, E. and Naldini, L., Lentiviral Vectors: Excellent Tools for Experimental Gene Transfer and Promising Candidates for Gene Therapy. *J. Gene Med.*, *2*, 308–316, **2000**, doi: 10.1002/1521-2254(200009/10)2:5<308::AID-JGM131>3.0.CO;2-3.
16. Ginn, S.L., Amaya, A.K., Alexander, I.E., Edelstein, M., Abedi, M.R., Gene Therapy Clinical Trials Worldwide to 2017: An Update. *J. Gene Med.*, *20*, e3015, **2018**, doi: 10.1002/jgm.3015.
17. Lundstrom, K., Viral Vectors in Gene Therapy. *Diseases*, *6*, 42, **2018**, doi: 10.3390/diseases6020042.
18. Kotterman, M.A., Chalberg, T.W., Schaffer, D.V., Viral Vectors for Gene Therapy: Translational and Clinical Outlook. *Annu. Rev. Biomed. Eng.*, 17, 63–89, 2015, doi: 10.1146/annurev-bioeng-071813-104938.
19. Samelson-Jones, B.J. and George, L.A., Adeno-Associated Virus Gene Therapy for Hemophilia. *Annu. Rev. Med.*, *74*, 231–247, **2023**, doi: 10.1146/annurev-med-043021-033013.
20. Fujino, H., Sonoda-Fukuda, E., Isoda, L., Kawabe, A., Takarada, T., Kasahara, N., Kubo, S., Retroviral Replicating Vectors Mediated Prodrug Activator Gene Therapy in a Gastric Cancer Model. *Int. J. Mol. Sci.*, *24*, 14823, ***2023***, doi: 10.3390/ijms241914823.
21. Ertl, H.C.J., Immunogenicity and Toxicity of AAV Gene Therapy. *Front. Immunol.*, *13*, 975803, **2022**, doi: 10.3389/fimmu.2022.975803.
22. Butt, M.H., Zaman, M., Ahmad, A., Khan, R., Mallhi, T.H., Hasan, M.M., Khan, Y.H., Hafeez, S., Massoud, E.E.S., Rahman, Md.H., *et al.*, Appraisal for the Potential of Viral and Nonviral Vectors in Gene Therapy: A Review. *Genes*, *13*, 8, 1370, **2022**, doi: 10.3390/genes13081370.

23. Gerfen, C.R., Economo, M.N., Chandrashekar, J., Long Distance Projections of Cortical Pyramidal Neurons. *J. Neurosci. Res.*, *96*, 1467–1475, **2018**, doi: 10.1002/jnr.23978.
24. Zhang, H., Zhan, Q., Huang, B., Wang, Y., Wang, X., AAV-Mediated Gene Therapy: Advancing Cardiovascular Disease Treatment. *Front. Cardiovasc. Med.*, *9*, 952755, **2022**, doi: 10.3389/fcvm.2022.952755.
25. Lamsfus-Calle, A., Daniel-Moreno, A., Ureña-Bailén, G., Raju, J., Antony, J.S., Handgretinger, R., Mezger, M., Hematopoietic Stem Cell Gene Therapy: The Optimal Use of Lentivirus and Gene Editing Approaches. *Blood Rev.*, *40*, 100641, **2020**, doi: https://doi.org/10.1016/j.blre.2019.100641.
26. Penaud-Budloo, M., Le Guiner, C., Nowrouzi, A., Toromanoff, A., Chérel, Y., Chenuaud, P., Schmidt, M., von Kalle, C., Rolling, F., Moullier, P., *et al.*, Adeno-Associated Virus Vector Genomes Persist as Episomal Chromatin in Primate Muscle. *J. Virol.*, *82*, 7875–7885, **2008**, doi: 10.1128/JVI.00649-08.
27. Chen, S.-H., Haam, J., Walker, M., Scappini, E., Naughton, J., Martin, N.P., Recombinant Viral Vectors as Neuroscience Tools. *Curr. Protoc. Neurosci.*, *87*, e67, **2019**, doi: 10.1002/cpns.67.
28. Jackson, D.A., Symons, R.H., Berg, P., Biochemical Method for Inserting New Genetic Information into DNA of Simian Virus 40: Circular SV40 DNA Molecules Containing Lambda Phage Genes and the Galactose Operon of Escherichia Coli. *Proc. Natl. Acad. Sci. U.S.A.*, *69*, 2904–2909, **1972**, doi: 10.1073/pnas.69.10.2904.
29. Travieso, T., Li, J., Mahesh, S., Mello, J. D. F. R. E., & Blasi, M. The use of viral vectors in vaccine development. *NPJ Vaccines*, 7, 1, 75, 2022, doi: 10.1038/s41541-022-00503-y.
30. Gleba, Y., Klimyuk, V., Marillonnet, S., Viral Vectors for the Expression of Proteins in Plants. *Curr. Opin. Biotechnol.*, *18*, 134–141, **2007**, doi: 10.1016/j.copbio.2007.03.002.
31. Lee, J.S., Hadjipanayis, A.G., Parker, M.D., Viral Vectors for Use in the Development of Biodefense Vaccines. *Adv. Drug Deliv. Rev.*, *57*, 1293–1314, **2005**, doi: 10.1016/j.addr.2005.01.011.
32. Centers for Disease Control and Prevention (CDC) Update: Investigation of Bioterrorism-Related Inhalational Anthrax–Connecticut 2001. *MMWR Morb. Mortal Wkly. Rep.*, *50*, 1049–1051, **2001**.
33. Mckinney, R.W., Berge, T.O., Sawyer, W.D., Tigertt, W.D., Crozier, D., Use of an Attenuated Strain of Venezuelan Equine Encephalomyelitis Virus For Immunization in Man. *Am. J. Trop. Med. Hyg.*, *12*, 597–603, **1963**, doi: 10.4269/ajtmh.1963.12.597.
34. Sakurai, F., Tachibana, M., Mizuguchi, H., Adenovirus Vector-Based Vaccine for Infectious Diseases. *Drug Metab. Pharmacokinet.*, *42*, 100432, **2022**, doi: https://doi.org/10.1016/j.dmpk.2021.100432.
35. Tahir, M., Ahmad, N., Lei, D., Ali, S., Emerging Role of Oncolytic Viruses and Stem Cells in Gene Therapy: Should They Be Integrated? *Drug Discov.*

Today, *27*, 2244–2251, **2022**, doi: https://doi.org/10.1016/j.drudis.2022.03.016.

36. Konno, A. and Hirai, H., Efficient Whole Brain Transduction by Systemic Infusion of Minimally Purified AAV-PHP.eB. *J. Neurosci. Methods*, *346*, 108914, **2020**, doi: https://doi.org/10.1016/j.jneumeth.2020.108914.
37. Zhong, G., Wang, H., He, W., Li, Y., Mou, H., Tickner, Z.J., Tran, M.H., Ou, T., Yin, Y., Diao, H., *et al.*, A Reversible RNA On-Switch That Controls Gene Expression of AAV-Delivered Therapeutics *in Vivo*. *Nat. Biotechnol.*, *38*, 169–175, **2020**, doi: 10.1038/s41587-019-0357-y.
38. Zhao, H., Li, Y., He, L., Pu, W., Yu, W., Li, Y., Wu, Y.-T., Xu, C., Wei, Y., Ding, Q., *et al.*, *In Vivo* AAV-CRISPR/Cas9–Mediated Gene Editing Ameliorates Atherosclerosis in Familial Hypercholesterolemia. *Circulation*, *141*, 67–79, **2020**, doi: 10.1161/CIRCULATIONAHA.119.042476.
39. Ghaleh, H.E.G., Bolandian, M., Dorostkar, R., Jafari, A., Pour, M.F., Concise Review on Optimized Methods in Production and Transduction of Lentiviral Vectors in Order to Facilitate Immunotherapy and Gene Therapy. *Biomed. Pharmacother.*, *128*, 110276, **2020**, doi: https://doi.org/10.1016/j.biopha.2020.110276.
40. Au, H.K.E., Isalan, M., Mielcarek, M., Gene Therapy Advances: A Meta-Analysis of AAV Usage in Clinical Settings. *Front. Med.*, *8*, 809118, **2022**, doi: 10.3389/fmed.2021.809118.
41. Ricobaraza, A., Gonzalez-Aparicio, M., Mora-Jimenez, L., Lumbreras, S., Hernandez-Alcoceba, R., High-Capacity Adenoviral Vectors: Expanding the Scope of Gene Therapy. *Int. J. Mol. Sci.*, *21*, 10, 3643, **2020**, doi: 10.3390/ijms21103643.
42. Ramlogan-Steel, C.A., Murali, A., Andrzejewski, S., Dhungel, B., Steel, J.C., Layton, C.J., Gene Therapy and the Adeno-Associated Virus in the Treatment of Genetic and Acquired Ophthalmic Diseases in Humans: Trials, Future Directions and Safety Considerations. *Clin. Exp. Ophthalmol.*, *47*, 521–536, **2019**, doi: https://doi.org/10.1111/ceo.13416.
43. Lin, Y.-Y., Belle, I., Blasi, M., Huang, M.-N., Buckley, A.F., Rountree, W., Klotman, M.E., Cara, A., Negri, D., Skeletal Muscle Is an Antigen Reservoir in Integrase-Defective Lentiviral Vector-Induced Long-Term Immunity. *Mol. Ther. Methods Clin. Dev.*, *17*, 532–544, **2020**, doi: 10.1016/j.omtm.2020.03.008.
44. Albershardt, T.C., Parsons, A.J., Reeves, R.S., Flynn, P.A., Campbell, D.J., ter Meulen, J., Berglund, P., Therapeutic Efficacy of PD1/PDL1 Blockade in B16 Melanoma Is Greatly Enhanced by Immunization with Dendritic Cell-Targeting Lentiviral Vector and Protein Vaccine. *Vaccine*, *38*, 3369–3377, **2020**, doi: https://doi.org/10.1016/j.vaccine.2020.02.034.
45. Li, S., Qiao, Y., Jiang, S., Wang, B., Kong, W., Shan, Y., Broad and Potent Bispecific Neutralizing Antibody Gene Delivery Using Adeno-Associated Viral Vectors for Passive Immunization against HIV-1. *J. Control. Release*, *338*, 633–643, **2021**, doi: https://doi.org/10.1016/j.jconrel.2021.09.006.

46. Warnock, J.N., Daigre, C., Al-Rubeai, M., Introduction to Viral Vectors, in: *Viral Vectors for Gene Therapy: Methods and Protocols*, O.-W. Merten, and M. Al-Rubeai, (Eds.), pp. 1–25, Humana Press, Totowa, NJ, 2011, ISBN 978-1-61779-095-9.
47. Chavda, V.P., Bezbaruah, R., Valu, D., Patel, B., Kumar, A., Prasad, S., Kakoti, B.B., Kaushik, A., Jesawadawala, M., Adenoviral Vector-Based Vaccine Platform for COVID-19: Current Status. *Vaccines*, *11*, 432, **2023**, doi: 10.3390/vaccines11020432.
48. Dyer, A., Di, Y., Calderon, H., Illingworth, S., Kueberuwa, G., Tedcastle, A., Jakeman, P., Chia, S.L., Brown, A., Silva, M.A., *et al.*, Oncolytic Group B Adenovirus Enadenotucirev Mediates Non-Apoptotic Cell Death with Membrane Disruption and Release of Inflammatory Mediators. *Mol. Ther. Oncolytics*, *4*, 18–30, **2017**, doi: 10.1016/j.omto.2016.11.003.
49. Spronck, E.A., Brouwers, C.C., Vallès, A., de Haan, M., Petry, H., van Deventer, S.J., Konstantinova, P., Evers, M.M., AAV5-miHTT Gene Therapy Demonstrates Sustained Huntingtin Lowering and Functional Improvement in Huntington Disease Mouse Models. *Mol. Ther. Methods Clin. Dev.*, *13*, 334–343, **2019**, doi: 10.1016/j.omtm.2019.03.002.
50. Sun, X., Yan, Z., Yi, Y., Li, Z., Lei, D., Rogers, C.S., Chen, J., Zhang, Y., Welsh, M.J., Leno, G.H., *et al.*, Adeno-Associated Virus–Targeted Disruption of the CFTR Gene in Cloned Ferrets. *J. Clin. Invest.*, *118*, 1578–1583, **2008**, doi: 10.1172/JCI34599.
51. Greig, J.A., Wang, Q., Reicherter, A.L., Chen, S.-J., Hanlon, A.L., Tipper, C.H., Clark, K.R., Wadsworth, S., Wang, L., Wilson, J.M., Characterization of Adeno-Associated Viral Vector-Mediated Human Factor VIII Gene Therapy in Hemophilia A Mice. *Hum. Gene Ther.*, *28*, 392–402, **2017**, doi: 10.1089/hum.2016.128.
52. Garcia-Gomez, M., Calabria, A., Garcia-Bravo, M., Benedicenti, F., Kosinski, P., López-Manzaneda, S., Hill, C., Del Mar Mañu-Pereira, M., Martín, M.A., Orman, I., *et al.*, Safe and Efficient Gene Therapy for Pyruvate Kinase Deficiency. *Mol. Ther.*, *24*, 1187–1198, **2016**, doi: 10.1038/mt.2016.87.
53. Hutson, T.H., Foster, E., Moon, L.D.F., Yáñez-Muñoz, R.J., Lentiviral Vector-Mediated RNA Silencing in the Central Nervous System. *Hum. Gene Ther. Methods*, *25*, 14–32, **2014**, doi: 10.1089/hgtb.2013.016.
54. Horvath, L., van Marion, I., Taï, K., Nielsen, T.T., Lundberg, C., Knockdown of GAD67 Protein Levels Normalizes Neuronal Activity in a Rat Model of Parkinson's Disease. *J. Gene Med.*, *13*, 188–197, **2011**, doi: 10.1002/jgm.1555.
55. Singer, O., Marr, R.A., Rockenstein, E., Crews, L., Coufal, N.G., Gage, F.H., Verma, I.M., Masliah, E., Targeting BACE1 with siRNAs Ameliorates Alzheimer Disease Neuropathology in a Transgenic Model. *Nat. Neurosci.*, *8*, 1343–1349, **2005**, doi: 10.1038/nn1531.
56. Sinnett, S.E. and Gray, S.J., Recent Endeavors in MECP2 Gene Transfer for Gene Therapy of Rett Syndrome. *Discov. Med.*, *24*, 153–159, **2017**.

57. Guggino, W.B., Benson, J., Seagrave, J., Yan, Z., Engelhardt, J., Gao, G., Conlon, T.J., Cebotaru, L., A Preclinical Study in Rhesus Macaques for Cystic Fibrosis to Assess Gene Transfer and Transduction by AAV1 and AAV5 with a Dual-Luciferase Reporter System. *Hum. Gene Ther. Clin. Dev.*, *28*, 145–156, **2017**, doi: 10.1089/humc.2017.067.
58. Thakur, V., Gonzalez, M., Pennington, K., Chattopadhyay, M., Viral Vector Mediated Continuous Expression of Interleukin-10 in DRG Alleviates Pain in Type 1 Diabetic Animals. *Mol. Cell. Neurosci.*, *72*, 46–53, **2016**, doi: 10.1016/j.mcn.2016.01.006.
59. Eissa, I.R., Naoe, Y., Bustos-Villalobos, I., Ichinose, T., Tanaka, M., Zhiwen, W., Mukoyama, N., Morimoto, T., Miyajima, N., Hitoki, H., *et al.*, Genomic Signature of the Natural Oncolytic Herpes Simplex Virus HF10 and Its Therapeutic Role in Preclinical and Clinical Trials. *Front. Oncol.*, *7*, 149, **2017**, doi: 10.3389/fonc.2017.00149.
60. Lundstrom, K., Oncolytic Alphaviruses in Cancer Immunotherapy. *Vaccines (Basel)*, *5*, 9, **2017**, doi: 10.3390/vaccines5020009.
61. Määttä, A.-M., Mäkinen, K., Ketola, A., Liimatainen, T., Yongabi, F.N., Vähä-Koskela, M., Pirinen, R., Rautsi, O., Pellinen, R., Hinkkanen, A., *et al.*, Replication Competent Semliki Forest Virus Prolongs Survival in Experimental Lung Cancer. *Int. J. Cancer*, *123*, 1704–1711, **2008**, doi: 10.1002/ijc.23646.
62. Roche, F.P., Sheahan, B.J., O'Mara, S.M., Atkins, G.J., Semliki Forest Virus-Mediated Gene Therapy of the RG2 Rat Glioma. *Neuropathol. Appl. Neurobiol.*, *36*, 648–660, **2010**, doi: 10.1111/j.1365-2990.2010.01110.x.
63. Ylösmäki, E., Martikainen, M., Hinkkanen, A., Saksela, K., Attenuation of Semliki Forest Virus Neurovirulence by microRNA-Mediated Detargeting. *J. Virol.*, *87*, 335–344, **2013**, doi: 10.1128/JVI.01940-12.
64. Lin, Y., Zhang, H., Liang, J., Li, K., Zhu, W., Fu, L., Wang, F., Zheng, X., Shi, H., Wu, S., *et al.*, Identification and Characterization of Alphavirus M1 as a Selective Oncolytic Virus Targeting ZAP-Defective Human Cancers. *Proc. Natl. Acad. Sci. U.S.A.*, *111*, E4504–4512, **2014**, doi: 10.1073/pnas.1408759111.
65. Hoang-Le, D., Smeenk, L., Anraku, I., Pijlman, G.P., Wang, X.J., de Vrij, J., Liu, W.J., Le, T.T., Schroder, W.A., Khromykh, A.A., *et al.*, A Kunjin Replicon Vector Encoding Granulocyte Macrophage Colony-Stimulating Factor for Intra-Tumoral Gene Therapy. *Gene Ther.*, *16*, 190–199, **2009**, doi: 10.1038/gt.2008.169.
66. Clarke, D.K., Cooper, D., Egan, M.A., Hendry, R.M., Parks, C.L., Udem, S.A., Recombinant Vesicular Stomatitis Virus as an HIV-1 Vaccine Vector. *Springer Semin. Immunopathol.*, *28*, 239–253, **2006**, doi: 10.1007/s00281-006-0042-3.
67. Zhang, L., Steele, M.B., Jenks, N., Grell, J., Suksanpaisan, L., Naik, S., Federspiel, M.J., Lacy, M.Q., Russell, S.J., Peng, K.-W., Safety Studies in Tumor and Non-Tumor-Bearing Mice in Support of Clinical Trials Using Oncolytic VSV-IFNβ-NIS. *Hum. Gene Ther. Clin. Dev.*, *27*, 111–122, **2016**, doi: 10.1089/humc.2016.061.

68. Hastie, E. and Grdzelishvili, V.Z., Vesicular Stomatitis Virus as a Flexible Platform for Oncolytic Virotherapy against Cancer. *J. Gen. Virol.*, *93*, 2529–2545, **2012**, doi: 10.1099/vir.0.046672-0.
69. Niu, Z., Bai, F., Sun, T., Tian, H., Yu, D., Yin, J., Li, S., Li, T., Cao, H., Yu, Q., *et al.*, Recombinant Newcastle Disease Virus Expressing IL15 Demonstrates Promising Antitumor Efficiency in Melanoma Model. *Technol. Cancer Res. Treat.*, *14*, 607–615, **2015**, doi: 10.7785/tcrt.2012.500414.
70. Bai, F.-L., Yu, Y.-H., Tian, H., Ren, G.-P., Wang, H., Zhou, B., Han, X.-H., Yu, Q.-Z., Li, D.-S., Genetically Engineered Newcastle Disease Virus Expressing Interleukin-2 and TNF-Related Apoptosis-Inducing Ligand for Cancer Therapy. *Cancer Biol. Ther.*, *15*, 1226–1238, **2014**, doi: 10.4161/cbt.29686.
71. Wu, Y., He, J., Geng, J., An, Y., Ye, X., Yan, S., Yu, Q., Yin, J., Zhang, Z., Li, D., Recombinant Newcastle Disease Virus Expressing Human TRAIL as a Potential Candidate for Hepatoma Therapy. *Eur. J. Pharmacol.*, *802*, 85–92, **2017**, doi: 10.1016/j.ejphar.2017.02.042.
72. Kim, D.-S., Kim, H., Shim, S.-H., Kim, C., Song, M., Kim, Y.-H., Jung, Y.-W., Nam, J.-H., Coxsackievirus B3 Used as a Gene Therapy Vector to Express Functional FGF2. *Gene Ther.*, *19*, 1159–1165, **2012**, doi: 10.1038/gt.2011.201.
73. Shafren, D.R., Au, G.G., Nguyen, T., Newcombe, N.G., Haley, E.S., Beagley, L., Johansson, E.S., Hersey, P., Barry, R.D., Systemic Therapy of Malignant Human Melanoma Tumors by a Common Cold-Producing Enterovirus, Coxsackievirus A21. *Clin. Cancer Res.*, *10*, 53–60, **2004**, doi: 10.1158/1078-0432.ccr-0690-3.
74. Berry, L.J., Au, G.G., Barry, R.D., Shafren, D.R., Potent Oncolytic Activity of Human Enteroviruses against Human Prostate Cancer. *Prostate*, *68*, 577–587, **2008**, doi: 10.1002/pros.20741.
75. Reddi, H.V., Madde, P., McDonough, S.J., Trujillo, M.A., Morris, J.C., Myers, R.M., Peng, K.W., Russell, S.J., McIver, B., Eberhardt, N.L., Preclinical Efficacy of the Oncolytic Measles Virus Expressing the Sodium Iodide Symporter in Iodine Non-Avid Anaplastic Thyroid Cancer: A Novel Therapeutic Agent Allowing Noninvasive Imaging and Radioiodine Therapy. *Cancer Gene Ther.*, *19*, 659–665, **2012**, doi: 10.1038/cgt.2012.47.
76. Hartkopf, A.D., Bossow, S., Lampe, J., Zimmermann, M., Taran, F.-A., Wallwiener, D., Fehm, T., Bitzer, M., Lauer, U.M., Enhanced Killing of Ovarian Carcinoma Using Oncolytic Measles Vaccine Virus Armed with a Yeast Cytosine Deaminase and Uracil Phosphoribosyltransferase. *Gynecol. Oncol.*, *130*, 362–368, **2013**, doi: 10.1016/j.ygyno.2013.05.004.
77. Lampe, J., Bossow, S., Weiland, T., Smirnow, I., Lehmann, R., Neubert, W., Bitzer, M., Lauer, U.M., An Armed Oncolytic Measles Vaccine Virus Eliminates Human Hepatoma Cells Independently of Apoptosis. *Gene Ther.*, *20*, 1033–1041, **2013**, doi: 10.1038/gt.2013.28.
78. Lange, S., Lampe, J., Bossow, S., Zimmermann, M., Neubert, W., Bitzer, M., Lauer, U.M., A Novel Armed Oncolytic Measles Vaccine Virus for the

Treatment of Cholangiocarcinoma. *Hum. Gene Ther.*, *24*, 554–564, **2013**, doi: 10.1089/hum.2012.136.

79. van der Loo, J.C.M., Swaney, W.P., Grassman, E., Terwilliger, A., Higashimoto, T., Schambach, A., Baum, C., Thrasher, A.J., Williams, D.A., Nordling, D.L., *et al.*, Scale-up and Manufacturing of Clinical-Grade Self-Inactivating γ-Retroviral Vectors by Transient Transfection. *Gene Ther.*, *19*, 246–254, **2012**, doi: 10.1038/gt.2011.102.
80. Thornhill, S.I., Schambach, A., Howe, S.J., Ulaganathan, M., Grassman, E., Williams, D., Schiedlmeier, B., Sebire, N.J., Gaspar, H.B., Kinnon, C., *et al.*, Self-Inactivating Gammaretroviral Vectors for Gene Therapy of X-Linked Severe Combined Immunodeficiency. *Mol. Ther.*, *16*, 590–598, **2008**, doi: 10.1038/sj.mt.6300393.
81. Sastry, L., Xu, Y., Cooper, R., Pollok, K., Cornetta, K., Evaluation of Plasmid DNA Removal from Lentiviral Vectors by Benzonase Treatment. *Hum. Gene Ther.*, *15*, 221–226, **2004**, doi: 10.1089/104303404772680029.
82. Jordan, M. and Wurm, F., Transfection of Adherent and Suspended Cells by Calcium Phosphate. *Methods*, *33*, 136–143, **2004**, doi: 10.1016/j.ymeth.2003.11.011.
83. Kuystermans, D. and Al-Rubeai, M., Bioreactor Systems for Producing Antibody from Mammalian Cells. Antibody Expression and Production. Cell Engineering, vol. 7, pp. 25–52, 2011, Springer, Dordrecht., doi:10.1007/978-94-007-1257-7_2.
84. Tomás, H.A., Rodrigues, A.F., Carrondo, M.J.T., Coroadinha, A.S., LentiPro26: Novel Stable Cell Lines for Constitutive Lentiviral Vector Production. *Sci. Rep.*, *8*, 5271, **2018**, doi: 10.1038/s41598-018-23593-y.
85. Thomas, C.E., Schiedner, G., Kochanek, S., Castro, M.G., Lowenstein, P.R., Preexisting Antiadenoviral Immunity Is Not a Barrier to Efficient and Stable Transduction of the Brain, Mediated by Novel High-Capacity Adenovirus Vectors. *Hum. Gene Ther.*, *12*, 839–846, **2001**, doi: 10.1089/104303401750148829.
86. DelloRusso, C., Scott, J.M., Hartigan-O'Connor, D., Salvatori, G., Barjot, C., Robinson, A.S., Crawford, R.W., Brooks, S.V., Chamberlain, J.S., Functional Correction of Adult *Mdx* Mouse Muscle Using Gutted Adenoviral Vectors Expressing Full-Length Dystrophin. *Proc. Natl. Acad. Sci.*, *99*, 12979–12984, **2002**, doi: 10.1073/pnas.202300099.
87. Ehrhardt, A. and Kay, M.A., A New Adenoviral Helper–Dependent Vector Results in Long-Term Therapeutic Levels of Human Coagulation Factor IX at Low Doses *in Vivo*. *Blood*, *99*, 3923–3930, **2002**, doi: 10.1182/blood.V99.11.3923.
88. Thomas, C.E., Birkett, D., Anozie, I., Castro, M.G., Lowenstein, P.R., Acute Direct Adenoviral Vector Cytotoxicity and Chronic, but Not Acute, Inflammatory Responses Correlate with Decreased Vector-Mediated Transgene Expression in the Brain. *Mol. Ther.*, *3*, 36–46, **2001**, doi: 10.1006/mthe.2000.0224.

89. Morral, N., O'Neal, W.K., Rice, K., Leland, M.M., Piedra, P.A., Aguilar-Córdova, E., Carey, K.D., Beaudet, A.L., Langston, C., Lethal Toxicity, Severe Endothelial Injury, and a Threshold Effect with High Doses of an Adenoviral Vector in Baboons. *Hum. Gene Ther.*, *13*, 143–154, **2002**, doi: 10.1089/10430340152712692.
90. Brockstedt, D.G., Podsakoff, G.M., Fong, L., Kurtzman, G., Mueller-Ruchholtz, W., Engleman, E.G., Induction of Immunity to Antigens Expressed by Recombinant Adeno-Associated Virus Depends on the Route of Administration. *Clin. Immunol.*, *92*, 67–75, **1999**, doi: 10.1006/clim.1999.4724.
91. Halbert, C.L., Rutledge, E.A., Allen, J.M., Russell, D.W., Miller, A.D., Repeat Transduction in the Mouse Lung by Using Adeno-Associated Virus Vectors with Different Serotypes. *J. Virol.*, *74*, 1524–1532, **2000**, doi: 10.1128/JVI.74.3.1524-1532.2000.
92. Lewandoski, M., Conditional Control of Gene Expression in the Mouse. *Nat. Rev. Genet.*, *2*, 743–755, **2001**, doi: 10.1038/35093537.
93. Somia, N. and Verma, I.M., Gene Therapy: Trials and Tribulations. *Nat. Rev. Genet.*, *1*, 91–99, **2000**, doi: 10.1038/35038533.
94. Gao, G.-P., Alvira, M.R., Wang, L., Calcedo, R., Johnston, J., Wilson, J.M., Novel Adeno-Associated Viruses from Rhesus Monkeys as Vectors for Human Gene Therapy. *Proc. Natl. Acad. Sci.*, *99*, 11854–11859, **2002**, doi: 10.1073/pnas.182412299.
95. Grimm, D. and Kay, M., From Virus Evolution to Vector Revolution: Use of Naturally Occurring Serotypes of Adeno-Associated Virus (AAV) as Novel Vectors for Human Gene Therapy. *Curr. Gene Ther.*, *3*, 281–304, **2003**, doi: 10.2174/1566523034578285.
96. Rabinowitz, J.E., Rolling, F., Li, C., Conrath, H., Xiao, W., Xiao, X., Samulski, R.J., Cross-Packaging of a Single Adeno-Associated Virus (AAV) Type 2 Vector Genome into Multiple AAV Serotypes Enables Transduction with Broad Specificity. *J. Virol.*, *76*, 791–801, **2002**, doi: 10.1128/JVI.76.2.791-801.2002.
97. Li, Z., Düllmann, J., Schiedlmeier, B., Schmidt, M., von Kalle, C., Meyer, J., Forster, M., Stocking, C., Wahlers, A., Frank, O., *et al.*, Murine Leukemia Induced by Retroviral Gene Marking. *Science*, *296*, 497–497, **2002**, doi: 10.1126/science.1068893.
98. Cavazzana-Calvo, M., Hacein-Bey, S., de Basile, G.S., Gross, F., Yvon, E., Nusbaum, P., Selz, F., Hue, C., Certain, S., Casanova, J.-L., *et al.*, Gene Therapy of Human Severe Combined Immunodeficiency (SCID)-X1 Disease. *Science*, *288*, 669–672, **2000**, doi: 10.1126/science.288.5466.669.
99. Hacein-Bey-Abina, S., von Kalle, C., Schmidt, M., Deist, F.L., Wulffraat, N., McIntyre, E., Radford, I., Villeval, J.-L., Fraser, C.C., Cavazzana-Calvo, M., *et al.*, A Serious Adverse Event after Successful Gene Therapy for X-Linked

Severe Combined Immunodeficiency. *N. Engl. J. Med.*, *348*, 255–256, **2003**, doi: 10.1056/NEJM200301163480314.

100. Baum, C., Düllmann, J., Li, Z., Fehse, B., Meyer, J., Williams, D.A., von Kalle, C., Side Effects of Retroviral Gene Transfer into Hematopoietic Stem Cells. *Blood*, *101*, 2099–2113, **2003**, doi: 10.1182/blood-2002-07-2314.
101. Kutner, R.H., Puthli, S., Marino, M.P., Reiser, J., Simplified Production and Concentration of HIV-1-Based Lentiviral Vectors Using HYPERFlask Vessels and Anion Exchange Membrane Chromatography. *BMC Biotech.*, *9*, 10, **2009**, doi: 10.1186/1472-6750-9-10.
102. Emmerling, V.V., Pegel, A., Milian, E.G., Venereo-Sanchez, A., Kunz, M., Wegele, J., Kamen, A.A., Kochanek, S., Hoerer, M., Rational Plasmid Design and Bioprocess Optimization to Enhance Recombinant Adeno-Associated Virus (AAV) Productivity in Mammalian Cells. *Biotechnol. J.*, *11*, 290–297, **2016**, doi: 10.1002/biot.201500176.
103. Lesch, H.P., Heikkilä, K.M., Lipponen, E.M., Valonen, P., Müller, A., Räsänen, E., Tuunanen, T., Hassinen, M.M., Parker, N., Karhinen, M., *et al.*, Process Development of Adenoviral Vector Production in Fixed Bed Bioreactor: From Bench to Commercial Scale. *Hum. Gene Ther.*, *26*, 560–571, **2015**, doi: 10.1089/hum.2015.081.
104. Wang, X., Olszewska, M., Qu, J., Wasielewska, T., Bartido, S., Hermetet, G., Sadelain, M., Rivière, I., Large-Scale Clinical-Grade Retroviral Vector Production in a Fixed-Bed Bioreactor. *J. Immunother.*, *38*, 127–135, **2015**, doi: 10.1097/CJI.0000000000000072.
105. van der Loo, J.C.M., Swaney, W.P., Grassman, E., Terwilliger, A., Higashimoto, T., Schambach, A., Hacein-Bey-Abina, S., Nordling, D.L., Cavazzana-Calvo, M., Thrasher, A.J., *et al.*, Critical Variables Affecting Clinical-Grade Production of the Self-Inactivating Gamma-Retroviral Vector for the Treatment of X-Linked Severe Combined Immunodeficiency. *Gene Ther.*, *19*, 872–876, **2012**, doi: 10.1038/gt.2012.37.
106. Feng, L., Guo, M., Zhang, S., Chu, J., Zhuang, Y., Zhang, S., Improvement in the Suspension-Culture Production of Recombinant Adeno-Associated Virus-LacZ in HEK-293 Cells Using Polyethyleneimine-DNA Complexes in Combination with Hypothermic Treatment. *Biotechnol. Appl. Biochem.*, *50*, 121–132, **2008**, doi: 10.1042/BA20070081.
107. Li, L.-H., Shivakumar, R., Feller, S., Allen, C., Weiss, J.M., Dzekunov, S., Singh, V., Holaday, J., Fratantoni, J., Liu, L.N., Highly Efficient, Large Volume Flow Electroporation. *Technol. Cancer Res. Treat.*, *1*, 341–350, **2002**, doi: 10.1177/153303460200100504.
108. Urabe, M., Ding, C., Kotin, R.M., Insect Cells as a Factory to Produce Adeno-Associated Virus Type 2 Vectors. *Hum. Gene Ther.*, *13*, 1935–1943, **2002**, doi: 10.1089/10430340260355347.
109. Cecchini, S., Virag, T., Kotin, R.M., Reproducible High Yields of Recombinant Adeno-Associated Virus Produced Using Invertebrate Cells in 0.02- to

200-Liter Cultures. *Hum. Gene Ther.*, *22*, 1021–1030, **2011**, doi: 10.1089/hum.2010.250.

110. Grieger, J.C., Soltys, S.M., Samulski, R.J., Production of Recombinant Adeno-Associated Virus Vectors Using Suspension HEK293 Cells and Continuous Harvest of Vector From the Culture Media for GMP FIX and FLT1 Clinical Vector. *Mol. Ther.*, *24*, 287–297, **2016**, doi: 10.1038/mt.2015.187.
111. Lundstrom, K., Latest Development in Viral Vectors for Gene Therapy. *Trends Biotechnol.*, *21*, 117–122, 2003.

3

The Role of Adjuvants in the Application of Viral Vector Vaccines

Vivek P. Chavda[1]*, Anjali P. Bedse[2] and Shilpa S. Raut[2]

[1]*Department of Pharmaceutics and Pharmaceutical Technology, L.M. College of Pharmacy, Ahmedabad, Gujarat, India*
[2]*Department of Pharmaceutics, K K Wagh College of Pharmacy, Nashik, Maharashtra, India*

Abstract

Viral vector vaccines have revolutionized modern vaccinology due to their ability to trigger robust cellular and humoral immune responses and their versatility against various pathogens. To maximize their effectiveness, the strategic use of adjuvants is essential. Adjuvants, which are substances incorporated into vaccines, enhance the body's immune response to the antigen, ensuring stronger and more durable immunity even with lower antigen doses. This chapter provides a detailed examination of adjuvants used alongside viral vector vaccines, their mechanisms of action, and their overall impact on vaccine efficacy. It begins with an overview of viral vector vaccines, tracing their history, development, and commonly utilized vectors such as adenovirus, lentivirus, and vesicular stomatitis virus. Following this, the chapter introduces adjuvants, covering a range of types from traditional ones like aluminum salts and oil-in-water emulsions to advanced formulations including saponins, liposomes, and nanoparticle-based adjuvants. The safety and regulatory considerations of using adjuvants in viral vector vaccines are also thoroughly reviewed. The chapter outlines the comprehensive testing and evaluation required to ensure that adjuvants do not introduce unacceptable toxicity or adverse effects, covering preclinical toxicity studies, clinical trial phases, and post-marketing surveillance. The regulatory environment, though complex and region-specific, is clearly outlined in terms of general principles and requirements. Challenges and future directions in the field are addressed, emphasizing the need for novel adjuvants that provide potent immunostimulatory effects while maintaining safety. Innovations such as TLR agonists, STING pathway activators, and

**Corresponding author*: vivek.chavda@lmcp.ac.in

Vivek P. Chavda and Vasso Apostolopoulos (eds.) Viral Vectors for Vaccine Delivery, (65–90) © 2025 Scrivener Publishing LLC

other innate immune modulators are discussed for their potential to significantly advance the field. The chapter also emphasizes the importance of understanding the molecular interactions between viral vectors and adjuvants to optimize vaccine formulations.

Keywords: Adjuvants, viral vector vaccines, vaccine development, immune response, antigen presentation, efficacy, safety

3.1 Introduction

Vaccines are essential instruments in healthcare, being essential to the prevention of infectious diseases and the preservation of public health. They have greatly decreased morbidity and death rates on a global scale, resulting in the saving of many lives and enhancing general well-being. Vaccines provide significant economic benefits in addition to their health advantages, as they reduce healthcare expenses and boost efficiency [1]. Vaccines encounter challenges including unequal worldwide distribution, financial obstacles restricting access in some areas, and the infrequent incidence of side effects, despite their significant significance. Although mild side effects such as redness or fever are frequent, severe adverse reactions are quite uncommon [2]. It is essential to address these difficulties by implementing fair distribution systems, improving accessibility, and continuously monitoring safety to enhance the benefits of vaccinations on the health and welfare of the world [3].

The development of viral vector vaccines for benign viruses allows them to transport genetic factors containing antigens into host cells, stimulating an immune reaction. Fighting against infectious diseases has been greatly facilitated by vaccines, such as COVID-19 and Ebola vaccinations. In 1972, the first viral vector was created, representing notable progress in vaccination science. Adenovirus, poxviruses, and lentiviruses are used as viral vectors to trigger strong immune reactions against particular infections [4]. The immunizations provide benefits such as strong antibody and cellular responses that are essential for eradicating pathogens. Viral vector vaccines stimulate robust immune responses by replicating natural infections, eliminating the necessity for adjuvants. Although effective, obstacles like as preexisting immunity to vectors and intricate production procedures are present. Ongoing research and advancement in viral vector vaccines show potential for improving vaccination approaches against several infectious illnesses [5–7].

Substances called adjuvants are used in vaccines to improve the body's immunity to the antigen. They are available in different forms, including mineral salts, emulsions, and immunological potentiators. Aluminum salts are a prevalent adjuvant that enhances the immunological response by prolonging and intensifying it. Additional adjuvants consist of Freund's adjuvant, MF59, and AS03 [8]. Adjuvants can act as transporters, reservoirs, and enhancers of immunological responses, aiding the immune system in identifying and reacting efficiently to the antigen. They are especially advantageous for subunit vaccinations that may have difficulty in eliciting a strong immunological response [9].

Adjuvants have a function in viral vector vaccine application by boosting and molding immune responses specific to antigens. Adjuvants are not necessary for significant immune responses evoked by viral vector vaccines because of their intrinsic characteristics. Adjuvants can enhance these responses, increasing their efficiency and effectiveness. Adjuvants can be utilized to enhance both humoral and cellular immune responses, which are essential for eradicating pathogens. Adjuvants in viral vector vaccines enhance immune responses, resulting in improved protection against diseases [10].

3.2 Viral Vector Vaccines: A Powerful Platform

Viral vector vaccines use harmless viruses to deliver genetic material encoding antigens into host cells, thereby stimulating an immune response. Examples of viral vectors include adenoviruses, poxviruses, and lentiviruses [11]. These vaccines provide potent antibody and cellular responses crucial for pathogen elimination. Unlike traditional subunit vaccines, viral vector vaccines require no adjuvant, as the vector itself triggers the immune response. Some challenges associated with viral vector vaccines include limited availability, cost-related issues, and the potential for side effects [12].

Adenoviruses, specifically Ad26 and Ad5, are commonly utilized in vaccine research because of their effective delivery of genetic material into host cells. Ad26-based vaccines have demonstrated potential in fighting diseases such as COVID-19, Ebola, and human immunodeficiency virus (HIV) [13]. Poxviruses, including modified vaccinia Ankara (MVA), are a prevalent type of viral vector utilized in vaccinations. Vaccines based on MVA have effectively immunized against smallpox and are under investigation to treat cancer and a variety of infectious diseases [14]. Lentiviral vectors, originating from HIV, have been modified to be incapable of reproduction and deemed safe for inclusion in vaccinations. These vectors are highly efficient in gene therapy and have demonstrated promise in developing vaccinations against diseases, including HIV and cancer. Each viral vector type has distinct benefits and difficulties, underscoring the significance of choosing the most appropriate vector for individual vaccination targets to achieve the best immune responses and safety profiles [15].

When compared to other immunization types, viral vector vaccines offer distinct benefits. An important advantage is that they can generate robust immune responses independently, as the vectors can effectively trigger the necessary immunological reactions without requiring adjuvants. Viral vector vaccines can trigger strong antibody and cellular responses essential for effectively fighting diseases. These vaccines induce strong immune responses by imitating natural illnesses, resulting in long-term protection against pathogens. Yet, viral vector vaccines have drawbacks, including an intricate production procedure and the potential for genetic integration [5]. Existing immunity to the viral vectors may weaken immune responses, requiring measures to address this obstacle for further immunizations. Viral vector vaccines provide benefits compared to conventional vaccination platforms, but they can have drawbacks. One major benefit is their capacity to trigger strong immunological responses by introducing genetic material encoding antigens directly into host cells, replicating natural infection and, therefore, activating both cellular and humoral defenses [16]. This method frequently leads to enduring immunity, providing the possibility of long-term defense against infectious illnesses. Viral vector vaccines can be modified to include various antigens or genetic changes to improve immune response or target specific immune pathways, making them useful for a wide range of infections. Additionally, viral vectors like adenoviruses and lentiviruses have natural adjuvant qualities, enhancing immune responses without requiring extra adjuvants [17]. Moreover, these vaccines usually exhibit great stability, making storage and distribution easier, which is essential for worldwide vaccination efforts, especially in areas with limited resources. However, viral vector vaccines have some drawbacks. Concerns about existing immunity to the viral vectors in the target population may reduce vaccine effectiveness, particularly if individuals have prior exposure or vaccination against the vector. Furthermore, immunological reactions unique to the vector may arise, which could reduce the efficacy of subsequent doses or booster shots [18]. The manufacturing procedure for viral vector vaccines is intricate and expensive, necessitating specific facilities and expertise. Safety problems, such as insertional mutagenesis or vector replication, require thorough consideration through rigorous preclinical and clinical testing. The minimal chance of negative effects caused by vectors highlights the need for ongoing monitoring and surveillance after vaccination. Ultimately, viral vector vaccines have notable benefits in terms of immune response, adaptability, and durability, but it is essential to overcome their drawbacks to fully utilize them as reliable and efficient methods in fighting infectious diseases [16].

Effective viral vector vaccines have been developed for COVID-19, Ebola, and other various infectious illnesses. These vaccines utilize benign viruses to transport genetic material containing antigens into host cells, triggering an immune response. Viral vector vaccines provide advantages such as robust antibody and cellular responses, less need for adjuvants, and the capacity to simulate natural infections, leading to enhanced immune reactions compared to other vaccination platforms. Nevertheless, they pose obstacles such as intricate production procedures, susceptibility to preexisting immunity, and the possibility of genetic integration.

3.3 Challenges Associated with Viral Vector Vaccines

3.3.1 Preexisting Immunity against the Viral Vector

Preexisting immunity to the vector, particularly neutralizing antibodies, restricts virus delivery into cells, effectively reducing the dose of vectored antigens delivered [19]. Adenoviral (AdV) infections in humans often lead to preexisting vector immunity, reducing vector efficiency. Clinical application of human adenovirus (HAd) serotype 5 is hindered by preexisting immunity [20]. This is facilitated by immune system components such as type I interferon (IFN)-activated NK cells, Ad-specific T cells, and neutralizing antibodies. Strategies such as capsid modification, vector encapsulation, heterologous viral vectors, and rare human or nonhuman AdVs have been created to overcome this. Knowing about the toxicity, immunity, and circumvention of AdV vectors can help optimize these vectors for therapeutic use [21]. Preexisting immunity in the human population has been overcome in large part by the invention of novel animal-based Ad vectors, especially those derived from simian sources. The complicated nature of T cell tests and the existence of TRM cells, which do not circulate in the bloodstream, have made it difficult to determine how Ad-specific T cells affect the potency of these vectors [21]. Understanding preexisting immunity to Ad vectors and choosing the best Ad vector for clinical usage require knowledge of both Ad-specific circulating and tissue-resident T cells [22].

Preclinical research indicates that preexisting Ad immunity can be circumvented by using different vaccination strategies. Ad vectors may be able to elicit protective immune responses using the airway as a means of dissemination (Figure 3.1). To ascertain the number of separate vaccinations that can be produced with a single antigenic Ad backbone, more studies are necessary to assess the viability of readministering Ad vectors, frequency, and regimen [23].

The key to overcoming preexisting Ad immunity is to optimize prime-boost regimens using Ad vectors. Useful information on ChAd/MVA prime-boost's capacity to overcome HAd immunity will be obtained from clinical studies. Later research ought to assess the impact of Ad-based vaccination regimens on HIV acquisition. This crucial problem will be addressed in upcoming clinical studies with high-risk people, ensuring the effectiveness of prime-boost regimens in overcoming HAd immunity [24].

3.3.2 Safety Concerns Related to Insertional Mutagenesis

Integrating gene delivery systems in mammalian cells improves transgene expression but risks insertional mutagenesis and malignant cell

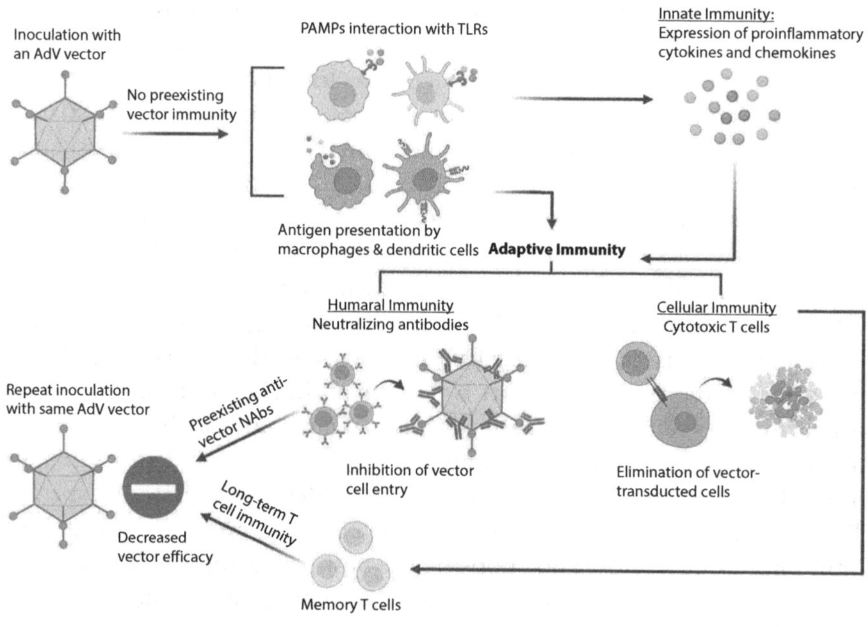

Figure 3.1 Activation of innate and adaptive immune responses in response to an adenoviral (AdV) vector. (Adopted under CC BY 4.0 from [21]).

transformation. Animal models using AAV-mediated gene transfer result in cancers, while Sleeping Beauty DNA transposon systems have been linked to insertional mutagenesis events in cell culture systems, calling for the development of safer gene delivery methods for genetic modification [25, 26].

For retroviridae-based gene delivery models, which include retroviral- and lentiviral-derived vector systems, there are two primary pathways that result in insertional mutagenesis. Two long terminal repeats (LTRs) containing enhancer and promoter elements are present in the genomes of the retroviral-derived vector systems at the 5′ and 3′ ends [27]. In the first mechanism, retroviridae-based vector integration into cellular chromosomes near the integration site causes short-range insertional mutagenesis. This integration can either enhance the expression of oncogenes or suppress the expression of tumor suppressor genes if the retroviridae-based vector integrates within an exon of a particular gene. The connection between a cellular promoter that drives the production of an endogenous oncogene and the enhancer element of a retroviral LTR is the second long-range mode of action [28].

Three key approaches will be used to address the problem of insertional mutagenesis-induced cancers in patients: Gene delivery models that are safer to use, improved transgene expression duration in transduced cells through the construction of episomal gene delivery systems, and the production of genetically altered meganucleases and zinc finger proteins for the repair of genetic defects are the three main areas of focus [29].

In order to reduce the likelihood of interactions between the transfer vector system and the host genome, safer integrated gene delivery models include self-inactivating retroviridae-derived vectors that are devoid of retroviral enhancers and promoter regions in the LTRs [30]. Cellular oncogenes that could be present close to the integration site cannot be stimulated to express themselves by the nontranscriptional 3′-LTR. Because it may activate cellular promoters of carcinogenic factors, the inclusion of an enhancer within the internal promoter of a self-inactivating retroviridae-derived vector still enhances the risk of insertional mutagenesis [31].

Another approach to preventing insertional mutagenesis involves creating episomal gene delivery models that have prolonged transgene expression. The genome of the transduced cell is not altered by episomal vector techniques because the chromosomal DNA does not fuse with them [21]. Meganucleases and genetically modified zinc finger proteins are gaining attention in gene transfer technology for their ability to precisely rectify defective genes or add genetic material into particular regions in transfected cell genomes [32, 33].

3.3.3 Scalability and Manufacturing Challenges

The vaccine production chain faces challenges such as limited space capacities, lack of tech-transfer experts and industrial facilities, inadequate arrangements, raw material shortages, supply chain delays, and adherence to regulatory requirements. Limited space can be addressed by outsourcing vaccine manufacturing to CDMOs or other pharma companies. The global demand for vaccines is high, but resources for production components and trained personnel are often low. Supply chain delays can occur due to the need for efficient cold chain handling and controlled environments. Adherence to regulatory requirements is crucial for the safety of the finished product. Manufacturing sites must adhere to current good manufacturing practices (cGMPs) to minimize contamination risks and regularly test products for quality and compliance with changing standards. To pinpoint shortfalls and oversee the proper distribution of available resources, a central governing body was certainly required. Additional proposed options included repurposing current facilities and increasing production process flexibility by allowing materials to be interchangeable. Geographical reorganization of processes could simplify the production chain. It is important to include improved durability and resilience in the vaccine production process so that low- and middle-income nations can manufacture vaccines on their own [34–36].

3.4 The Role of Adjuvants in Overcoming Challenges

3.4.1 Mechanisms of Action of Adjuvants

Vaccine adjuvants play a crucial role in boosting adaptive immunity through the stimulation of innate immune cells [37]. Through the activation of antigen-presenting cells (APCs), they provide co-stimulatory and antigen presentation signals. These signals, which include inflammatory cytokines, co-stimulatory molecules, antigen peptides–major histocompatibility complexes (MHC), and naïve T cell activation, result in an improved adaptive immune response [38]. PAMPs and DAMPs are typical immunostimulants that may provoke these signals. Delivery systems like lipid nanoparticles facilitate antigen presentation.

3.4.2 Innate Immune Stimulation

Adjuvants, which fall under the category of immunostimulants and delivery systems, act by targeting specific receptors in order to promote the maturation and activation of APCs. They induce an innate immune response by acting as PAMPs, DAMPs, or mimics [39]. Mature APCs enhance antigen presentation and express co-stimulatory signals, enhancing adaptive immune responses. The release of cytokines is a key factor in determining adaptive immune responses, and it is triggered by various immunostimulant types that communicate through distinct PRRs [40].

3.4.3 Adaptive Immune Response Enhancement

Immunostimulants interact with Toll-like receptors (TLRs) on APCs, leading to increased cytokine production, co-stimulatory signal upregulation, and antigen presentation, all of which improve adaptive immune responses. Via diverse TLR signaling, several immunostimulant types mediate various adaptive immunological responses. When TLRs on the cell surface identify components of the microbial membrane, pro-inflammatory cytokines such as IL-1β, TNF-α, and IL-6 are produced. Type I IFNs are produced by intracellular TLRs expressed in intracellular vesicles, and they help in T helper type 1 (T_H1) cell development and function [41]. Immunostimulants attached to TLR2 heterodimers initiate signaling via the MyD88 pathway, which activates NF-κB and promotes the production of cytokines that promote inflammation. Through the MyD88 pathway, TLR4 and TLR5 activate signaling, which activates NF-κB and polarizes naïve T cells into T_H1-type cells. APCs produce type I IFNs and pro-inflammatory cytokines in response to TLR7/8/9 targets activating NF-κB and IRF7 through the MyD88 pathway [42]. Carbohydrate-structured immunostimulants activate CLRs, triggering APCs to internalize, process, and present antigens, and enhancing adaptive immune responses. They also activate signaling pathways and control naive T cell polarization [43].

The injection causes tissue damage, attracting immune system sentinel cells. The concentration and penetration of aluminum ions are reduced because aluminum salts are not very soluble across cell membrane concentration, preventing intracellular accumulation. Sentinel cells with phagocytic properties will internalize the adjuvant particles, forming an intracellular aluminum depot [44]. The aluminum adjuvant that is phagocytosed develops into a phagolysosome and destroys pathogens. Aluminum adjuvant, on the other hand, is inert and forms a long-lasting availability of aluminum ions [45–49].

3.4.4 Different Classes of Adjuvants Used with Viral Vector Vaccines

3.4.4.1 Classes of Adjuvants

Delivery aids, such as virosomes or traditional liposomes including non-immunostimulatory components, can serve as adjuvants, improving the manner in which the immune system gets acquainted with antigens and assisting in distributing immunomodulatory substances, vaccination antigens, or both in an efficient manner [50]. Immunomodulatory molecules, including RIG-I–like receptors, C-type lectins, NOD-like receptors, and ligands of innate immune receptors such as TLRs, can directly activate these receptors, with advanced compounds like TLR4 ligand MPL and TLR9 ligand CpG oligodeoxynucleotide (ODN) used in human papillomavirus (HPV) vaccines [51, 52].

Other classes of adjuvants include a combination of both adjuvant and immunostimulatory components. The RTS,S malaria vaccine from GlaxoSmithKline (GSK) includes MPL and QS21, with adjuvant systems AS01 and AS04 classified as combination systems [53–55]. MF59 recruits monocytes and neutrophils to immunization sites through a chemokine gradient, reliant on the ASC and Myd88 signaling pathways, and aluminum salts serve as carriers [56, 57].

3.4.4.1.1 Aluminum-Based Adjuvants

Aluminum salts were first presented by Glenny as adjuvants in 1926 and have been utilized in vaccine formulations for nearly a century. The initial vaccines were created by combining a base with antigen precipitation [58]. Aluminum-adsorbed vaccines, a kind of vaccination that acts by primarily adsorbing antigens on hydrated gels made of aluminum salts, replace the heterogeneous preparations of alum precipitation vaccines [59, 60]. Aluminum hydroxyphosphate and aluminum oxyhydroxide are the two primary forms of hydrated aluminum gels utilized in approved vaccinations [61]. The solubility of aluminum hydroxyphosphate and aluminum oxyhydroxide is minimal at pH 5 to 7, increasing sharply below pH 5 and at pH 6, respectively. With increasing pH, aluminum salt solubility and aluminum ion concentration both increase, resulting in micrometer-sized aggregates in vaccine formulations and administration sites [62, 63].

3.4.4.1.2 Toll-Like Receptor (TLR) Agonists

Immunostimulants engage with TLRs on APCs, stimulating them to boost antigen presentation, increase co-stimulatory signals, induce cytokine production, and trigger adaptive immune responses [64, 65]. TLRs, situated on the outermost layer of the cell, distinguish the components of microbial membranes. Stimulation by immunostimulants produces inflammatory cytokines resulting in T_H1 or T_H2 immunological responses [66].

TLR3 and TLR7 are intracellular TLRs that react with nucleic acids. Activation by immunostimulants produces type I IFNs, which promote T_H1 cell differentiation and function. These IFNs also stimulate $CD8^+$ T cell proliferation. Immunostimulants activate TLRs through the MyD88 pathway, triggering the production of pro-inflammatory cytokines like IL12 [67]. Immunostimulants targeting TLR2 and TLR3 trigger T_H2- and T_H1-type adaptive responses respectively, while those targeting TLR4 and TLR5 activate NF-κB, promoting T_H1-type differentiation and IRF3 generation. TLR7/8/9 targets TLR7 in the endosome, activating NF-κB and IRF7, producing inflammatory cytokines and type I IFNs, and stimulating T_H1 and CTL responses [33].

3.4.5 Targeting CLR Pathway

C-type lectin receptors (CLRs) are antigen receptors found on cell membranes. They are activated by carbohydrate-structured immunostimulants, triggering APCs to internalize, process, and present antigens, enhancing adaptive immune responses and controlling naive T cell polarization [68–70].

3.4.6 Saponins

There has been a lot of interest in saponins' potential as vaccine adjuvants because they may stimulate the mammalian immune system [71, 72]. Quil A and QS-21 are lead saponin adjuvants used in vaccine formulations for HIV, cancer, malaria, respiratory syncytial virus, cytomegalovirus, *Toxoplasma gondii*, and visceral leishmaniasis [73–78]. Quil A and QS-21 are ideal for subunit and intracellular pathogen vaccines, as they stimulate the T_H1 immune response and produce CTLs against antigens. However, they have drawbacks like high toxicity and instability.

3.4.7 Cytokines and Chemokines

Innate and adaptive immunity are both regulated by cytokines, including interleukin-2 (IL-2), type I IFNs, IFN-γ, and IL-12. The use of recombinant cytokine homologs as adjuvants in vaccines has been limited due to the short half-life. These problems have been effectively resolved by encapsulating DNA vaccines into liposomes and using cytokine expression vectors in conjunction with DNA vaccinations [37, 79].

3.4.8 Case Studies of Specific Adjuvants Used with Viral Vector Vaccines

Among the most advanced compounds are the TLR9 ligand CpG ODN, which is the adjuvant in the Heplisav vaccine candidate for hepatitis B from Dynavax that has successfully completed a phase 3 clinical trial, and the TLR4 ligand MPL, which is a component of the adjuvant system in the Cervarix HPV vaccine (from GSK) [80–84].

Though MPL and QS21 are components of the GSK RTS,S malaria vaccine that was evaluated in a phase 3 clinical investigation, these are also the part of the adjuvant system AS01 and AS04 (Cervarix vaccine). Quil A and its derivatives QS-21 have been used as adjuvants in vaccine formulations for several diseases in different animal models and humans, including HIV, cancer, malaria, respiratory syncytial virus, cytomegalovirus, *Toxoplasma gondii*, and visceral leishmaniasis. Quil A and QS-21 have a unique capacity to elicit the T_H1 immune response and the production of CTLs against external antigens, making them well-suited for subunit vaccines, vaccines targeting intracellular pathogens, and cancer vaccines [80–84].

3.5 Optimizing Adjuvant Design for Viral Vector Vaccines

3.5.1 Importance of Adjuvant Selection and Formulation

Adjuvant selection in vaccines is critical to ensuring vaccination potency. Factors such as the vaccine antigen's physical and chemical properties, desired immune response, target population age, and administration routes are considered [85]. Modern adjuvant studies strive to boost vaccine-induced responses while ensuring safety. Human vaccination adjuvants include aluminum salts, oil-in-water emulsions, virosomes, and AS04 [8].

3.5.2 Adjuvant Formulation Development

Adjuvant formulation development predominantly focuses on micro- and nanoparticle systems such as aluminum salts, liposomes, and emulsions. Aluminum salts are highly charged, facilitating antigen adsorption. Formulation parameters like particle size and surface characteristics can affect shelf-life stability and biological activity in antigen delivery to APCs or immune cell stimulation [86, 87]. These factors can influence uptake by APCs, lymphatic trafficking, immune response quality, potency, and toxicity. The chemical structure of the oil in vaccine emulsion formulations has a critical role in the immunological responses. Immunostimulants administered as particle formulations can improve localized immune response, reduce systemic exposure and inflammation, and improve adjuvant safety [88–91].

3.5.3 Adjuvant Formulations for the Development of New Vaccines

Immunomodulatory substances can elicit diverse immunological responses depending on their formulation. For instance, a malaria vaccine candidate formulated with AS02 (an oil-in-water emulsion containing MPL and QS21) protected six of seven recipients from infection. In contrast, the same antigen formulated with AS03 or AS04 protected only two of seven and one of eight recipients, respectively. Switching from an oil-in-water emulsion to a liposome formulation (AS01) with the same antigen and immunostimulants enhanced efficacy, T_H1 cell–mediated immunity, and antigen-specific humoral immunity in both mice and humans [91].

The addition of MPL to aluminum hydroxide (AS04) significantly enhanced anti-HPV antibody titers in both vaccinated mice and humans compared to a vaccine adjuvant containing aluminum hydroxide alone [90]. Vaccine formulations must be safe and effective for all age groups, with metabolizable components being preferable. Adjuvant activity should be localized and limited, avoiding direct influence on lymphocytes and nonspecific responses in B or T cells. To induce an effective immune response tailored to the target pathogen, careful selection of both the immunostimulant and adjuvant formulation components is crucial [56, 92, 93].

3.5.4 Strategies for Optimizing Adjuvant Design

3.5.4.1 Dose Sparing

Danielle and colleagues have introduced a dose-sparing approach for vaccines that involves the development of an adjuvant dermal patch. This method uses *E. coli* heat-labile enterotoxin protein (LT) as an adjuvant and administers a dry LT-IS patch to the vaccine injection site. The dry LT-IS patch is an excellent choice for mass production and stockpiling in the event of a flu epidemic due to its formulation properties, which include inherent stability and use as a dose-sparing strategy, which allows a lower dose of injected vaccine to produce an effective immune response [94].

Recombinant vaccines provide important manufacturing benefits, but they have low immunogenicity independently. Adjuvants combined with recombinant pandemic influenza protein can significantly decrease the required antigen quantity to achieve desired antibody levels, impacting manufacturing efficiency. The incorporation of the adjuvant glucopyranosyl lipid adjuvant-stable emulsion (GLA-SE) reduced the required quantity of recombinant influenza H5 protein by more than 30 times to achieve a 40% seroconversion rate following a single immunization compared to using the antigen alone [95].

3.5.4.2 Enabling a More Rapid Immune Response

A single-dose vaccination is the best option for a variety of applications, including biodefense vaccines for pandemic flu, anthrax, and other potential bioterrorism weapons. Adjuvants can be introduced to specific antigens to increase their efficiency, such as the AS04 adjuvant added to the hepatitis B antigen in GSK's Fendrix, which reduces the regimen from three to two doses [96, 97].

3.5.4.3 Antibody Response Broadening

Several diseases, including HIV, influenza viruses, HPV, and the malaria parasite, exhibit significant antigenic drift, strain changes, or both. Therefore, the capacity of adjuvants to expand the range of immunological response profiles may be essential for the effectiveness of vaccinations targeting those specific areas. Research using massively parallel sequencing has shown experimentally that adjuvants' flaring impact may be mediated by an increase in B cell diversity rather than just higher titers. In clinical settings, adjuvants have been observed to increase the antibody response to influenza and HPV vaccines [98–100].

3.5.4.4 Antibody Response Magnitude and Functionality

Commonly used adjuvants like aluminum salts or oil-in-water emulsions are known to enhance the antibody responses to vaccination antigens. Adjuvants are increasingly recognized for the ability to increase overall antibody titers as well as the number of functional antibodies, antibodies with a higher affinity for vaccine antigens, or both [101, 102].

3.5.5 Delivery Systems

3.5.5.1 Targeting Specific Immune Cell Populations

Several vaccines are being developed to target T cell responses that are not effectively stimulated by frequently used adjuvants. The new generation frequently uses agonists for TLRs and other innate immune receptors to boost T helper cell responses, especially when creating vaccines against diseases that can be controlled by cellular immune responses [85].

3.5.5.2 Combination Adjuvants

Combination adjuvants have the potential to significantly improve vaccine-induced immune responses, which might be extremely beneficial. Concurrent administration of TLR-3 agonist poly I:C and TLR-9 agonist CpG ODN with a DNA-encoded HIV Gag vaccine enhanced the $CD8^+$ T cell response by boosting the number of IFN-γ– and IL-2–producing $CD8^+$ T cells. Combining an HIV surface peptide with 2-kDa macrophage-activating lipopeptide (MALP2; TLR-2 agonist), poly I:C (TLR-3 agonist), and CpG ODN (TLR-9 agonist) improved vaccine efficacy significantly. Administering a combination of these three TLR agonists improved immunity against viral exposure in mice more than any combination of two TLRs. This combination enhanced T cell reactivity and increased IL-15 production by DCs [103].

Microparticle adjuvant combinations may strengthen immune responses by encapsulating or adsorbing CpG ODN on their surfaces. Microparticles can be resuspended in adjuvant solutions, such as PLG microparticles in QS-21 solution. These combinations not only increase formulation efficacy but also reduce possible adverse effects of severe adjuvant exposure, such as MDP's pyrogenicity [104–106].

3.5.5.3 *Challenges and Future Directions in Adjuvant Development for Viral Vector Vaccines*

Advancements in studying innate immunity and its impact on stimulating antigen-specific responses and memory of immune responses have contributed to enhancing research and development initiatives related to adjuvant design and discovery. Earlier alternatives, such as CpG, monophosphoryl lipid-A, and imidazoquinolines, have shown efficacy in animal studies and phase 1 human trials. Vaccine development has changed from traditional whole-cell or viral vaccines to subunit shots due to isolated antigens lacking immunogenicity, necessitating the addition of potent adjuvants. A dearth of vaccinations for major illnesses such as HIV, hepatitis C virus, herpes simplex virus, and *Neisseria meningitidis* emphasizes the need for new vaccine adjuvants that can boost the immune response to protective levels against these types of infections. The primary goal should be to distinguish possible increases in immune toxicity from greater immunogenicity given by vaccination adjuvants. The long-term objective should be selecting appropriate platforms and discovering essential innate immune targets for eliciting strong yet safe immune responses [107].

3.6 Conclusion

Viral vector vaccines are a promising method for avoiding infectious diseases by demonstrating efficiency against a variety of diseases, including viruses, bacteria, and parasites. Researchers are improving viral vector vaccines by integrating adjuvants to enhance their immunogenicity and efficacy, showing tremendous promise for the future. Yet, numerous obstacles and possibilities still exist, influencing the course of viral vector vaccine advancement and distribution.

In viral vector vaccine research, the main focus is improving vaccination safety, efficacy, and scalability through optimizing vector design and delivery mechanisms. Progress in genetic engineering methods, like rational vector design and modular vector platforms, allow for the creation of improved vectors that have increased immunogenicity and decreased reactogenicity. Exploring new delivery methods such as intranasal, oral, and mucosal administration shows potential for enhancing strong mucosal immunity, which is crucial for defending against respiratory and gastrointestinal infections [108].

Adjuvants in viral vector vaccine formulations are increasingly recognized for their vital function in boosting immune responses and improving vaccine effectiveness. Adjuvants can influence both innate and adaptive immune responses, extend the presence of antigens, and enhance the development of APCs, ultimately boosting the immunological reaction to viral vector vaccines. Adjuvants such as aluminum salts, oil-in-water emulsions, and TLR agonists have been successfully added to viral vector vaccine formulations to improve immune response and protective immunity.

Although there have been breakthroughs, there are still significant hurdles in the development and implementation of viral vector vaccines and adjuvants. Concerns about safety, such as immunological responses caused by vectors, genetic mutations from insertion, and shedding of vectors, require comprehensive evaluation before clinical trials to reduce any dangers. Furthermore, it is crucial to address manufacturing scalability, cost-effectiveness, and regulatory issues to guarantee the widespread availability and cost of viral vector vaccines, particularly in countries with low or middle incomes.

The rise of novel infectious diseases including pandemic influenza, coronaviruses, and emerging variations highlights the necessity for quick vaccine development methods that can adjust to changing viral threats. Viral vector vaccine platforms provide flexibility and diversity, enabling quick development and distribution of vaccinations for new infectious illnesses. Moreover, creating universal adjuvants that can boost immune responses for many vaccine types has the potential to speed up vaccine development and enhance vaccine effectiveness against difficult infections.

Ultimately, the future of viral vector vaccines and adjuvants will be shaped by ongoing advancements, partnerships, and financial support for research and development. Viral vector vaccines have the ability to transform global vaccination efforts by overcoming current obstacles and taking advantage of new opportunities. They provide effective solutions for fighting infectious illnesses and protecting public health on a global scale.

References

1. Pollard, A.J. and Bijker, E.M., A Guide to Vaccinology: From Basic Principles to New Developments. *Nat. Rev. Immunol.*, *21*, 83–100, **2021**, doi: 10.1038/s41577-020-00479-7.
2. Dhamanti, I., Suwantika, A.A., Adlia, A., Yamani, L.N., Yakub, F., Adverse Reactions of COVID-19 Vaccines: A Scoping Review of Observational Studies. *IJGM*, *16*, 609–618, **2023**, doi: 10.2147/IJGM.S400458.
3. Jalilian, H., Amraei, M., Javanshir, E., Jamebozorgi, K., Faraji-Khiavi, F., Ethical Considerations of the Vaccine Development Process and Vaccination:

A Scoping Review. *BMC Health Serv. Res.*, *23*, 255, **2023**, doi: 10.1186/s12913-023-09237-6.

4. Deng, S., Liang, H., Chen, P., Li, Y., Li, Z., Fan, S., Wu, K., Li, X., Chen, W., Qin, Y., *et al.*, Viral Vector Vaccine Development and Application during the COVID-19 Pandemic. *Microorganisms*, *10*, 1450, **2022**, doi: 10.3390/microorganisms10071450.
5. Wang, S., Liang, B., Wang, W., Li, L., Feng, N., Zhao, Y., Wang, T., Yan, F., Yang, S., Xia, X., Viral Vectored Vaccines: Design, Development, Preventive and Therapeutic Applications in Human Diseases. *Signal Transduction Targeted Ther.*, *8*, 149, **2023**, doi: 10.1038/s41392-023-01408-5.
6. El-Maradny, Y.A., Ramadan, A.A., Chavda, V.P., Balar, P.C., Redwan, E.M., The Fast-Track Development of COVID-19 Vaccines, in: *Advanced Vaccination Technologies for Infectious and Chronic Diseases*, pp. 415–440, Elsevier, Amsterdam, 2024, ISBN 978-0-443-18564-9.
7. Chavda, V.P., Balar, P.C., Apostolopoulos, V., History of Vaccination, in: *Advanced Vaccination Technologies for Infectious and Chronic Diseases*, pp. 1–12, Elsevier, Amsterdam, 2024, ISBN 978-0-443-18564-9.
8. Facciolà, A., Visalli, G., Laganà, A., Di Pietro, A., An Overview of Vaccine Adjuvants: Current Evidence and Future Perspectives. *Vaccines*, *10*, 819, **2022**, doi: 10.3390/vaccines10050819.
9. Bachmann, M.F. and Jennings, G.T., Vaccine Delivery: A Matter of Size, Geometry, Kinetics and Molecular Patterns. *Nat. Rev. Immunol.*, *10*, 787–796, **2010**, doi: 10.1038/nri2868.
10. Retnakumar, S.V., Bonam, S.R., Hu, H., Bayry, J., THEME: Vaccines and Vaccine Adjuvants/Immunomodulators for Infectious Diseases. *Vaccines*, *11*, 383, **2023**, doi: 10.3390/vaccines11020383.
11. Travieso, T., Li, J., Mahesh, S., Mello, J.D.F.R.E., Blasi, M., The Use of Viral Vectors in Vaccine Development. *npj Vaccines*, *7*, 1, 75, **2022**, doi: 10.1038/s41541-022-00503-y.
12. Liu, M.A., Immunologic Basis of Vaccine Vectors. *Immunity*, *33*, 504–515, **2010**, doi: 10.1016/j.immuni.2010.10.004.
13. Mendonça, S.A., Lorincz, R., Boucher, P., Curiel, D.T., Adenoviral Vector Vaccine Platforms in the SARS-CoV-2 Pandemic. *npj Vaccines*, *6*, 97, **2021**, doi: 10.1038/s41541-021-00356-x.
14. Orlova, O.V., Glazkova, D.V., Bogoslovskaya, E.V., Shipulin, G.A., Yudin, S.M., Development of Modified Vaccinia Virus Ankara-Based Vaccines: Advantages and Applications. *Vaccines*, *10*, 1516, **2022**, doi: 10.3390/vaccines10091516.
15. Munis, A.M., Gene Therapy Applications of Non-Human Lentiviral Vectors. *Viruses*, *12*, 1106, **2020**, doi: 10.3390/v12101106.
16. Ura, T., Okuda, K., Shimada, M., Developments in Viral Vector-Based Vaccines. *Vaccines*, *2*, 624–641, **2014**, doi: 10.3390/vaccines2030624.

17. Sasso, E., D'Alise, A.M., Zambrano, N., Scarselli, E., Folgori, A., Nicosia, A., New Viral Vectors for Infectious Diseases and Cancer. *Semin. Immunol.*, *50*, 101430, **2020**, doi: 10.1016/j.smim.2020.101430.
18. Ghaemmaghamian, Z., Zarghami, R., Walker, G., O'Reilly, E., Ziaee, A., Stabilizing Vaccines via Drying: Quality by Design Considerations. *Adv. Drug Deliv. Rev.*, *187*, 114313, **2022**, doi: 10.1016/j.addr.2022.114313.
19. Saxena, M., Van, T.T.H., Baird, F.J., Coloe, P.J., Smooker, P.M., Pre-Existing Immunity against Vaccine Vectors – Friend or Foe? *Microbiology*, *159*, 1–11, **2013**, doi: 10.1099/mic.0.049601-0.
20. Bangari, D.S. and Mittal, S.K., Development of Nonhuman Adenoviruses as Vaccine Vectors. *Vaccine*, *24*, 849–862, **2006**, doi: 10.1016/j.vaccine.2005.08.101.
21. Wang, W.-C., Sayedahmed, E.E., Mittal, S.K., Significance of Preexisting Vector Immunity and Activation of Innate Responses for Adenoviral Vector-Based Therapy. *Viruses*, *14*, 2727, **2022**, doi: 10.3390/v14122727.
22. Shirley, J.L., de Jong, Y.P., Terhorst, C., Herzog, R.W., Immune Responses to Viral Gene Therapy Vectors. *Mol. Ther.*, *28*, 709–722, **2020**, doi: 10.1016/j.ymthe.2020.01.001.
23. Wold, W.S.M. and Toth, K., Adenovirus Vectors for Gene Therapy, Vaccination and Cancer Gene Therapy. *Curr. Gene Ther.*, *13*, 421–433, **2013**, doi: 10.2174/1566523213666131125095046.
24. Fausther-Bovendo, H. and Kobinger, G.P., Pre-Existing Immunity against Ad Vectors: Humoral, Cellular, and Innate Response, What's Important? *Hum. Vaccin. Immunother.*, *10*, 2875–2884, **2014**, doi: 10.4161/hv.29594.
25. Hackett, P.B., Largaespada, D.A., Switzer, K.C., Cooper, L.J.N., Evaluating Risks of Insertional Mutagenesis by DNA Transposons in Gene Therapy. *Transl. Res.*, *161*, 265–283, **2013**, doi: 10.1016/j.trsl.2012.12.005.
26. Izsvák, Z., Hackett, P.B., Cooper, L.J., Ivics, Z., Translating Sleeping Beauty Transposition into Cellular Therapies: Victories and Challenges. *Bioessays*, 32, 9, 756–67, 2010 Sep, Doi: 10.1002/Bies.201000027.
27. Dufait, I., Liechtenstein, T., Lanna, A., Bricogne, C., Laranga, R., Padella, A., Breckpot, K., Escors, D., Retroviral and Lentiviral Vectors for the Induction of Immunological Tolerance. *Scientifica (Cairo)*, 2012, 694137, 2012 Dec, Doi: 10.6064/2012/694137.
28. Romano, G., Gene Transfer in Experimental Medicine. *Drug News Perspect.*, *16*, 267, **2003**, doi: 10.1358/dnp.2003.16.5.829314.
29. Chavda, V.P., Ghali, E.N.H.K., Balar, P.C., Chauhan, S.C., Tiwari, N., Shukla, S., Athalye, M., Patravale, V., Apostolopoulos, V., Yallapu, M.M., Protein Subunit Vaccines: Promising Frontiers against COVID-19. *J. Control. Release*, *366*, 761–782, **2024**, doi: 10.1016/j.jconrel.2024.01.017.
30. Yu, S.F., von Rüden, T., Kantoff, P.W., Garber, C., Seiberg, M., Rüther, U., Anderson, W.F., Wagner, E.F., Gilboa, E., Self-Inactivating Retroviral Vectors Designed for Transfer of Whole Genes into Mammalian Cells. *Proc. Natl. Acad. Sci.*, *83*, 3194–3198, **1986**, doi: 10.1073/pnas.83.10.3194.

31. Ramezani, A., Hawley, T.S., Hawley, R.G., Reducing the Genotoxic Potential of Retroviral Vectors, in: *Gene Therapy Protocols: Design and Characterization of Gene Transfer Vectors*, J.M. Le Doux, (Ed.), pp. 183–203, Humana Press, Totowa, NJ, 2008, ISBN 978-1-60327-248-3.
32. Romano, G., Development of Safer Gene Delivery Systems to Minimize the Risk of Insertional Mutagenesis-Related Malignancies: A Critical Issue for the Field of Gene Therapy. *ISRN Oncol.*, *2012*, 1–14, **2012**, doi: 10.5402/2012/616310.
33. Paques, F. and Duchateau, P., Meganucleases and DNA Double-Strand Break-Induced Recombination: Perspectives for Gene Therapy. *CGT*, *7*, 49–66, **2007**, doi: 10.2174/156652307779940216.
34. Feddema, J.J., Fernald, K.D.S., Schikan, H.G.C.P., Van De Burgwal, L.H.M., Upscaling Vaccine Manufacturing Capacity - Key Bottlenecks and Lessons Learned. *Vaccine*, *41*, 4359–4368, **2023**, doi: 10.1016/j.vaccine.2023.05.027.
35. Strategies, I. @ of M. (US) C. on the C.V.I.P.A., Mitchell, V.S., Philipose, N.M., Sanford, J.P., Regulatory Aspects of Vaccine Development, Manufacture, and Distribution, in: *The Children's Vaccine Initiative: Achieving the Vision*, National Academies Press (US), Washington, 1993.
36. Manufacturing,SafetyandQualityControlofVaccines,Availableonline:https://www.who.int/news-room/feature-stories/detail/manufacturing-safety-and-quality-control (accessed on 2 March 2024).
37. Awate, S., Babiuk, L.A., Mutwiri, G., Mechanisms of Action of Adjuvants. *Front. Immunol.*, *4*, 114, **2013**, doi: 10.3389/fimmu.2013.00114.
38. Zhao, T., Cai, Y., Jiang, Y., He, X., Wei, Y., Yu, Y., Tian, X., Vaccine Adjuvants: Mechanisms and Platforms. *Signal Transduction Targeted Ther.*, *8*, 283, **2023**, doi: 10.1038/s41392-023-01557-7.
39. Bergmann-Leitner, E.S. and Leitner, W.W., Adjuvants in the Driver's Seat: How Magnitude, Type, Fine Specificity and Longevity of Immune Responses Are Driven by Distinct Classes of Immune Potentiators. *Vaccines*, *2*, 252–296, **2014**, doi: 10.3390/vaccines2020252.
40. Pulendran, B., Arunachalam, P.S., O'Hagan, D.T., Emerging Concepts in the Science of Vaccine Adjuvants. *Nat. Rev. Drug Discov.*, *20*, 454–475, **2021**, doi: 10.1038/s41573-021-00163-y.
41. Goulopoulou, S., McCarthy, C.G., Webb, R.C., Toll-like Receptors in the Vascular System: Sensing the Dangers Within. *Pharmacol. Rev.*, *68*, 142, **2016**, doi: 10.1124/pr.114.010090.
42. Venugopal, P.G., Nutman, T.B., Semnani, R.T., Activation and Regulation of Toll-Like Receptors (TLRs) by Helminth Parasites. *Immunol. Res.*, *43*, 252–263, **2009**, doi: 10.1007/s12026-008-8079-0.
43. Wilson-Welder, J.H., Torres, M.P., Kipper, M.J., Mallapragada, S.K., Wannemuehler, M.J., Narasimhan, B., Vaccine Adjuvants: Current Challenges and Future Approaches. *J. Pharm. Sci.*, *98*, 1278–1316, **2009**, doi: 10.1002/jps.21523.

44. Pauwels, A.-M., Trost, M., Beyaert, R., Hoffmann, E., Patterns, Receptors, and Signals: Regulation of Phagosome Maturation. *Trends Immunol.*, *38*, 407–422, **2017**, doi: 10.1016/j.it.2017.03.006.
45. Mold, M., Eriksson, H., Siesjö, P., Darabi, A., Shardlow, E., Exley, C., Unequivocal Identification of Intracellular Aluminium Adjuvant in a Monocytic THP-1 Cell Line. *Sci. Rep.*, *4*, 6287, **2014**, doi: 10.1038/srep06287.
46. Mile, I., Svensson, A., Darabi, A., Mold, M., Siesjö, P., Eriksson, H., Al Adjuvants Can Be Tracked in Viable Cells by Lumogallion Staining. *J. Immunol. Methods*, *422*, 87–94, **2015**, doi: 10.1016/j.jim.2015.04.008.
47. Lu, F., Boutselis, I., Borch, R.F., HogenEsch, H., Control of Antigen-Binding to Aluminum Adjuvants and the Immune Response with a Novel Phosphonate Linker. *Vaccine*, *31*, 4362–4367, **2013**, doi: 10.1016/j.vaccine.2013.07.019.
48. Morefield, G.L., Tammariello, R.F., Purcell, B.K., Worsham, P.L., Chapman, J., Smith, L.A., Alarcon, J.B., Mikszta, J.A., Ulrich, R.G., An Alternative Approach to Combination Vaccines: Intradermal Administration of Isolated Components for Control of Anthrax, Botulism, Plague and Staphylococcal Toxic Shock. *J. Immune Based Ther. Vaccines*, *6*, 5, **2008**, doi: 10.1186/1476-8518-6-5.
49. Gherardi, R.K., Aouizerate, J., Cadusseau, J., Yara, S., Authier, F.J., Aluminum Adjuvants of Vaccines Injected into the Muscle: Normal Fate, Pathology and Associated Disease. *Morphologie*, *100*, 85–94, **2016**, doi: 10.1016/j.morpho.2016.01.002.
50. Tretiakova, D.S. and Vodovozova, E.L., Liposomes as Adjuvants and Vaccine Delivery Systems. *Biochem. (Mosc.) Suppl. Ser. A: Membr. Cell Biol.*, *16*, 1–20, **2022**, doi: 10.1134/S1990747822020076.
51. The RTS,S Clinical Trials Partnership, First Results of Phase 3 Trial of RTS,S/AS01 Malaria Vaccine in African Children. *N. Engl. J. Med.*, *365*, 1863–1875, **2011**, doi: 10.1056/NEJMoa1102287.
52. Eng, N.F., Bhardwaj, N., Mulligan, R., Diaz-Mitoma, F., The Potential of 1018 ISS Adjuvant in Hepatitis B Vaccines: HEPLISAV™ Review. *Hum. Vaccin. Immunother.*, *9*, 1661–1672, **2013**, doi: 10.4161/hv.24715.
53. Mosca, F., Tritto, E., Muzzi, A., Monaci, E., Bagnoli, F., Iavarone, C., O'Hagan, D., Rappuoli, R., De Gregorio, E., Molecular and Cellular Signatures of Human Vaccine Adjuvants. *Proc. Natl. Acad. Sci. U.S.A.*, *105*, 10501–10506, **2008**, doi: 10.1073/pnas.0804699105.
54. Fox, C.B., Baldwin, S.L., Duthie, M.S., Reed, S.G., Vedvick, T.S., Immunomodulatory and Physical Effects of Oil Composition in Vaccine Adjuvant Emulsions. *Vaccine*, *29*, 9563–9572, **2011**, doi: 10.1016/j.vaccine.2011.08.089.
55. Morel, S., Didierlaurent, A., Bourguignon, P., Delhaye, S., Baras, B., Jacob, V., Planty, C., Elouahabi, A., Harvengt, P., Carlsen, H., Adjuvant System AS03 Containing α-Tocopherol Modulates Innate Immune Response and Leads to Improved Adaptive Immunity. *Vaccine*, *29*, 2461–2473, **2011**, doi: 10.1016/j.vaccine.2011.01.011.

56. O'Hagan, D.T., Ott, G.S., De Gregorio, E., Seubert, A., The Mechanism of Action of MF59 – An Innately Attractive Adjuvant Formulation. *Vaccine, 30,* 4341–4348, **2012**, doi: 10.1016/j.vaccine.2011.09.061.
57. Seubert, A., Monaci, E., Pizza, M., O'Hagan, D.T., Wack, A., The Adjuvants Aluminum Hydroxide and MF59 Induce Monocyte and Granulocyte Chemoattractants and Enhance Monocyte Differentiation toward Dendritic Cells. *J. Immunol., 180,* 5402–5412, **2008**, doi: 10.4049/jimmunol.180.8.5402.
58. Glenny, A.T., Pope, C.G., Waddington, H., Wallace, U., Immunological Notes. XVII–XXIV. *J. Pathol., 29,* 31–40, **1926**, doi: 10.1002/path.1700290106.
59. Lindblad, E.B., Aluminium Adjuvants—in Retrospect and Prospect. *Vaccine, 22,* 3658–3668, **2004**, doi: 10.1016/j.vaccine.2004.03.032.
60. Gupta, R., Aluminum Compounds as Vaccine Adjuvants. *Adv. Drug Deliv. Rev., 32,* 155–172, **1998**, doi: 10.1016/S0169-409X(98)00008-8.
61. Shirodkar, S., Hutchinson, R.L., Perry, D.L., White, J.L., Hem, S.L., Aluminum Compounds Used as Adjuvants in Vaccines. *Pharm. Res., 07,* 1282–1288, **1990**, doi: 10.1023/A:1015994006859.
62. Danielsson, R. and Eriksson, H., Aluminium Adjuvants in Vaccines – A Way to Modulate the Immune Response. *Semin. Cell Dev. Biol., 115,* 3–9, **2021**, doi: 10.1016/j.semcdb.2020.12.008.
63. Rinella, J.V., White, J.L., Hem, S.L., Effect of pH on the Elution of Model Antigens from Aluminum-Containing Adjuvants. *J. Colloid Interface Sci., 205,* 161–165, **1998**, doi: 10.1006/jcis.1998.5648.
64. Pulendran, B., Modulating Vaccine Responses with Dendritic Cells and Toll-like Receptors. *Immunol. Rev., 199,* 227–250, **2004**, doi: 10.1111/j.0105-2896.2004.00144.x.
65. Lind, N.A., Rael, V.E., Pestal, K., Liu, B., Barton, G.M., Regulation of the Nucleic Acid-Sensing Toll-like Receptors. *Nat. Rev. Immunol., 22,* 224–235, **2022**, doi: 10.1038/s41577-021-00577-0.
66. Kleinhaus, A.L., Electrophysiological Actions of Convulsants and Anticonvulsants on Neurons of the Leech Subesophageal Ganglion. *Comp. Biochem. Physiol. C Comp. Pharmacol., 52,* 27–34, **1975**, doi: 10.1016/0306-4492(75)90008-8.
67. Kawai, T. and Akira, S., The Role of Pattern-Recognition Receptors in Innate Immunity: Update on Toll-like Receptors. *Nat. Immunol., 11,* 373–384, **2010**, doi: 10.1038/ni.1863.
68. Smirnov, D., Schmidt, J.J., Capecchi, J.T., Wightman, P.D., Vaccine Adjuvant Activity of 3M-052: An Imidazoquinoline Designed for Local Activity without Systemic Cytokine Induction. *Vaccine, 29,* 5434–5442, **2011**, doi: 10.1016/j.vaccine.2011.05.061.
69. Robertson, B., Lindh, B., Aldskogius, H., WGA-HRP and Choleragenoid-HRP as Anterogradely Transported Tracers in Vagal Visceral Afferents and Binding of WGA and Choleragenoid to Nodose Ganglion Neurons in Rodents. *Brain Res., 590,* 207–212, **1992**, doi: 10.1016/0006-8993(92)91097-x.

70. García García, M.J., López-Herce Cid, J., Martínez Bermejo, A., Perdikidi Olivieri, L., Rubio de la Iglesia, F., Hernández González, J., [Treatment of refractory status convulsivus with chlormethiazole]. *An. Esp. Pediatr.*, *29*, 324–326, **1988**.
71. Bomford, R., Stapleton, M., Winsor, S., McKNIGHT, A., Andronova, T., The Control of the Antibody Isotype Response to Recombinant Human Immunodeficiency Virus Gp120 Antigen by Adjuvants. *AIDS Res. Hum. Retrovir.*, *8*, 1765–1771, **1992**, doi: 10.1089/aid.1992.8.1765.
72. Skene, C.D. and Sutton, P., Saponin-Adjuvanted Particulate Vaccines for Clinical Use. *Methods*, *40*, 53–59, **2006**, doi: 10.1016/j.ymeth.2006.05.019.
73. Oliveira-Freitas, E., Casas, C.P., Borja-Cabrera, G.P., Santos, F.N., Nico, D., Souza, L.O.P., Tinoco, L.W., da Silva, B.P., Palatnik, M., Parente, J.P., *et al.*, Acylated and Deacylated Saponins of Quillaja Saponaria Mixture as Adjuvants for the FML-Vaccine against Visceral Leishmaniasis. *Vaccine*, *24*, 3909–3920, **2006**, doi: 10.1016/j.vaccine.2006.02.034.
74. Sjölander, S., Hansen, J.-E.S., Lövgren-Bengtsson, K., Åkerblom, L., Morein, B., Induction of Homologous Virus Neutralizing Antibodies in Guinea-Pigs Immunized with Two Human Immunodeficiency Virus Type 1 Glycoprotein Gp120-Iscom Preparations. A Comparison with Other Adjuvant Systems. *Vaccine*, *14*, 344–352, **1996**, doi: 10.1016/0264-410X(95)00163-U.
75. Evans, T.G., McElrath, M.J., Matthews, T., Montefiori, D., Weinhold, K., Wolff, M., Keefer, M.C., Kallas, E.G., Corey, L., Gorse, G.J., *et al.*, QS-21 Promotes an Adjuvant Effect Allowing for Reduced Antigen Dose during HIV-1 Envelope Subunit Immmunization in Humans. *Vaccine*, *19*, 2080–2091, **2001**, doi: 10.1016/S0264-410X(00)00415-1.
76. Chapman, P.B., Morrissey, D.M., Panageas, K.S., Hamilton, W.B., Zhan, C., Destro, A.N., Williams, L., Israel, R.J., Livingston, P.O., Induction of Antibodies against GM2 Ganglioside by Immunizing Melanoma Patients Using GM2-Keyhole Limpet Hemocyanin + QS21 Vaccine: A Dose-Response Study. *Clin. Cancer Res.*, *6*, 874–879, **2000**.
77. Moreno, C.A., Rodriguez, R., Oliveira, G.A., Ferreira, V., Nussenzweig, R.S., Moya Castro, Z.R., Calvo-Calle, J.M., Nardin, E., Preclinical Evaluation of a Synthetic Plasmodium Falciparum MAP Malaria Vaccine in Aotus Monkeys and Mice. *Vaccine*, *18*, 89–99, **1999**, doi: 10.1016/s0264-410x(99)00184-x.
78. Britt, W., Fay, J., Seals, J., Kensil, C., Formulation of an Immunogenic Human Cytomegalovirus Vaccine: Responses in Mice. *J. Infect. Dis.*, *171*, 18–25, **1995**, doi: 10.1093/infdis/171.1.18.
79. Egan, M.A. and Israel, Z.R., The Use of Cytokines and Chemokines as Genetic Adjuvants for Plasmid DNA Vaccines. *Clin. Appl. Immunol. Rev.*, *2*, 255–287, **2002**, doi: 10.1016/S1529-1049(02)00051-X.
80. Waite, D.C., Jacobson, E.W., Ennis, F.A., Edelman, R., White, B., Kammer, R., Anderson, C., Kensil, C.R., Three Double-Blind, Randomized Trials Evaluating the Safety and Tolerance of Different Formulations of the

Saponin Adjuvant QS-21. *Vaccine, 19*, 3957–3967, **2001**, doi: 10.1016/s0264-410x(01)00142-6.
81. Takahashi, H., Takeshita, T., Morein, B., Putney, S., Germain, R.N., Berzofsky, J.A., Induction of CD8+ Cytotoxic T Cells by Immunization with Purified HIV-1 Envelope Protein in ISCOMs. *Nature, 344*, 873–875, **1990**, doi: 10.1038/344873a0.
82. Soltysik, S., Wu, J.Y., Recchia, J., Wheeler, D.A., Newman, M.J., Coughlin, R.T., Kensil, C.R., Structure/Function Studies of QS-21 Adjuvant: Assessment of Triterpene Aldehyde and Glucuronic Acid Roles in Adjuvant Function. *Vaccine, 13*, 1403–1410, **1995**, doi: 10.1016/0264-410x(95)00077-e.
83. Schetters, T.P., Kleuskens, J., Scholtes, N., Bos, H.J., Vaccination of Dogs against Babesia Canis Infection Using Parasite Antigens from *in Vitro* Culture. *Parasite Immunol., 14*, 295–305, **1992**, doi: 10.1111/j.1365-3024.1992.tb00469.x.
84. Cox, S.J., Barnett, P.V., Dani, P., Salt, J.S., Emergency Vaccination of Sheep against Foot-and-Mouth Disease: Protection against Disease and Reduction in Contact Transmission. *Vaccine, 17*, 1858–1868, **1999**, doi: 10.1016/s0264-410x(98)00486-1.
85. Reed, S.G., Orr, M.T., Fox, C.B., Key Roles of Adjuvants in Modern Vaccines. *Nat. Med., 19*, 1597–1608, **2013**, doi: 10.1038/nm.3409.
86. Owusu-Agyei, S., Ansong, D., Asante, K., Kwarteng Owusu, S., Owusu, R., Wireko Brobby, N.A., Dosoo, D., Osei Akoto, A., Osei-Kwakye, K., Adjei, E.A., *et al.*, Randomized Controlled Trial of RTS,S/AS02D and RTS,S/AS01E Malaria Candidate Vaccines Given According to Different Schedules in Ghanaian Children. *PLoS One, 4*, e7302, **2009**, doi: 10.1371/journal.pone.0007302.
87. Stewart, V.A., McGrath, S.M., Walsh, D.S., Davis, S., Hess, A.S., Ware, L.A., Kester, K.E., Cummings, J.F., Burge, J.R., Voss, G., *et al.*, Pre-Clinical Evaluation of New Adjuvant Formulations to Improve the Immunogenicity of the Malaria Vaccine RTS,S/AS02A. *Vaccine, 24*, 6483–6492, **2006**, doi: 10.1016/j.vaccine.2006.06.033.
88. Polhemus, M.E., Remich, S.A., Ogutu, B.R., Waitumbi, J.N., Otieno, L., Apollo, S., Cummings, J.F., Kester, K.E., Ockenhouse, C.F., Stewart, A., *et al.*, Evaluation of RTS,S/AS02A and RTS,S/AS01B in Adults in a High Malaria Transmission Area. *PLoS One, 4*, e6465, **2009**, doi: 10.1371/journal.pone.0006465.
89. Kester, K.E., Cummings, J.F., Ofori-Anyinam, O., Ockenhouse, C.F., Krzych, U., Moris, P., Schwenk, R., Nielsen, R.A., Debebe, Z., Pinelis, E., *et al.*, Randomized, Double-Blind, Phase 2a Trial of Falciparum Malaria Vaccines RTS,S/AS01B and RTS,S/AS02A in Malaria-Naive Adults: Safety, Efficacy, and Immunologic Associates of Protection. *J. Infect. Dis., 200*, 337–346, **2009**, doi: 10.1086/600120.
90. Mettens, P., Dubois, P.M., Demoitié, M.-A., Bayat, B., Donner, M.-N., Bourguignon, P., Stewart, V.A., Heppner, D.G., Garçon, N., Cohen, J.,

Improved T Cell Responses to Plasmodium Falciparum Circumsporozoite Protein in Mice and Monkeys Induced by a Novel Formulation of RTS,S Vaccine Antigen. *Vaccine, 26,* 1072–1082, **2008**, doi: 10.1016/j.vaccine.2007.12.018.

91. Stoute, J.A., Slaoui, M., Heppner, D.G., Momin, P., Kester, K.E., Desmons, P., Wellde, B.T., Garçon, N., Krzych, U., Marchand, M., *et al.*, A Preliminary Evaluation of a Recombinant Circumsporozoite Protein Vaccine against *Plasmodium Falciparum Malaria. N. Engl. J. Med., 336,* 86–91, **1997**, doi: 10.1056/NEJM199701093360202.
92. Sham, J.S., Sawyer, W.H., Pang, P.K., Direct Cardiac Stimulation by Arginine Vasotocin in Bullfrogs (Rana Catesbeiana). *Am. J. Physiol., 256,* R187–192, **1989**, doi: 10.1152/ajpregu.1989.256.1.R187.
93. Orr, M.T., Fox, C.B., Baldwin, S.L., Sivananthan, S.J., Lucas, E., Lin, S., Phan, T., Moon, J.J., Vedvick, T.S., Reed, S.G., *et al.*, Adjuvant Formulation Structure and Composition Are Critical for the Development of an Effective Vaccine against Tuberculosis. *J. Control. Release, 172,* 190–200, **2013**, doi: 10.1016/j.jconrel.2013.07.030.
94. Smyla, D., Guebre-Xabier, M., Glenn, G., Lai, Y.-H., Look, J.L., Frech, S., Butler, B., Yu, J., Zhang, C.X., Ellingsworth, L., *et al.*, The Adjuvant Patch: A Universal Dose Sparing Approach for Pandemic and Conventional Vaccines. *BioPharm Int., 2007 Supplement,* **2007**.
95. Girard, M.P., Katz, J.M., Pervikov, Y., Hombach, J., Tam, J.S., Report of the 7th Meeting on Evaluation of Pandemic Influenza Vaccines in Clinical Trials, World Health Organization, Geneva, 17–18 February 2011. *Vaccine, 29,* 7579–7586, **2011**, doi: 10.1016/j.vaccine.2011.08.031.
96. Levie, K., Gjorup, I., Skinhøj, P., Stoffel, M., A 2-Dose Regimen of a Recombinant Hepatitis B Vaccine with the Immune Stimulant AS04 Compared with the Standard 3-Dose Regimen of Engerix-B in Healthy Young Adults. *Scand. J. Infect. Dis., 34,* 610–614, **2002**, doi: 10.1080/00365540110080881.
97. Chiew Tong, N.K., Beran, J., Kee, S.A., Miguel, J.L., SanNchez, C., Bayas, J.M., Vilella, A., De Juanes, J.R., Arrazola, P., Calbo-Torrecillas, F., *et al.*, Immunogenicity and Safety of an Adjuvanted Hepatitis B Vaccine in Pre-Hemodialysis and Hemodialysis Patients. *Kidney Int., 68,* 2298–2303, **2005**, doi: 10.1111/j.1523-1755.2005.00689.x.
98. Khurana, S., Verma, N., Yewdell, J.W., Hilbert, A.K., Castellino, F., Lattanzi, M., Del Giudice, G., Rappuoli, R., Golding, H., MF59 Adjuvant Enhances Diversity and Affinity of Antibody-Mediated Immune Response to Pandemic Influenza Vaccines. *Sci. Transl. Med., 3,* 85ra48, **2011**, doi: 10.1126/scitranslmed.3002336.
99. Draper, E., Bissett, S.L., Howell-Jones, R., Waight, P., Soldan, K., Jit, M., Andrews, N., Miller, E., Beddows, S., A Randomized, Observer-Blinded Immunogenicity Trial of Cervarix® and Gardasil® Human Papillomavirus Vaccines in 12-15 Year Old Girls. *PLoS One, 8,* e61825, **2013**, doi: 10.1371/journal.pone.0061825.

100. Galli, G., Hancock, K., Hoschler, K., DeVos, J., Praus, M., Bardelli, M., Malzone, C., Castellino, F., Gentile, C., McNally, T., *et al.*, Fast Rise of Broadly Cross-Reactive Antibodies after Boosting Long-Lived Human Memory B Cells Primed by an MF59 Adjuvanted Prepandemic Vaccine. *Proc. Natl. Acad. Sci. U.S.A.*, *106*, 7962–7967, **2009**, doi: 10.1073/pnas.0903181106.
101. McCluskie, M.J., Pryde, D.C., Gervais, D.P., Stead, D.R., Zhang, N., Benoit, M., Robertson, K., Kim, I.-J., Tharmanathan, T., Merson, J.R., *et al.*, Enhancing Immunogenicity of a 3′aminomethylnicotine-DT-Conjugate Anti-Nicotine Vaccine with CpG Adjuvant in Mice and Non-Human Primates. *Int. Immunopharmacol.*, *16*, 50–56, **2013**, doi: 10.1016/j.intimp.2013.03.021.
102. Kasturi, S.P., Skountzou, I., Albrecht, R.A., Koutsonanos, D., Hua, T., Nakaya, H.I., Ravindran, R., Stewart, S., Alam, M., Kwissa, M., *et al.*, Programming the Magnitude and Persistence of Antibody Responses with Innate Immunity. *Nature*, *470*, 543–547, **2011**, doi: 10.1038/nature09737.
103. Grossmann, C., Tenbusch, M., Nchinda, G., Temchura, V., Nabi, G., Stone, G.W., Kornbluth, R.S., Überla, K., Enhancement of the Priming Efficacy of DNA Vaccines Encoding Dendritic Cell-Targeted Antigens by Synergistic Toll-like Receptor Ligands. *BMC Immunol.*, *10*, 43, **2009**, doi: 10.1186/1471-2172-10-43.
104. Levast, B., Awate, S., Babiuk, L., Mutwiri, G., Gerdts, V., Van Drunen Littel-van Den Hurk, S., Vaccine Potentiation by Combination Adjuvants. *Vaccines*, *2*, 297–322, **2014**, doi: 10.3390/vaccines2020297.
105. Oahagan, D., Synergistic Adjuvant Activity of Immunostimulatory DNA and Oil/Water Emulsions for Immunization with HIV P55 Gag Antigen. *Vaccine*, *20*, 3389–3398, **2002**, doi: 10.1016/S0264-410X(02)00272-4.
106. Cleland, J.L., Barrón, L., Daugherty, A., Eastman, D., Kensil, C., Lim, A., Weissburg, R.P., Wrin, T., Vennari, J., Powell, M.F., Development of a Single-Shot Subunit Vaccine for HIV-1. 3. Effect of Adjuvant and Immunization Schedule on the Duration of the Humoral Immune Response to Recombinant MN Gp120. *J. Pharm. Sci.*, *85*, 1350–1357, **1996**, doi: 10.1021/js960329b.
107. Petrovsky, N. and Aguilar, J.C., Vaccine Adjuvants: Current State and Future Trends. *Immunol. Cell Biol.*, *82*, 488–496, **2004**, doi: 10.1111/j.0818-9641.2004.01272.x.
108. Kumar, A., Vaghela, D.A., Balar, P.C., Bhavisker, K., Bezbaruah, R., Nongrang, L., Bedse, A.P., Chavda, V.P., Nasal Vaccine for the Control of Emerging Variants of SARS-CoV-2, in: *SARS-CoV-2 Variants and Global Population Vulnerability*, Apple Academic Press, Florida, 2024, ISBN 978-1-00-346793-9.

4

Replication-Competent Viral Vectors for Vaccine Delivery

Vivek P. Chavda[1*], Pankti C. Balar[2], Dixa A. Vaghela[2], Divya Teli[3], Amit Chaudhari[3] and Shahnaz Alom[4,5]

[1]*Department of Pharmaceutics and Pharmaceutical Technology, L.M. College of Pharmacy, Ahmedabad, Gujarat, India*
[2]*Pharmacy Section, L.M. College of Pharmacy, Ahmedabad, Gujarat, India*
[3]*Department of Pharmaceutical Chemistry, L.M. College of Pharmacy, Ahmedabad, Gujarat, India*
[4]*Girijananda Chowdhury Institute of Pharmaceutical Sciences, Girijananda Chowdhury University, Tezpur Campus, Tezpur, Sonitpur, Assam, India*
[5]*Department of Pharmaceutical Sciences, Dibrugarh University, Dibrugarh, Assam, India*

Abstract
The exciting world of replication-competent viral vectors is revolutionizing vaccine delivery. These vectors, inspired by nature's immune triggers, offer unique advantages and open doors to combating a myriad of diseases. Crafted from diverse viruses like adenoviruses, poxviruses, and measles viruses, these vectors carry the blueprint for desired antigens (disease-fighting molecules) from target pathogens. Unlike their inert counterparts, they possess the remarkable ability to replicate within host cells, mimicking natural viral infections in a controlled manner. This replication unleashes a cascade of immune activation. Expressed antigens raise red flags for the immune system, prompting robust responses from both innate and adaptive arms. Compared to conventional vaccines, this prolonged antigen presentation translates to stronger, more durable immunity, encompassing both antibody and cellular defenses. The beauty of these vectors lies in their adaptability. They can be tailored to express antigens from a vast array of pathogens, from viruses and bacteria to even parasites and some cancers. Their potential to trigger immunity at mucosal surfaces, the entry points for many infections, adds another layer of promise. Of course, unleashing nature's power requires careful control.

**Corresponding author*: vivek.chavda@lmcp.ac.in

Vivek P. Chavda and Vasso Apostolopoulos (eds.) Viral Vectors for Vaccine Delivery, (91–124) © 2025 Scrivener Publishing LLC

The potential for uncontrolled replication and unforeseen side effects remains a top priority in research and development. Scientists are tirelessly working on refining these vectors, ensuring safety while preserving their potent immunogenicity. Replication-competent viral vectors stand as a beacon of hope in the fight against infectious diseases. Their ability to generate potent and lasting immunity, combined with their versatility and adaptability, makes them invaluable tools in the vaccinologist's arsenal. By addressing safety concerns and further optimizing their design, these vectors hold the potential to revolutionize vaccine development and protect us from a wide spectrum of threats.

***Keywords*:** Replication-competent viral vectors, vaccine, immunization

4.1 Introduction

Vaccination is the most effective medical intervention for preventing morbidity and mortality against virus diseases. They work by exposing the body to an inactive form of a virus, which triggers the immune system to develop antibodies and other immune defenses. These defenses can quickly fight off the virus if it ever enters the body [1]. Viral vaccines are categorized as live attenuated vaccines, inactivated vaccines, viral subunit vaccines, viral vector vaccines, etc. Live attenuated viral vaccines including smallpox, oral polio vaccine, hepatitis vaccine, influenza vaccine, measles, mumps, and rubella vaccines are under clinical trials [2, 3].

Viral vectors play a vital role in vaccine development by overexpressing proteins or knockdown specific genes to study specific cell types *in vivo* [4]. It is capable of manipulating therapeutic gene expression. Among various viral vectors, replication-competent viral vectors (RCVVs) are a type of gene therapy vector that can replicate within the host cell and increase immunization. This offers several advantages over replication-deficient viral vectors (RDVVs), which cannot replicate on their own [5]. RCVVs enhance transgene expression within target cells, leading to more sustained expression compared to RDVVs. This can be effective for long-term transgene expression. RCVVs can spread to neighboring cells and increase treatment area, which can be beneficial for viral diseases, can trigger a strong immune response against transgene products, and can be beneficial for vaccine development for stimulating antitumor immunity in cancer therapy. Moreover, RCVVs require low doses because of their ability to replicate themselves. It could reduce potential side effects and make treatment cost-effective [6].

Despite having many advantages, RCVVs also have some limitations such as RCVVs may revert to their wild-type form and cause diseases; therefore, safety testing is crucial. Then, the body's immune system can attack the RCVVs itself, and controlling its replication is crucial for preventing unwanted side effects [7].

Overall, RCVVs offer a promising approach for vaccine delivery and gene therapy. This chapter mainly emphasizes the use of RCVVs as a different viral vaccine delivery. However, careful research and safety concerns are also addressed in this chapter to prevent unwanted side effects and develop more prominent vaccine delivery by using RCVVs.

4.2 Types of Replication-Competent Viral Vectors

4.2.1 Adenoviruses (AdVs)

Adenovirus vectors are also divided into replicating and nonreplicating virus vectors. Among them, replication-competent AdVs have almost common features as nonreplicant ADVs, but the difference is that the E3 region is being deleted, and as a result, it has a limited clone capacity of 3 to 4 kb compared to replication-defective AdV [8, 9]. Replicating AdVs possess a "dose-sparring" effect. The estimated dosage of replicating AdV recombinant is two to three logs lower than nonreplicating viral vectors. Due to this feature, it offers a practical advantage in experiments *in vivo* [5].

Replicating AdV recombinants have a major scientific benefit in that it mimics a natural AdV infection, inducing co-stimulatory chemicals and cytokines that have a strong adjuvant impact. All things considered, the replicating vector can elicit a full immune response, encompassing humoral, cellular, and mucosal immune responses in addition to components of innate immunity, which is crucial for a prompt reaction to an invasive invader. Based on the documented safety record of oral wild-type Ad4 and Ad7 vaccinations, which have been utilized by the US Military for more than 25 years, It is anticipated that replication-competent vaccines based on Ad4 and Ad7 vectors, which are now in development, will be just as safe [8].

4.2.2 Vesicular Stomatitis Viruses (VSVs)

Recombinant VSV–based vaccines encode viral glycoproteins. ERVEBO® is a replicant VSV vaccine and expresses the EBOV glycoprotein. ERVEBO® is currently used in humans and manufactured by Merck.

VSV-based replicating RNA vaccines can be effective in single-dose administration and stimulate both humoral and cellular immunity. These recombinant VSVs grow in mammalian cell culture, allowing for large-scale production [9]. The absence of homologous recombination and the non-segmented genomic structure of VSV, which inhibit mutations and improve its safety profile, are further benefits of the virus as a vaccination vector [10]. The immunogenicity of several severe acute respiratory syndrome coronavirus 2 (SARS-CoV-2) vaccine candidates has been investigated. High levels of inhibitory antibodies were evoked by our VSV-eGFP-SARS-CoV-2 vaccination, with median and mean serum neutralizing titers of greater than 1/5,000. In the same strain of mice, two doses of VSV-eGFP-SARS-CoV-2 produced greater neutralizing titers with a quicker onset than the comparable dosage of an inactivated SARS-CoV-2 vaccine [11]. Further research is required to evaluate the durability of VSV-eGFP-SARS-CoV-2 for inducing immunity.

4.2.3 Modified Vaccinia Ankara (MVA)

MVA is a promising viral vector for vaccine development. The first smallpox vaccine was developed using the MVA strain due to its high safety profile; it was used for children, the elderly, and people who have weakened immune systems [12]. The adverse effects of first- and second-generation smallpox vaccines are also overcome by using the MVA strain. Because of its high *in vivo* immunogenicity, its capacity to integrate up to 25 kb of foreign DNA into its genome, and its capacity to express a variety of transgenes with appropriate post-translational modification, MVA is regarded as a promising viral vector [13]. A large number of candidate vaccines such as HIV, tuberculosis, malaria, Ebola, RSV, MERS, CMV, and influenza are developed using the MVA vector. MVA is also an effective viral vector for the development of recombinant veterinary vaccines [14].

4.2.4 Measles Virus (MV)

MV replicant viral vectors are gaining traction as a novel platform for developing vaccines and gene therapy treatments. Unlike some vectors, MV vectors can replicate inside host cells, amplifying the delivered gene expression and potentially leading to stronger immune responses. They are derived from live-attenuated measles virus (MV) strains, making them safe and nonpathogenic in humans. MV vectors can accommodate relatively large gene inserts, allowing for the delivery of complex therapeutic genes [15].

Vaccination against measles can lead to preexisting immunity, potentially hindering the efficacy of MV vectors. Researchers are developing strategies to overcome this challenge, including using different MV strains or combining MV vectors with other immunomodulatory agents. Although attenuated, MV vectors still retain some of the virus's natural properties, raising concerns about potential side effects. Careful safety testing and monitoring are essential during development and clinical trials [16].

4.2.5 Influenza Virus (IV)

Influenza viral vectors have demonstrated efficacy in eliciting both systemic and mucosal immune responses. A pivotal study conducted by Efferson *et al.* investigated a recombinant influenza virus engineered to express the immunodominant HER-2 cytotoxic T lymphocyte (CTL) epitope, KIF (E75), situated within the stalk region of the neuraminidase (NA) protein. This research marked a significant advancement in the field, as it was the first to provide evidence that live, attenuated recombinant influenza vectors could successfully induce human epitope-specific CTLs targeting tumor-associated antigens.

The study's findings underscore the potential of utilizing recombinant influenza viruses as a platform for cancer immunotherapy. Specifically, the incorporation of the HER-2 CTL epitope into the viral vector not only facilitated the generation of a robust immune response but also highlighted the capacity of such vectors to activate CTLs against specific tumor markers. This approach represents a promising strategy for developing vaccines aimed at enhancing antitumor immunity, particularly in cancers associated with overexpression of HER-2. Moreover, the implications of this research extend beyond immediate therapeutic applications. The ability to harness viral vectors for targeted immune responses opens avenues for further exploration into multi-epitope vaccine designs and combination therapies that could improve patient outcomes in oncology. Future studies will be essential to evaluate the long-term efficacy and safety of these innovative vaccination strategies in clinical settings, paving the way for novel interventions in cancer treatment [17]. Ferko *et al.* developed a hyperattenuated recombinant influenza virus containing 137 C-terminal amino acid residues of human immunodeficiency virus type 1 Nef protein within the NS gene. Animal studies showed that hybrid influenza virus can induce $CD8^+$ T cell responses [18]. The modular nature of the influenza virus genome makes it easy to insert different foreign genes into the vector. Influenza virus replication vector (IVRVs) is a promising tool for gene therapy, vaccine development, and other applications. Research is ongoing to improve the safety and efficacy of IVRVs [19]. A brief overview is described in Table 4.1.

Table 4.1 Overview of replication-competent viral vector.

Viral vector	Insert	Advantage	Disadvantage	Reference
Adenoviruses (AdVs)	3–4 kb	It provides persistent immunity, low dose mucosal delivery, and induce effective immune response	Due to its small size, it is a concern for intranasal administration.	[20]
Vesicular stomatitis viruses (VSVs)	11 kb	VSVs express high transgene expression, broad tropism, and minimum risk of insertional mutagenesis and potent immunostimulatory properties.	Safety measures are required, certain strains of VSVs have a natural tropism for nerve cells, and they accommodate smaller transgenes only.	[21]
Modified vaccinia Ankara (MVA)	25 kb	MVA is highly attenuated, meaning it cannot replicate in human cells and has a very low risk of causing serious side effects. Trigger strong immune response, versatility and genetic stability	MVA's inability to replicate in human cells can limit its potency as a vaccine vector, sometimes requiring booster doses. It may induce cytotoxic effects and complexity of production	[22]
Measles virus (MV)	>5 kb	It provides persistent immunity, infects dendritic cells and macrophages, and has genetic stability	Prior immunity has been required	[23]
Poxviruses	>10 kb	It can able to produce excellent immunogenicity for eradicating smallpox	Safety concerns required for immunocompromised persons	[24]
Vesicular stomatitis virus	>5 kb	It is able to produce a high level of expression, production is also easy, and no previous immunity is required	Due to a high level of expression, safety concern is required.	[10]

4.3 Mechanisms of RCVV-Mediated Vaccination

A practical way to deliver vaccine antigens to specific target cells or tissues is by viral vectors. Historically, the best defense against viral infection and illness has come from live attenuated, replicating vaccines rather than inactivated preparations. Measles, mumps, rubella, vaccinia, polio, and yellow fever are a few of the vaccinations that fall under this category [5]. Interestingly, these immunizations produce practically a lifetime of protective immunity.

Among various sophisticated methods for vaccine development, the viral vector–based vaccination is one of the best. It contains disease-unrelated attenuated viruses that have been altered to act as vectors, delivering genetic material (DNA) to human cells where it produces a viral protein that fights off a specific infection. The body recognizes this as a foreign substance and, as with the body's natural defense mechanism, develops an immunological response against it [25, 26]. The virus effectively exposes antigens to immune cells and activates strong immune systems by infecting antigen-presenting dendritic cells, macrophages, and co-stimulatory chemicals that function as adjuvants [27, 28]. It also triggers cytokine and chemokine responses.

Viral vector–based vaccinations come in two varieties: replicating (also known as self-replicating or replication-competent) and nonreplicating (also known as replication-incompetent or replication-deficient). Replicating viral vector vaccines generate new viral entities after they infect cells, whereas RDVVs are altered so they are unable to generate new viral entities. The host cell mechanism is responsible for the creation of new viral entities, which subsequently infect other host cells to generate more viral antigens [25]. In contrast to nonreplicating viral vaccines, which remove both the E1 and E3 regions of the gene to make room for a foreign gene, replicating viral vector vaccines only remove the E3 region of the viral vector's genetic material.

The presence of early region 1 generally distinguishes replication-competent AdV vectors from replication-defective AdV vectors. Polypeptides that are essential for independent replication, suppressing host interferon reactions, and avoiding premature cell death, are encoded by the E1 gene [29, 30]. Although E1's presence in the viral vector genome allows it to replicate autonomously, it also occupies genomic space that is often used for foreign gene insertion. Typically, deletions are made in the E3 and E4 genes, which encode multiple proteins that are crucial for immune evasion, such as inactivating the intracellular antiviral response (E4) and down-regulating MHC class I expression (E3) [29].

Replicating viral vectors, by mimicking natural infections, induce cytokines and other stimulatory molecules with potent adjuvant effects. These vectors can elicit innate, humoral, cellular, and mucosal immune responses (Figure 4.1). However, their replication capacity is limited to 3-5 kb compared to replication-defective viral vectors. The *in vivo* multiplication of replicating viral vectors enhances antigen presentation, leading to strong immune responses. This dose-sparing effect suggests that even low doses may be sufficient to confer protection against infection, potentially reducing the need for multiple doses [26, 31].

One of the most often used vectors for vaccine development is the adenovirus (Ad). The exploration of adenoviral vectors for gene therapy has significantly advanced our understanding of virology and molecular biology, providing valuable insights that could enhance future vaccination strategies. Adenovirus type 26 (Ad26), in particular, has emerged as a compelling candidate for vaccine development due to several advantageous characteristics. Its ability to effectively infect both dividing and nondividing cells allows for versatile applications in gene delivery. Furthermore, Ad26 exhibits high levels of transgene expression and can be produced in large quantities *in vitro*, making it suitable for widespread use. Importantly, Ad26 does not integrate into the host genome, which reduces potential risks associated with genomic alterations. Its inherent physical and genetic stability further contributes to its appeal as a vaccine vector. The mechanism by which Ad26 induces immune responses is particularly noteworthy; it plays a critical role in antigen presentation by infecting dendritic cells. This interaction leads to the upregulation of co-stimulatory molecules and the activation of cytokine and chemokine responses, thereby promoting robust immune activation.

Research has demonstrated that vaccines utilizing Ad26 vectors can elicit strong immune responses, making them effective tools in combating infectious diseases and, potentially, cancer. The ability to present antigens efficiently enhances the likelihood of generating both humoral and cellular immunity, which are essential components of a comprehensive immune response [33]. AdV target epithelial cells make them excellent candidates for inducing systemic and mucosal immunity. Ad vectors have been developed for a wide range of vaccine applications, incorporating numerous DNA and single-stranded RNA viruses in addition to HIV and SIV [8].

Replication-competent AdV vectors are distinct from replication-defective AdV vectors in that they are deleted exclusively in the E3 region, which results in a clone capacity that is 3 to 5 kb smaller. However, these

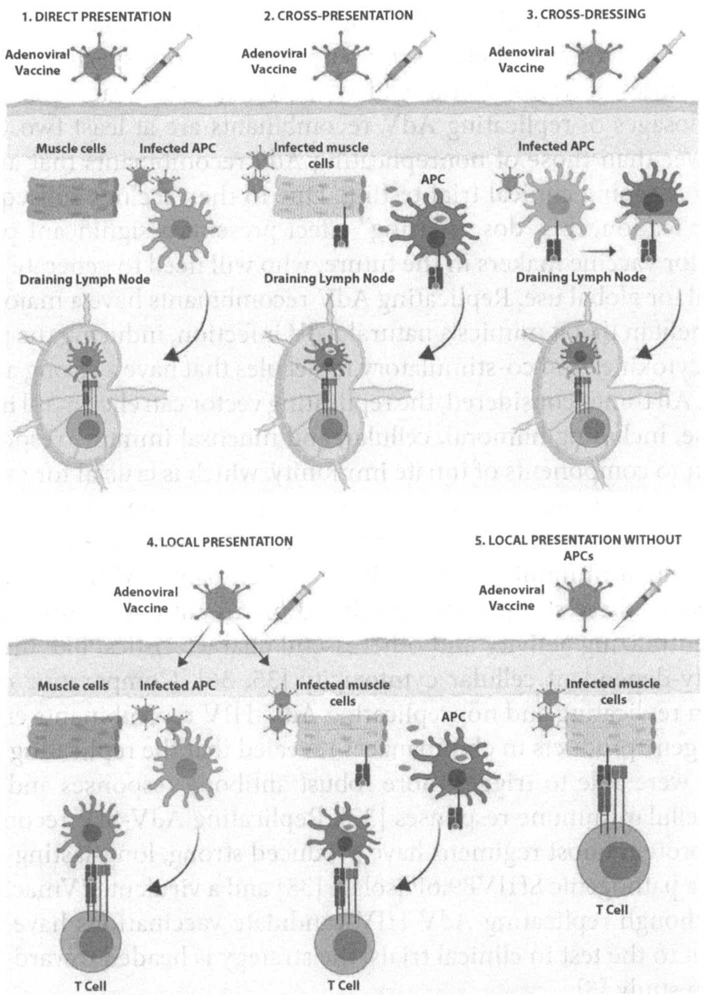

Figure 4.1 Mechanisms of antigen presentation following intramuscular vaccination with vaccines containing an adenoviral vector. (1) **Direct presentation:** At the injection site, the adenoviral vaccine transduces antigen-presenting cells (APCs). When APCs move to draining lymph nodes (dLNs), they give T cells processed vaccination antigens. (2) **Cross-presentation:** At the injection site, skilled APCs phagocytose vaccine antigen debris from AdV vaccine–transduced cells. APCs then transport the debris to draining lymph nodes (dLNs) and present it to lymphocytes. (3) **Cross-dressing:** Peptide: Trogocytosis, a process of membrane gnawing, may transfer MHC complexes from AdV-transduced APCs to naive APCs. (4) **Local presentation:** T cells may be directly presented with antigen by APCs residing at or invading the injection site. (5) **Local presentation without APCs:** Outside of secondary lymphoid organs, nonprofessional APCs, such as parenchymal cells near the injection site (muscle cells are used as an example), can convey antigenic peptide on MHC I to invading $CD8^{+}$ T lymphocytes. (Taken from [32] under the Creative Commons Attribution License (CC BY 4).

drawbacks are outweighed by the additional benefits that vectors have. They have several useful effects, one of which is "dose-sparing." Based on the safe doses of licensed oral wild-type Ad4 and Ad7 vaccines, the projected dosages of replicating AdV recombinants are at least two to three logs lower than those of nonreplicating Ad5 recombinants that are presently undergoing clinical trial testing. Due to the vaccine's subsequent *in vivo* replication, this "dose-sparing" effect presents a significant practical benefit for vaccine makers in the future, who will need to generate enough material for global use. Replicating AdV recombinants have a major scientific benefit in that it mimics a natural AdV infection, inducing the production of cytokines and co-stimulatory molecules that have a strong adjuvant impact. All things considered, the replicating vector can elicit a full immune response, including humoral, cellular, and mucosal immune responses in addition to components of innate immunity, which is crucial for establishing a prompt defense against an invasive invader. Preclinical investigations employing replicating AdV-HIV and SIV recombinants have demonstrated strong cellular immunity so far [34], and when paired with envelope subunit boosts, these studies have produced broad antibody responses with both neutralizing activity and other useful characteristics, like mediating antibody-dependent cellular cytotoxicity [35, 36]. Comparative research between replicating and nonreplicating AdV-HIV recombinants encoding similar gene products in chimpanzees revealed that the replicating recombinants were able to trigger more robust antibody responses and induce larger cellular immune responses [37]. Replicating AdV-SIV recombinant prime/protein boost regimens have produced strong, long-lasting defense against a pathogenic SHIV89.6P isolate [38] and a virulent SIVmac251 [34, 39]. Although replicating AdV-HIV candidate vaccinations have not yet been put to the test in clinical trials, the strategy is headed toward a phase I human study [5].

In the case of RCVVs for COVID-19, the genetic material (DNA) for the S protein (spike protein) of the SARS-CoV-2 virus is altered and inserted into an appropriate unrelated viral vector, which, upon entry into the cells, transfers the SARS-CoV-2 virus's genetic material to the host cells. This stimulates and directs the body's cells to replicate the spike protein. The body's immune system produces antibodies in response to these spike protein copies that are exposed on the surfaces of cells. Therefore, the antibodies will fight against the COVID-19 virus if the person has it. Because the transferred genes do not merge with the host's DNA and the viral vectors are transformed into harmless through genetic modification, neither the SARS-CoV-2 virus nor the viral vector can infect the recipient [25].

4.4 Applications of Replication-Competent Viral Vectors

Formerly, the best defense against viral sickness and infection has come from live attenuated, replicating vaccinations as opposed to inactivated versions. Recombinant viral vectors have transferred antigens from certain pathogens [40]. As the most closely related method of displaying and delivering conformational epitopes with enhanced production of antibodies and immune response, virus-like particles are a potent tool for developing immunizations. To trigger immunological responses against the proteins produced by the encoded transgenes, several kinds of additional viruses, including lentiviruses, adenoviruses (Adv), poxviruses, rhabdoviruses, herpesviruses, alphaviruses, and VSVs, have been included in vaccination vectors [41]. It is possible to design viral vectors to deliver vaccination antigens onto specific cells or locations. Multiple viral vectors have undergone genetic engineering to become replication-deficient to raise their safety profile and decrease reactogenicity. Viral vectors may generate substantial immune responses—sometimes even after only a single dose—and significant immunogenicity [42]. The viruses being utilized as platforms for replication-competent vectors differ greatly from one another, and their separate features permit the testing of multiple vaccine design ideas and the simulation of different elements of HIV infection [43]. Preclinical and clinical experiments have employed viral vectors as vaccines against infectious illnesses, including malaria, SARS-CoV-2, Ebola, and HIV. Regarding immunogenicity, safety, and effectiveness, they all have positive and negative aspects of their own. The several viral vector systems that have been employed in therapeutics are explained below.

4.4.1 Prophylactic Vaccines

The stunning development of viral vectors has made it possible to create new therapeutic and prophylactic vaccine candidates. Traditional whole-cell vaccines gave rise to preventive vaccinations for better subunit immunizations. There are two human papillomavirus (HPV) prophylactic vaccinations that are approved for use in multiple nations. They both rely on L1, the main HPV virion protein, and its virus-like particles. Right now, there are three preventive HPV vaccines on the market: nonvalent, bivalent, tetravalent, and non-based on recombinant DNA technology [44]. Influenza virus vectors might be an effective option for utilization in human medicine because humans lack inherent immunity. After recombinant influenza vaccination viral subtypes H5N1 and H1N1, which express the protective antigen of Brucella, were found to strongly stimulate the cellular immune system and have a protective impact [45]. The Epstein-Barr virus is the first known cancerous virus that infects individuals chronically. In preclinical tests, Epstein-Barr virus glycoproteins, such as gH/gL, gp42, and gB, exhibit superior immunogenicity compared to the previously preferred gp350 antigen [46]. Prophylactic vaccination of even modest percentages of healthcare personnel and the general public might significantly reduce the effect of an Ebola virus (EBOV) disease outbreak, according to one mean-field compartmental stochastic model research [47].

4.4.2 Therapeutic Vaccines

Numerous viruses have been considered for use in vaccination strategies since the vaccinia virus was discovered to be transformed into a vaccine vector. The immunogenicity and effectiveness of currently used vectors, such as those based on Adv, have significantly risen. In addition, attractive novel vectors have surfaced that take advantage of viruses including VSV and the cytomegalovirus (CMV). Studying CMV-induced T cell immunity may also inform alternative vector-based vaccine strategies. When a peptide is located in the C-terminal region of viral proteins, it becomes much more accessible for proteasomal processing, which leads to the development of protective peptide-specific T cell memory [48].

4.4.2.1 Vesicular Stomatitis Virus

Belonging to the Rhabdovirus family, the enveloped bullet-shaped VSV has a negative-sense RNA genome. Rose and associates invented the use of the VSV as a vaccine vector in 1990 [49]. An attenuated replication-competent recombinant VSV gag vaccine has developed a potential vaccination platform to treat HIV-1 and other important human illnesses, and it has a tolerable safety profile [50]. The viral RNA is bound by the nucleoprotein of VSV, which also performs transcription, replication, and assembly [51]. In many preclinical investigations, VSV vaccination vectors have been shown to elicit strong cellular and humoral immune responses, resulting in protection in numerous animal models of pathogen challenge, often following a single vector dose [52]. Recently, the recombinant viral vector against Ebola (rVSV-ZEBOV) based on the VSV was licensed for use in humans [53]. Replication-competent vaccines based on attenuated recombinant vectors of the virus that express the glycoprotein of either the Marburg virus or the EBOV are being developed at the Public Health Agency of Canada [54]. This recombinant VSV–Zaire EBOV is the most developed contender for an Ebola vaccine and is being utilized to stop the spread of the infection. All participants in the EBOV clinical trials had a moderate $CD8^+$ response and a strong production of neutralizing antibodies, in line with an analysis of immunogenicity in clinical research [55]. Vaccines based on VSV vector have been demonstrated to be very efficient against the Marburg virus, providing protection even when given after viral exposure [56].

4.4.2.2 Cytomegalovirus

Human CMV also termed human herpesvirus 5 is a beta herpesvirus with two strands of DNA that is linear and falls to the Herpesviridae family [57]. A natural human CMV infection results in broad T cell responses that cover approximately 10% of the total $CD4^+$ and $CD8^+$ T cell memory compartments and are directed against a wide range of antigens [58]. Human CMV-specific T cell responses are persistent, and they are more common in elderly individuals. Recombinant mCMV-based constructs were initially used to study the immunogenicity which crucially protected against a heterologous virus infection by inducing an increase of T cells that were reactive to peptides generated from heterologous antigens [59]. To stop the EBOV from spreading across animal populations, a CMV-based vaccination strategy may be used to "disseminate" CMV-based EBOV vaccines [60]. A CMV-based vector encoding an epitope from the Zaire EBOV nucleoprotein—the antigen of EBOV—was evaluated in preclinical investigations. Mice immunized with the MCMV vector carrying the antigen for EBOV NP developed strong CD8+ T cell responses against EBOV NP, providing total protection against the deadly EBOV challenge [61]. Primate recipients of a rhesus CMV vector–producing EBOV glycoproteins strategy produced a robust IgG response and successfully protected vaccinated animals against fatal EBOV infections [62]. More proof that the virus has the potential to be a vaccine vector comes from studies looking at CMV viral vector vaccinations against EBOV viruses. Single-cycle replication murine CMV and rhesus CMV vectors have been developed as a viable option to live-attenuated viruses, with a comfortable safety profile [63]. These serve in a broad range of fields, including genetic research and medical treatment, and are well known for being extremely effective gene transfer agents [64].

4.4.2.3 Measles Virus

Initiated in the late 1990s, the MV was developed as a vaccine vector [65]. Even after a single vaccination, the majority of recipients still develop incredibly strong, protective antibody- and T cell–mediated immunity via the most attenuated strains and have excellent safety profiles [66]. This might have significant effects on MV vector platforms that are being considered for vaccine development. Both fundamental research on MV virology and the investigation of MV as a vaccine vector were expedited in 1995 by the creation of reverse genetics instruments and the extraction of MV from cloned DNA [67]. The research found excellent cargo capacity and a superb stimulation of both humoral and cellular immune reactions against transgenes that are encoded [68]. The investigation was performed for the immunogenicity of an HIV-1 subtype C MV vaccine in cynomolgus macaques using prime or prime-boost regimens. The vaccine expresses HIV-1 Gag, RT, and Nef as a fusion protein [69]. This vaccination provided a significant amount of antibodies reactive to exogenous antigens and MV-encoded proteins, which were further increased upon boosting, as well as strong antigen-specific $CD4^+$ and moderate $CD8^+$ T cell responses. A potential chikungunya vaccine based on the MV developed with excellent immunogenicity even in the face of anti-vector immunity [70]. Several clinical outcomes that demonstrated a tolerable safety profile and an adequate generation of chikungunya-neutralizing antibodies following one or two vaccinations pointed to MV vector-based vaccines as a viable option [71].

4.4.2.4 Adenoviral Vectors

Many viruses have been investigated for use in vaccination techniques since the vaccinia virus was discovered in 1984 and developed into a vaccine vector. Significant advancements in immunogenicity and effectiveness have been made in recent years to establish vectors, such as those based on adenovirus. Since 2003, adenoviruses have been employed in several clinical immunization studies and investigated as viral vectors [72, 73]. AdV vector vaccines ingested via the intramuscular (i.m.) route may generate both systemic humoral immunity and certain types of mucosal humoral immunity. Systemic AdV vector immunization can stimulate $CD8^+$ T cell responses via IFN-β promoter stimulator-1 and type-I IFN signaling which may be specific to the antigen in both the mucosal and systemic divisions [74]. Immunization with replicating single-cycle Adv vector and protein increases produced favorable mucosal immune responses in animal models. When combined with single-cycle Adv-expressing genetic adjuvants, vaginal antibody responses were significantly increased following a single vaccination via the intranasal or intramuscular methods, expressing the HIV envelope [75]. Clinical experiments have examined a replication-incompetent Adv5 vector that expresses hemagglutinin, a chimpanzee Adv-based vector that expresses nucleoprotein, and matrix protein-1 as a potential new platform for influenza virus vaccinations [76]. To enable vaccination against Zika virus infection, genes encoding the membrane protein and envelop protein were inserted into the AdV vector genome during the active development phase of Zika virus vaccines. In a clinical experiment, an Ad26 vector vaccine produced significant levels of neutralizing anti-Zika virus antibodies without causing serious adverse effects [77]. Zika virus–like particles were produced in a mouse model by expressing the Zika virus proteins with an Adv vector system. An adjuvanted formulation can develop long-lasting neutralizing antibodies and memory B cells that can last up to 6 months with only one dosage [78]. Since the EBOV was first identified, a lot of work has been done on designing vaccines. The European Union has licensed an Ad26-based vector that expresses the glycoprotein of the EBOV [79]. A substantial humoral immune response was elicited by i.m. injection of Ad5-EBOV, according to comparative immunogenicity studies, due to greater antigen expression and germinal center reaction. At the same time, intradermal injection produced a more robust polyfunctional cellular immune response by engaging more dermal dendritic cells [80].

4.4.2.5 Applications of Replication-Competent Viral Vectors against COVID-19

The development of vaccines against the COVID-19 pandemic–causing SARS-CoV-2 surpassed all previous vaccination initiatives. With 199 vaccine candidates in preclinical and 183 in clinical trials of which 25 are based on nonreplicating viral vectors and 4 on replicating viral vectors in the clinical phase [81]. Viral vector vaccines have been a key component of the strategy to contain the SARS-CoV-2 pandemic over the past few years, especially in middle- and low-income nations. In the worldwide vaccination campaign against COVID-19, Adv-vectored vaccines are proving to be highly effective. AdV vectors that are highly immunogenic, easily adjustable, and quickly produced have shown to be a good fit for the pandemic response [82].

The Ad26 vector–based vaccine, known as Ad26.COV2.S, has received emergency use authorization to address the COVID-19 pandemic. This vaccine utilizes a recombinant, replication-incompetent human Ad26 vector that encodes the full-length spike protein of the SARS-CoV-2 virus in a prefusion-stabilized conformation. Its design is aimed at eliciting a robust immune response while minimizing the risk of replication in the host. Clinical trials have demonstrated that a single dose of Ad26.COV2.S provides significant protection against symptomatic COVID-19 and severe disease. Specifically, efficacy rates reported in phase 3 trials indicate that the vaccine is approximately 66.9% effective against moderate to severe COVID-19, with even higher efficacy observed against severe cases. For instance, the vaccine showed an efficacy of 76.7% against severe disease occurring at least 14 days after vaccination. Moreover, the safety profile of Ad26.COV2.S appears comparable to other vaccines in its class, with most adverse effects being mild to moderate and transient. Serious adverse events were balanced between vaccinated individuals and those receiving a placebo, indicating that the vaccine is generally well-tolerated.

The unique advantage of using the Ad26 vector lies in its lower seroprevalence compared to more commonly used adenoviral vectors, such as Ad5. This characteristic reduces the likelihood of preexisting immunity interfering with vaccine efficacy. Additionally, the single-dose regimen simplifies logistics for vaccination campaigns, particularly in resource-limited settings or during public health emergencies. With the introduction of the ChAdOx1 nCov-19 vaccine against SARS-CoV-2, chimpanzee Adv vaccinations have gained interest. In a phase III experiment, this vaccination proved to be both safe and effective in avoiding both symptomatic and severe cases of COVID-19 in a variety of population trends, including elderly persons [83]. A very effective MV-based prefusion S protein vaccine option has been identified that expresses the whole S protein and can completely protect animal models against lung pathology and severe SARS-CoV-2 infection [84]. V591 is a measles vector–based SARS-CoV-2 vaccine candidate reported with the development of spike-binding antibodies in 81% of participants receiving two injections. Despite good toleration of the vaccine, the study findings indicate inadequate immunogenicity [85]. Several preclinical investigations using integrase-defective lentiviral vectors against HIV, Zika, malaria, and SARS-CoV-2 have shown strong immunogenicity and long-lasting, protective immune responses in mice and rhesus monkeys. Several completed clinical studies of COVID-19 vaccine candidates are listed in Table 4.2.

Table 4.2 Specifics of COVID-19 vaccine candidates based on viral vectors: Finished clinical trials.

Viral vector	Phase	Study design	Number enrolled	NCT number	Sponsor
Recombinant SARS-CoV-2 Ad5	Phase 4	Randomized, observer-blind, parallel-controlled study	300	NCT04952727	Jiangsu Province Centers for Disease Control and Prevention
Intranasal parainfluenza virus type 5 SARS CoV-2 S vaccine (CVXGA1)	Phase 1	Open-label, dose-ranging Trial	72	NCT04954287	CyanVac LLC
Heterologous prime-boost of recombinant COVID-19 vaccine (Ad5 vector) and RBD-based protein subunit vaccine	Phase 4	A randomized, observer-blind, placebo-controlled study	120	NCT04833101	Jiangsu Province Centers for Disease Control and Prevention
Tetravalent influenza virus lysis vaccine	Phase 3	NA	299	NCT05107375	Anhui Zhifei Longcom Biologic Pharmacy Co., Ltd.

(Continued)

Table 4.2 Specifics of COVID-19 vaccine candidates based on viral vectors: Finished clinical trials. (*Continued*)

Viral vector	Phase	Study design	Number enrolled	NCT number	Sponsor
Adenovirus type 5–vectored COVID-19 vaccine	Phase 1	Single-center, open-label phase I clinical trial	89	NCT04568811	Jiangsu Province Centers for Disease Control and Prevention
Simian adenovirus expressing SARS-CoV-2 S protein	Phase 3	Parallel, double-blind, active-controlled, non-inferiority study	4065	NCT05710783	Laboratorio Avi-Mex, S.A. de C.V.
Recombinant novel coronavirus vaccine (adenovirus type 5 vector)	Phase 2	Randomized, double-blind, placebo-controlled IIb clinical trial	480	NCT04566770	CanSino Biologics Inc.
Recombinant novel coronavirus vaccine (adenovirus type 5 vector)	Phase 1	Single-center, open-label, dose-escalating trial	108	NCT04313127	CanSino Biologics Inc.

(*Continued*)

Table 4.2 Specifics of COVID-19 vaccine candidates based on viral vectors: Finished clinical trials. (*Continued*)

Viral vector	Phase	Study design	Number enrolled	NCT number	Sponsor
Recombinant novel coronavirus vaccine (adenovirus type 5 vector)	Phase 3	Global multicentered, randomized, double-blind, placebo-controlled, adaptive-designed clinical trial	44247	NCT04526990	CanSino Biologics Inc.
Recombinant adenovirus type 26 component of Gam-COVID-Vac vaccine	Phase 2	Prospective, single-center, open-label, non-comparative, non-randomized single-arm study	100	NCT04686773	R-Pharm
Recombinant novel coronavirus vaccine (adenovirus type 5 vector)	Phase 2	Randomized, double-blinded, and placebo-controlled clinical trial	508	NCT04341389	Institute of Biotechnology, Academy of Military Medical Sciences, PLA of China

(*Continued*)

Table 4.2 Specifics of COVID-19 vaccine candidates based on viral vectors: Finished clinical trials. (*Continued*)

Viral vector	Phase	Study design	Number enrolled	NCT number	Sponsor
Recombinant SARS-CoV-2 Ad5–vectored vaccine	Phase 4	Randomized, observer-blind, parallel-controlled study	300	NCT04952727	Jiangsu Province Centers for Disease Control and Prevention
Recombinant Ad5-vectored COVID-19 vaccine	Phase 4	A randomized, observer-blind, placebo-controlled study	120	NCT04833101	Jiangsu Province Centers for Disease Control and Prevention
Ad26.COV2.S	Phase 1	Open-label clinical trial	867	NCT04889209	National Institute of Allergy and Infectious Diseases (NIAID)

4.4.3 Cancer Immunotherapy

Gene therapy is a type of therapy that involves inserting foreign genes into malignant cells or the tissues around them to target and kill cancer cells. Viral vectors are an exciting approach to improving foreign gene delivery because they can target particular cells that have superior gene transduction efficiency [86]. Adv type 5 and the poxviral-based vaccination are significant vectors that work as immunological mediators to immunize against tumor-associated antigens [87]. Numerous viruses, including Adv, herpes simplex virus (HSV), MV, vaccinia virus, myxoma virus, VSV, and New Castle disease virus, have been investigated for use as immunotherapies [88]. Interleukin 2 (IL-2) functions as a flexible master pro-inflammatory anticancer cytokine by boosting the cytotoxic activity of natural killer and cytotoxic T cells, which is essential for T cell development and survival. Numerous investigations have shown that oncolytic viruses may effectively deliver IL-2 to the tumor microenvironment without endangering patient safety [89].

Adv vectors are perfect for oncolytic vectors and gene transfer because they have a non-enveloped, icosahedral capsid that is around 90 nm in diameter and contains a linear double-stranded DNA genome. Gene treatments based on AdV amplify the initial antiviral response and retarget tumor cells or elements of the tumor microenvironment, therefore inducing anticancer immune responses [90]. IL-2, Fms-like tyrosine kinase 3 ligand (Flt3L), interferon-α (IFN-α), and IFN-β were all boosted by immunostimulatory Adv cancer gene therapy [91]. The challenge of preexisting immunity to adenovirus serotype 5 (Ad5) has led researchers to explore alternative adenoviral vectors derived from less prevalent serotypes, including those from both human and animal origins, such as chimpanzee adenovirus and Ad26. Notably, Ad26 exhibits a lower seroprevalence compared to Ad5, making it a promising candidate for vaccine development. Research has demonstrated that Ad26 is not only safe for use but also capable of eliciting robust humoral and cell-mediated immune responses [92].

A significant study investigated the safety and immunogenicity of a mosaic Ad26-based vaccine in both humans and rhesus monkeys. This innovative vaccine utilized an Ad26 vector designed to produce a combination of Env, Gag, and Pol antigens in a mosaic format. The results indicated that the mosaic Ad26 vaccination was well tolerated and generated a strong immune response, highlighting its potential as an effective platform for immunization [92].

These findings suggest that utilizing less common adenoviral vectors like Ad26 could circumvent the limitations posed by preexisting immunity

Table 4.3 Viral vaccine vectors candidates for cancer immunotherapy: Finished clinical trials.

Viral vector	Phase	Study design	Number enrolled	NCT number	Sponsor
Ad5 [E1-, E2b-]-CEA(6D)or ETBX-011	Phase1 Phase 2	Single group assignment	35	NCT01147965	Etubics Corporation
Recombinant vaccinia virus vector vaccine, recombinant fowlpox virus vector vaccine	Phase 2	Randomized parallel assignment	97	NCT02649439	National Cancer Institute
Anti-MAGE-A3-DP4 T cell receptor (TCR) peripheral blood lymphocytes	Phase1 Phase 2	Non-randomized sequential assignment	21	NCT02111850	National Cancer Institute
Recombinant vaccinia-PSA(L155)/TRICOM (PROSTVAC-V/TRICOM)	Phase 1	Interventional	21	NCT00096551	National Cancer Institute
Adenoviral vector engineered to express the herpes thymidine kinase gene (AdV-tk)	Phase 1	Non-randomized single group assignment	27	NCT00638612	Candel Therapeutics, Inc.
Dendritic cell–targeting lentiviral vector ID-LV305	Phase 1	Non-randomized parallel assignment	15	NCT03450122	M.D. Anderson Cancer Center

(Continued)

Table 4.3 Viral vaccine vectors candidates for cancer immunotherapy: Finished clinical trials. (*Continued*)

Viral vector	Phase	Study design	Number enrolled	NCT number	Sponsor
AVX901	Phase 1	Single group assignment	22	NCT01526473	H. Kim Lyerly
PROSTVAC-V/TRICOM	Phase 2	Randomized Parallel Assignment	64	NCT00450463	National Cancer Institute
BCG intravesical live combined with PANVAC Versus	Phase 2	Randomized parallel assignment	32	NCT02015104	National Cancer Institute
Adenoviral vector Ad-RTS-hIL-12 and veledimex	Phase 2	Randomized parallel assignment	12	NCT01703754	Alaunos Therapeutics
Adenoviral vector delivery of IL-12 gene	Phase 1	Non-randomized single group assignment	4	NCT00406939	Baylor College of Medicine
Oncolytic adenoviral vector NG-350A	Phase 1	Sequential assignment	28	NCT03852511	Akamis Bio

(*Continued*)

Table 4.3 Viral vaccine vectors candidates for cancer immunotherapy: Finished clinical trials. (*Continued*)

Viral vector	Phase	Study design	Number enrolled	NCT number	Sponsor
Retroviral replicating vector Toca 511	Phase 1	Single group assignment	58	NCT01470794	Tocagen Inc.
Retroviral replicating vector Toca 511 vector/Toca FC	Phase 1	Single group assignment	17	NCT01985256	Ocagen Inc.
Adenoviral vector encoding rat Her-2/neu	Phase 1	Non-randomized parallel assignment	8	NCT00307229	Ontario Clinical Oncology Group
Adenoviral serotype 5 vector AdCD40L	Phase 1 Phase 2	Single group assignment	30	NCT01455259	Uppsala University
PROSTVAC®-VF/TRICOM™	Phase 2	Randomize, double-blind, controlled study	120	NCT00078585	Bavarian Nordic

to more widely recognized serotypes. The ability of Ad26 to induce both antibody-mediated and cellular immune responses positions it as a valuable tool in the design of vaccines targeting various infectious diseases and potentially cancer therapies. Future research should focus on optimizing the formulation and delivery methods of these novel adenoviral vectors to enhance their efficacy and broaden their applications in clinical settings.

An animal model was used to demonstrate how a single immunization with integrase-defective lentiviral vectors may produce a functional antitumor immunity that might stop tumor development, suggesting that this would be an effective and appropriate approach for cancer immunotherapy [93]. Oncolytic virotherapy employing HSV-1–derived mutants has considerable potential as an anticancer. HSV vector–based gene treatments have mostly been utilized in clinical settings to treat cancer due to their inherent oncolytic capacity [94]. Several completed clinical studies of viral vector–based vaccines for cancer are listed in Table 4.3.

4.5 Conclusion

The field of RCVVs for vaccine delivery is experiencing an exciting renaissance. Their ability to trigger robust and lasting immune responses against diverse pathogens has propelled them to the forefront of vaccine development. As this area blossoms, several critical frontiers beckon, promising advancements in RCVV platforms, safety and efficacy, and application breadth. Harnessing genetic engineering, scientists are crafting tailored vectors with enhanced immunogenicity, controlled replication, and targeted antigen expression. Combining adjuvants or exploring new viral backbones further expands the disease spectrum RCVVs can tackle. The surge in mRNA technology opens doors for mRNA-based RCVVs, potentially offering speedier development, easier manufacturing, and reduced mutagenic risks. Merging these technologies holds immense promise for future vaccine innovation. Balancing potency with safety is crucial. Targeted modifications and genetic engineering, including codon optimization, gene deletions, and replication control, pave the way for safer, more manageable RCVVs. Refining dosing strategies and administration routes can maximize efficacy while minimizing side effects. Ongoing surveillance and post-marketing studies ensure long-term safety in diverse populations. RCVVs engineered to target tumor antigens hold immense potential for cancer treatment, stimulating potent antitumor immune responses and warranting further preclinical and clinical exploration. RCVVs offer a rapid response platform for swiftly developing vaccines against novel zoonotic diseases and global pandemics. Strengthening international collaborations and preparedness frameworks can enable the timely deployment of RCVVs in outbreak scenarios, potentially curbing widespread disease transmission. The evolution of RCVVs redefines the vaccine landscape, harnessing the innate power of viruses for immunization strategies. By continuously refining RCVV platforms, bolstering safety and efficacy, and exploring a wider range of applications, we can usher in transformative advancements in preventive medicine. Through multidisciplinary research, stringent regulatory oversight, and global cooperation, we can unlock the full potential of RCVVs to tackle existing and emerging health challenges, paving the way for a future with safer, more effective, and broader vaccine options.

References

1. Schleiss, M.R., Viral Vaccines, in: *Encyclopedia of Infection and Immunity*, pp. 545–55, 2022, https://doi.org/10.1016/B978-0-12-818731-9.00225-1.
2. Bharati, K. and Vrati, S., Viral Vaccines in India: An Overview. *Proc. Natl. Acad. Sci., India, Sect. B Biol. Sci.*, 82, 181–98, 2012, https://doi.org/10.1007/s40011-011-0014-9.
3. Chavda, V., Zajac, K.K., Gunn, J.L., Balar, P., Khadela, A., Vaghela, D., *et al.*, Ethnic differences in hepatocellular carcinoma prevalence and therapeutic outcomes. *Cancer Rep. (Hoboken)*, 6, Suppl 1, e1821, 2023, https://doi.org/10.1002/cnr2.1821.
4. Warnock, J.N., Daigre, C., Al-Rubeai, M., Introduction to viral vectors. *Methods Mol. Biol.*, 737, 1–25, 2011, https://doi.org/10.1007/978-1-61779-095-9_1.
5. Robert-Guroff, M., Replicating and non-replicating viral vectors for vaccine development. *Curr. Opin. Biotechnol.*, 18, 546–56, 2007, https://doi.org/10.1016/j.copbio.2007.10.010.
6. Dalba, C., Bellier, B., Kasahara, N., Klatzmann, D., Replication-competent Vectors and Empty Virus-like Particles: New Retroviral Vector Designs for Cancer Gene Therapy or Vaccines. *Mol. Ther.*, 15, 457–66, 2007, https://doi.org/10.1038/sj.mt.6300054.
7. Ghosh, S., Brown, A.M., Jenkins, C., Campbell, K., Viral Vector Systems for Gene Therapy: A Comprehensive Literature Review of Progress and Biosafety Challenges. *Appl. Biosaf.*, 25, 7–18, 2020, https://doi.org/10.1177/1535676019899502.
8. Shiver, J.W., R-G, M., Nabel, G.J., Replication-Defective and Competent Adenovirus Recombinants as Vaccine Vectors, in: *New Generation Vaccines*, 4th ed., p. 9, CRC Press, Boca Raton, 2010.
9. Huttner, A., Dayer, J.-A., Yerly, S., Combescure, C., Auderset, F., Desmeules, J., *et al.*, The effect of dose on the safety and immunogenicity of the VSV Ebola candidate vaccine: a randomised double-blind, placebo-controlled

phase 1/2 trial. *Lancet Infect. Dis.*, 15, 1156–66, 2015, https://doi.org/10.1016/S1473-3099(15)00154-1.

10. Case, J.B., Rothlauf, P.W., Chen, R.E., Kafai, N.M., Fox J.M., Smith, B.K., *et al.*, Replication-Competent Vesicular Stomatitis Virus Vaccine Vector Protects against SARS-CoV-2-Mediated Pathogenesis in Mice. *Cell Host Microbe*, 28, e4, 465–474, 2020, https://doi.org/10.1016/j.chom.2020.07.018.
11. Gao, Q., Bao, L., Mao, H., Wang, L., Xu, K., Yang, M., *et al.*, Development of an inactivated vaccine candidate for SARS-CoV-2. *Science*, 369, 77–81, 2020, https://doi.org/10.1126/science.abc1932.
12. Orlova, O.V., Glazkova, D.V., Bogoslovskaya, E.V., Shipulin, G.A., Yudin, S.M., Development of Modified Vaccinia Virus Ankara-Based Vaccines: Advantages and Applications. *Vaccines (Basel)*, 10, 1516, 2022, https://doi.org/10.3390/vaccines10091516.
13. Guerra, S., González, J.M., Climent, N., Reyburn, H., López-Fernández, L.A., Nájera, J.L., *et al.*, Selective Induction of Host Genes by MVA-B, a Candidate Vaccine against HIV/AIDS. *J. Virol.*, 84, 8141–52, 2010, https://doi.org/10.1128/JVI.00749-10.
14. Alberca, B., Bachanek-Bankowska, K., Cabana, M., Calvo-Pinilla, E., Viaplana, E., Frost, L., *et al.*, Vaccination of horses with a recombinant modified vaccinia Ankara virus (MVA) expressing African horse sickness (AHS) virus major capsid protein VP2 provides complete clinical protection against challenge. *Vaccine*, 32, 3670–4, 2014, https://doi.org/10.1016/j.vaccine.2014.04.036.
15. Ebenig, A., Lange, M.V., Mühlebach, M.D., Versatility of live-attenuated measles viruses as platform technology for recombinant vaccines. *npj Vaccines*, 7, 1–12, 2022, https://doi.org/10.1038/s41541-022-00543-4.
16. Nzounza, P., Martin, G., Dereuddre-Bosquet, N., Najburg, V., Gosse, L., Ruffié, C., *et al.*, A recombinant measles virus vaccine strongly reduces SHIV viremia and virus reservoir establishment in macaques. *npj Vaccines*, 6, 1–11, 2021, https://doi.org/10.1038/s41541-021-00385-6.
17. Efferson, C.L., Schickli, J., Ko, B.K., Kawano, K., Mouzi, S., Palese, P., *et al.*, Activation of Tumor Antigen-Specific Cytotoxic T Lymphocytes (CTLs) by Human Dendritic Cells Infected with an Attenuated Influenza A Virus Expressing a CTL Epitope Derived from the HER-2/neu Proto-Oncogene. *J. Virol.*, 77, 7411–24, 2003, https://doi.org/10.1128/JVI.77.13.7411-7424.2003.
18. Ferko, B., Stasakova, J., Sereinig, S., Romanova, J., Katinger, D., Niebler, B., *et al.*, Hyperattenuated Recombinant Influenza A Virus Nonstructural-Protein-Encoding Vectors Induce Human Immunodeficiency Virus Type 1 Nef-Specific Systemic and Mucosal Immune Responses in Mice. *J. Virol.*, 75, 8899–908, 2001, https://doi.org/10.1128/JVI.75.19.8899-8908.2001.
19. Li, J., Arévalo, M.T., Zeng, M., Engineering influenza viral vectors. *Bioengineered*, 4, 9–14, 2013, https://doi.org/10.4161/bioe.21950.

20. Thorner, A.R., Lemckert, A.A.C., Goudsmit, J., Lynch, D.M., Ewald, B.A., Denholtz, M., *et al.*, Immunogenicity of Heterologous Recombinant Adenovirus Prime-Boost Vaccine Regimens Is Enhanced by Circumventing Vector Cross-Reactivity. *J. Virol.*, 80, 12009–16, 2006, https://doi.org/10.1128/JVI.01749-06.
21. Daaboul, G.G., Lopez, C.A., Chinnala, J., Goldberg, B.B., Connor, J.H., Ünlü, M.S., Digital Sensing and Sizing of Vesicular Stomatitis Virus Pseudotypes in Complex Media; A Model for Ebola and Marburg Detection. *ACS Nano*, 8, 6047–55, 2014, https://doi.org/10.1021/nn501312q.
22. Altenburg, A.F., van de Sandt, C.E., Li, B.W.S., MacLoughlin, R.J., Fouchier, R.A.M., van Amerongen, G., *et al.*, Modified Vaccinia Virus Ankara Preferentially Targets Antigen Presenting Cells *In Vitro*, *Ex Vivo* and *In Vivo*. *Sci. Rep.*, 7, 8580, 2017, https://doi.org/10.1038/s41598-017-08719-y.
23. Wang, Q., Vossen, A., Ikeda, Y., Devaux, P., Measles vector as a multigene delivery platform facilitating iPSC reprogramming. *Gene Ther.*, 26, 151–64, 2019, https://doi.org/10.1038/s41434-019-0058-7.
24. Conrad, S. and Liu, J., Poxviruses as Gene Therapy Vectors: Generating Poxviral Vectors Expressing Therapeutic Transgenes. *Methods Mol. Biol.*, 1937, 189–209, 2019, https://doi.org/10.1007/978-1-4939-9065-8_11.
25. Chavda, V.P., Bezbaruah, R., Athalye, M., Parikh, P.K., Chhipa, A.S., Patel, S., *et al.*, Replicating Viral Vector-Based Vaccines for COVID-19: Potential Avenue in Vaccination Arena. *Viruses*, 14, 759, 2022, https://doi.org/10.3390/v14040759.
26. Kyriakidis, N.C., López-Cortés, A., González, E.V., Grimaldos, A.B., Prado, E.O., SARS-CoV-2 vaccines strategies: a comprehensive review of phase 3 candidates. *npj Vaccines*, 6, 28, 2021, https://doi.org/10.1038/s41541-021-00292-w.
27. Awate, S., Babiuk, L.A., Mutwiri, G., Mechanisms of Action of Adjuvants. *Front. Immunol.*, 4, 114, 2013, https://doi.org/10.3389/fimmu.2013.00114.
28. Pulendran, B., Arunachalam, P.S., O'Hagan, D.T., Emerging concepts in the science of vaccine adjuvants. *Nat. Rev. Drug Discov.*, 20, 454–75, 2021, https://doi.org/10.1038/s41573-021-00163-y.
29. Parks, C.L., Replication-Competent Viral Vectors for Vaccine Delivery, in: *Human Vaccines*, pp. 25–63, Elsevier, 2017, https://doi.org/10.1016/B978-0-12-802302-0.00001-7.
30. Hendrickx, R., Stichling, N., Koelen, J., Kuryk, L., Lipiec, A., Greber, U.F., Innate immunity to adenovirus. *Hum. Gene Ther.*, 25, 265–84, Mary Ann Liebert, Inc., 2014, https://doi.org/10.1089/hum.2014.001.
31. Van Riel, D. and De Wit, E., Next-generation vaccine platforms for COVID-19. *Nat. Mater.*, 19, 810–2, 2020, https://doi.org/10.1038/s41563-020-0746-0.
32. Coughlan, L., Factors Which Contribute to the Immunogenicity of Non-replicating Adenoviral Vectored Vaccines. *Front. Immunol.*, 11, 909, 2020, https://doi.org/10.3389/fimmu.2020.00909.

33. Banchereau, J. and Steinman, R.M., Dendritic cells and the control of immunity. *Nature*, 392, 245–52, 1998, https://doi.org/10.1038/32588.
34. Patterson, L.J., Malkevitch, N., Pinczewski, J., Venzon, D., Lou, Y., Peng, B., *et al.*, Potent, persistent induction and modulation of cellular immune responses in rhesus macaques primed with Ad5hr-simian immunodeficiency virus (SIV) env/rev, gag, and/or nef vaccines and boosted with SIV gp120. *J. Virol.*, American Society for Microbiology, 77, 8607–20, American Society for Microbiology, 2003, https://doi.org/10.1128/jvi.77.16.8607-8620.2003.
35. Gómez-Román, V.R., Patterson, L.J., Venzon, D., Liewehr, D., Aldrich, K., Florese, R., *et al.*, Vaccine-Elicited Antibodies Mediate Antibody-Dependent Cellular Cytotoxicity Correlated with Significantly Reduced Acute Viremia in Rhesus Macaques Challenged with SIVmac251. *J. Immunol.*, 174, 2185–9, 2005, https://doi.org/10.4049/jimmunol.174.4.2185.
36. Gomez-Roman, V.R., Florese, R.H., Peng, B., Montefiori, D.C., Kalyanaraman, V.S., Venzon, D., *et al.*, An Adenovirus-Based HIV Subtype B Prime/Boost Vaccine Regimen Elicits Antibodies Mediating Broad Antibody-Dependent Cellular Cytotoxicity Against Non-Subtype B HIV Strains. *JAIDS J. Acquir. Immune Defic. Syndr.*, 43, 270–7, 2006, https://doi.org/10.1097/01.qai.0000230318.40170.60.
37. Peng, B., Wang, L.R., Gómez-Román, V.R., Davis-Warren, A., Montefiori, D.C., Kalyanaraman, V.S., *et al.*, Replicating rather than nonreplicating adenovirus-human immunodeficiency virus recombinant vaccines are better at eliciting potent cellular immunity and priming high-titer antibodies. *J. Virol.*, 79, 10200–9, 2005, https://doi.org/10.1128/JVI.79.16.10200-10209.2005.
38. Demberg, T., Florese, R.H., Heath, M.J., Larsen, K., Kalisz, I., Kalyanaraman, V.S., *et al.*, A replication-competent adenovirus-human immunodeficiency virus (Ad-HIV) tat and Ad-HIV env priming/Tat and envelope protein boosting regimen elicits enhanced protective efficacy against simian/human immunodeficiency virus SHIV89.6P challenge in rhesus macaques. *J. Virol.*, 81, 3414–27, 2007, https://doi.org/10.1128/JVI.02453-06.
39. Malkevitch, N.V., Patterson, L.J., Aldrich, M.K., Wu, Y., Venzon, D., Florese, R.H., *et al.*, Durable protection of rhesus macaques immunized with a replicating adenovirus-SIV multigene prime/protein boost vaccine regimen against a second SIVmac251 rectal challenge: Role of SIV-specific CD8+ T cell responses. *Virology*, 353, 83–98, 2006, https://doi.org/10.1016/j.virol.2006.05.012.
40. Draper, S.J. and Heeney, J.L., Viruses as vaccine vectors for infectious diseases and cancer. *Nat. Rev. Microbiol.*, 8, 62–73, 2010, https://doi.org/10.1038/nrmicro2240.
41. Lundstrom, K., RNA Viruses as Tools in Gene Therapy and Vaccine Development. *Genes*, 10, 189, 2019, https://doi.org/10.3390/genes10030189.
42. Henao-Restrepo, A.M., Camacho, A., Longini, I.M., Watson, C.H., Edmunds, W.J., Egger, M., *et al.*, Efficacy and effectiveness of an rVSV-vectored vaccine in preventing Ebola virus disease: final results from the Guinea ring

vaccination, open-label, cluster-randomised trial (Ebola Ça Suffit!). *Lancet*, 389, 505–18, 2017, https://doi.org/10.1016/S0140-6736(16)32621-6.
43. Parks, C.L., Picker, L.J., King, C.R., Development of replication-competent viral vectors for HIV vaccine delivery. *Curr. Opin. HIV AIDS*, 8, 402–11, 2013, https://doi.org/10.1097/COH.0b013e328363d389.
44. Garbuglia, A.R., Lapa, D., Sias, C., Capobianchi, M.R., Del Porto, P., The Use of Both Therapeutic and Prophylactic Vaccines in the Therapy of Papillomavirus Disease. *Front. Immunol.*, 11, 188, 2020, https://doi.org/10.3389/fimmu.2020.00188.
45. Tabynov, K., Sansyzbay, A., Kydyrbayev, Z., Yespembetov, B., Ryskeldinova, S., Zinina, N., *et al.*, Influenza viral vectors expressing the Brucella OMP16 or L7/L12 proteins as vaccines against B. abortus infection. *Virol. J.*, 11, 69, 2014, https://doi.org/10.1186/1743-422X-11-69.
46. Zhong, L., Krummenacher, C., Zhang, W., Hong, J., Feng, Q., Chen, Y., *et al.*, Urgency and necessity of Epstein-Barr virus prophylactic vaccines. *npj Vaccines*, 7, 159, 2022, https://doi.org/10.1038/s41541-022-00587-6.
47. Potluri, R., Kumar, A., Maheshwari, V., Smith, C., Oriol Mathieu, V., Luhn, K., *et al.*, Impact of prophylactic vaccination strategies on Ebola virus transmission: A modeling analysis. *PLoS One*, 15, e0230406, 2020, https://doi.org/10.1371/journal.pone.0230406.
48. Dekhtiarenko, I., Ratts, R.B., Blatnik, R., Lee, L.N., Fischer, S., Borkner, L., *et al.*, Peptide Processing Is Critical for T-Cell Memory Inflation and May Be Optimized to Improve Immune Protection by CMV-Based Vaccine Vectors. *PLoS Pathog.*, 12, e1006072, 2016, https://doi.org/10.1371/journal.ppat.1006072.
49. Roberts, A., Kretzschmar, E., Perkins, A.S., Forman, J., Price, R., Buonocore, L., *et al.*, Vaccination with a Recombinant Vesicular Stomatitis Virus Expressing an Influenza Virus Hemagglutinin Provides Complete Protection from Influenza Virus Challenge. *J. Virol.*, 72, 4704–11, 1998, https://doi.org/10.1128/JVI.72.6.4704-4711.1998.
50. Fuchs, J.D., Frank, I., Elizaga, M.L., Allen, M., Frahm, N., Kochar, N., *et al.*, First-in-Human Evaluation of the Safety and Immunogenicity of a Recombinant Vesicular Stomatitis Virus Human Immunodeficiency Virus-1 gag Vaccine (HVTN 090). *Open Forum Infect. Dis.*, 2, ofv082, 2015, https://doi.org/10.1093/ofid/ofv082.
51. Green, T.J., Zhang, X., Wertz, G.W., Luo, M., Structure of the Vesicular Stomatitis Virus Nucleoprotein-RNA Complex. *Science*, 313, 357–60, 2006, https://doi.org/10.1126/science.1126953.
52. Rose, J.K. and Clarke, D.K., Rhabdoviruses as Vaccine Vectors: From Initial Development to Clinical Trials, in: *Biology and Pathogenesis of Rhabdo- and Filoviruses*, World Scientific Publishing Co Pte Ltd, Singapore, pp. 199–230, WORLD SCIENTIFIC, 2015, https://doi.org/10.1142/9789814635349_0009.
53. Ollmann Saphire, E., A Vaccine against Ebola Virus. *Cell*, 181, 6, 2020, https://doi.org/10.1016/j.cell.2020.03.011.

54. Jones, S.M., Feldmann, H., Ströher, U., Geisbert, J.B., Fernando, L., Grolla, A., *et al.*, Live attenuated recombinant vaccine protects nonhuman primates against Ebola and Marburg viruses. *Nat. Med.*, 11, 786–90, 2005, https://doi.org/10.1038/nm1258.
55. Dahlke, C., Kasonta, R., Lunemann, S., Krähling, V., Zinser, M.E., Biedenkopf, N., *et al.*, Dose-dependent T-cell Dynamics and Cytokine Cascade Following rVSV-ZEBOV Immunization. *EBioMedicine*, 19, 107–18, 2017, https://doi.org/10.1016/j.ebiom.2017.03.045.
56. Zaheer, A., Advancements in Marburg Virus Vaccine Development: Unravelling Recent Findings. A Narrative Review. *SJHR*, 5, 19, 2024, https://doi.org/10.51168/sjhrafrica.v5i3.1015.
57. Gugliesi, F., Coscia, A., Griffante, G., Galitska, G., Pasquero, S., Albano, C., *et al.*, Where do we Stand after Decades of Studying Human Cytomegalovirus? *Microorganisms*, 8, 685, 2020, https://doi.org/10.3390/microorganisms8050685.
58. Sylwester, A.W., Mitchell, B.L., Edgar, J.B., Taormina, C., Pelte, C., Ruchti, F., *et al.*, Broadly targeted human cytomegalovirus-specific CD4 + and CD8 + T cells dominate the memory compartments of exposed subjects. *J. Exp. Med.*, 202, 673–85, 2005, https://doi.org/10.1084/jem.20050882.
59. Karrer, U., Wagner, M., Sierro, S., Oxenius, A., Hengel, H., Dumrese, T., *et al.*, Expansion of Protective CD8+ T-Cell Responses Driven by Recombinant Cytomegaloviruses. *J. Virol.*, 78, 2255–64, 2004, https://doi.org/10.1128/JVI.78.5.2255-2264.2004.
60. Tsuda, Y., Caposio, P., Parkins, C.J., Botto, S., Messaoudi, I., Cicin-Sain, L., *et al.*, A Replicating Cytomegalovirus-Based Vaccine Encoding a Single Ebola Virus Nucleoprotein CTL Epitope Confers Protection against Ebola Virus. *PLoS Negl. Trop. Dis.*, 5, e1275, 2011, https://doi.org/10.1371/journal.pntd.0001275.
61. Tsuda, Y., Parkins, C.J., Caposio, P., Feldmann, F., Botto, S., Ball, S., *et al.*, A cytomegalovirus-based vaccine provides long-lasting protection against lethal Ebola virus challenge after a single dose. *Vaccine*, 33, 2261–6, 2015, https://doi.org/10.1016/j.vaccine.2015.03.029.
62. Marzi, A., Murphy, A.A., Feldmann, F., Parkins, C.J., Haddock, E., Hanley, P.W., *et al.*, Cytomegalovirus-based vaccine expressing Ebola virus glycoprotein protects nonhuman primates from Ebola virus infection. *Sci. Rep.*, 6, 21674, 2016, https://doi.org/10.1038/srep21674.
63. Valencia, S., Gill, R.B., Dowdell, K.C., Wang, Y., Hornung, R., Bowman, J.J., *et al.*, Comparison of vaccination with rhesus CMV (RhCMV) soluble gB with a RhCMV replication-defective virus deleted for MHC class I immune evasion genes in a RhCMV challenge model. *Vaccine*, 37, 333–42, 2019, https://doi.org/10.1016/j.vaccine.2018.08.043.
64. Warnock, J.N., Daigre, C., Al-Rubeai, M., Introduction to Viral Vectors, in: *Viral Vectors for Gene Therapy*, vol. 737, O.-W. Merten and M.

Al-Rubeai (Eds.), pp. 1–25, Humana Press, Totowa, NJ, 2011, https://doi.org/10.1007/978-1-61779-095-9_1.
65. Berche, P., History of measles. *Presse Méd.*, 51, 104149, 2022, https://doi.org/10.1016/j.lpm.2022.104149.
66. Ovsyannikova, I.G., Dhiman, N., Jacobson, R.M., Vierkant, R.A., Poland, G.A., Frequency of Measles Virus-Specific CD4$^+$ and CD8$^+$ T Cells in Subjects Seronegative or Highly Seropositive for Measles Vaccine. *Clin. Vaccine Immunol.*, 10, 411–6, 2003, https://doi.org/10.1128/CDLI.10.3.411-416.2003.
67. Radecke, F., Spielhofer, P., Schneider, H., Kaelin, K., Huber, M., Dötsch, C., *et al.*, Rescue of measles viruses from cloned DNA. *EMBO J.*, 14, 5773–84, 1995, https://doi.org/10.1002/j.1460-2075.1995.tb00266.x.
68. Zuniga, A., Wang, Z., Liniger, M., Hangartner, L., Caballero, M., Pavlovic, J., *et al.*, Attenuated measles virus as a vaccine vector. *Vaccine*, 25, 2974–83, 2007, https://doi.org/10.1016/j.vaccine.2007.01.064.
69. Stebbings, R., Li, B., Lorin, C., Koutsoukos, M., Février, M., Mee, E.T., *et al.*, Immunogenicity of a recombinant measles HIV-1 subtype C vaccine. *Vaccine*, 31, 6079–86, 2013, https://doi.org/10.1016/j.vaccine.2013.09.072.
70. Ramsauer, K., Schwameis, M., Firbas, C., Müllner, M., Putnak, R.J., Thomas, S.J., *et al.*, Immunogenicity, safety, and tolerability of a recombinant measles-virus-based chikungunya vaccine: a randomised, double-blind, placebo-controlled, active-comparator, first-in-man trial. *Lancet Infect. Dis.*, 15, 519–27, 2015, https://doi.org/10.1016/S1473-3099(15)70043-5.
71. Gerke, C., Frantz, P.N., Ramsauer, K., Tangy, F., Measles-vectored vaccine approaches against viral infections: a focus on Chikungunya. *Expert Rev. Vaccines*, 18, 393–403, 2019, https://doi.org/10.1080/14760584.2019.1562908.
72. Chang, J., Adenovirus Vectors: Excellent Tools for Vaccine Development. *Immune Netw.*, 21, e6, 2021, https://doi.org/10.4110/in.2021.21.e6.
73. Priddy, F.H., Brown, D., Kublin, J., Monahan, K., Wright, D.P., Lalezari, J., *et al.*, Safety and Immunogenicity of a Replication-Incompetent Adenovirus Type 5 HIV-1 Clade B gag/pol/nef Vaccine in Healthy Adults. *Clin. Infect. Dis.*, 46, 1769–81, 2008, https://doi.org/10.1086/587993.
74. Shoji, M., Tachibana, M., Katayama, K., Tomita, K., Tsuzuki, S., Sakurai, F., *et al.*, Type-I IFN signaling is required for the induction of antigen-specific CD8+ T cell responses by adenovirus vector vaccine in the gut-mucosa. *Biochem. Biophys. Res. Commun.*, 425, 89–93, 2012, https://doi.org/10.1016/j.bbrc.2012.07.056.
75. Matchett, W.E., Malewana, G.B.R., Mudrick, H., Medlyn, M.J., Barry, M.A., Genetic Adjuvants in Replicating Single-Cycle Adenovirus Vectors Amplify Systemic and Mucosal Immune Responses against HIV-1 Envelope. *Vaccines*, 8, 64, 2020, https://doi.org/10.3390/vaccines8010064.
76. Coughlan, L., Sridhar, S., Payne, R., Edmans, M., Milicic, A., Venkatraman, N., *et al.*, Heterologous Two-Dose Vaccination with Simian Adenovirus

and Poxvirus Vectors Elicits Long-Lasting Cellular Immunity to Influenza Virus A in Healthy Adults. *EBioMedicine*, 29, 146–54, 2018, https://doi.org/10.1016/j.ebiom.2018.02.011.

77. Salisch, N.C., Stephenson, K.E., Williams, K., Cox, F., Van Der Fits, L., Heerwegh, D., *et al.*, A Double-Blind, Randomized, Placebo-Controlled Phase 1 Study of Ad26.ZIKV.001, an Ad26-Vectored Anti–Zika Virus Vaccine. *Ann. Intern. Med.*, 174, 585–94, 2021, https://doi.org/10.7326/M20-5306.
78. Carrera, J., Aktepe, T.E., Earnest, L., Christiansen, D., Wheatley, A.K., Tan, H.-X., *et al.*, Adenovirus vector produced Zika virus-like particles induce a long-lived neutralising antibody response in mice. *Vaccine*, 41, 4888–98, 2023, https://doi.org/10.1016/j.vaccine.2023.06.068.
79. Volkmann, A., Williamson, A.-L., Weidenthaler, H., Meyer, T.P.H., Robertson, J.S., Excler, J.-L., *et al.*, The Brighton Collaboration standardized template for collection of key information for risk/benefit assessment of a Modified Vaccinia Ankara (MVA) vaccine platform. *Vaccine*, 39, 3067–80, 2021, https://doi.org/10.1016/j.vaccine.2020.08.050.
80. Zhang, Z., Zhao, Z., Wang, Y., Wu, S., Wang, B., Zhang, J., *et al.*, Comparative immunogenicity analysis of intradermal versus intramuscular immunization with a recombinant human adenovirus type 5 vaccine against Ebola virus. *Front. Immunol.*, 13, 963049, 2022, https://doi.org/10.3389/fimmu.2022.963049.
81. COVID-19 vaccine tracker and landscape, https://www.who.int/publications/m/item/draft-landscape-of-covid-19-candidate-vaccines (accessed March 11, 2024).
82. Jacob-Dolan, C. and Barouch, D.H., COVID-19 Vaccines: Adenoviral Vectors. *Annu. Rev. Med.*, 73, 41–54, 2022, https://doi.org/10.1146/annurev-med-012621-102252.
83. Falsey, A.R., Sobieszczyk, M.E., Hirsch, I., Sproule, S., Robb, M.L., Corey, L., *et al.*, Phase 3 Safety and Efficacy of AZD1222 (ChAdOx1 nCoV-19) Covid-19 Vaccine. *N. Engl. J. Med.*, 385, 2348–60, 2021, https://doi.org/10.1056/NEJMoa2105290.
84. Lu, M., Dravid, P., Zhang, Y., Trivedi, S., Li, A., Harder, O., *et al.*, A safe and highly efficacious measles virus-based vaccine expressing SARS-CoV-2 stabilized prefusion spike. *Proc. Natl. Acad. Sci. U.S.A.*, 118, e2026153118, 2021, https://doi.org/10.1073/pnas.2026153118.
85. Launay, O., Artaud, C., Lachâtre, M., Ait-Ahmed, M., Klein, J., Luong Nguyen, L.B., *et al.*, Safety and immunogenicity of a measles-vectored SARS-CoV-2 vaccine candidate, V591/TMV-083, in healthy adults: results of a randomized, placebo-controlled Phase I study. *eBioMedicine*, 75, 103810, 2022, https://doi.org/10.1016/j.ebiom.2021.103810.
86. Sultan, H., Fesenkova, V.I., Addis, D., Fan, A.E., Kumai, T., Wu, J., *et al.*, Designing therapeutic cancer vaccines by mimicking viral infections.

Cancer Immunol., Immunother., 66, 203–13, 2017, https://doi.org/10.1007/s00262-016-1834-5.

87. Boettcher, A.N., Usman, A., Morgans, A., VanderWeele, D.J., Sosman, J., Wu, J.D., Past, Current, and Future of Immunotherapies for Prostate Cancer. *Front. Oncol.*, 9, 884, 2019, https://doi.org/10.3389/fonc.2019.00884.
88. Zolaly, M.A., Mahallawi, W., Khawaji, Z.Y., Alahmadi, M.A., The Clinical Advances of Oncolytic Viruses in Cancer Immunotherapy. *Cureus*, 15, 6, 2023, https://doi.org/10.7759/cureus.40742.
89. Wang, H., Borlongan, M., Hemminki, A., Basnet, S., Sah, N., Kaufman, H.L., *et al.*, Viral Vectors Expressing Interleukin 2 for Cancer Immunotherapy. *Hum. Gene Ther.*, 34, 878–95, 2023, https://doi.org/10.1089/hum.2023.099.
92. Biegert, G.W.G., Rosewell Shaw, A., Suzuki, M., Current development in adenoviral vectors for cancer immunotherapy. *Mol. Ther. Oncolytics*, 23, 571–81, 2021, https://doi.org/10.1016/j.omto.2021.11.014.
91. Shaw, A.R. and Suzuki, M., Immunology of Adenoviral Vectors in Cancer Therapy. *Mol. Ther. Methods Clin. Dev.*, 15, 418–29, 2019, https://doi.org/10.1016/j.omtm.2019.11.001.
92. Barouch, D.H., Tomaka, F.L., Wegmann, F., Stieh, D.J., Alter, G., Robb, M.L., *et al.*, Evaluation of a mosaic HIV-1 vaccine in a multicentre, randomised, double-blind, placebo-controlled, phase 1/2a clinical trial (APPROACH) and in rhesus monkeys (NHP 13-19). *Lancet*, 392, 232–43, 2018, https://doi.org/10.1016/S0140-6736(18)31364-3.
93. Morante, V., Borghi, M., Farina, I., Michelini, Z., Grasso, F., Gallinaro, A., *et al.*, Integrase-Defective Lentiviral Vector Is an Efficient Vaccine Platform for Cancer Immunotherapy. *Viruses*, 13, 355, 2021, https://doi.org/10.3390/v13020355.
94. Kaur, B., Antonio Chiocca, E., Cripe, T.P., Oncolytic HSV-1 Virotherapy: Clinical Experience and Opportunities for Progress. *CPB*, 13, 1842–51, 2012, https://doi.org/10.2174/138920112800958814.

5

Nonreplicating Viral Vectors for Vaccine Delivery

Pankti C. Balar[1] and Vivek P. Chavda[2]*

[1]Pharmacy Section, L.M. College of Pharmacy, Ahmedabad, Gujarat, India
[2]Department of Pharmaceutics and Pharmaceutical Technology, L.M. College of Pharmacy, Ahmedabad, Gujarat, India

Abstract
Nonreplicating viral vectors have garnered attention due to their enhanced safety profile. Unlike replicating vectors, which can multiply within host cells, nonreplicating vectors do not replicate, mitigating the risk of uncontrolled spread and potential adverse effects. This paper aims to explore the versatility of nonreplicating viral vectors in vaccine delivery, emphasizing their design principles, applications, and future prospects. Nonreplicating viral vectors are typically derived from viruses rendered replication-deficient through genetic modifications. These modifications disable key viral replication machinery while retaining the ability to infect host cells and express desired genes. Commonly utilized nonreplicating viral vectors include adenoviruses, adeno-associated viruses (AAVs), lentiviruses, and alphaviruses. The design of nonreplicating viral vectors entails several critical considerations. First, selecting the viral backbone is crucial, considering factors such as tropism, immunogenicity, and safety. For example, adenoviral vectors efficiently transduce a variety of cell types, while AAVs exhibit low immunogenicity and enable long-term transgene expression. Nonreplicating viral vectors have demonstrated utility across various vaccine applications, including infectious diseases, cancer immunotherapy, and emerging pathogens. Adenoviral vectors, for instance, show promise in developing vaccines against malaria, HIV, and Ebola virus by efficiently delivering antigenic payloads to antigen-presenting cells, eliciting robust immune responses. Furthermore, nonreplicating viral vectors serve as a versatile platform for cancer immunotherapy. By encoding tumor-associated antigens or immune checkpoint inhibitors, viral vectors mobilize the immune system to recognize and eliminate cancer cells. Clinical trials employing viral

**Corresponding author*: vivek.chavda@lmcp.ac.in

Vivek P. Chavda and Vasso Apostolopoulos (eds.) Viral Vectors for Vaccine Delivery, (125–148) © 2025 Scrivener Publishing LLC

vector–based cancer vaccines have shown promising results, underscoring their potential in cancer treatment. During emerging infectious disease outbreaks like the COVID-19 pandemic, nonreplicating viral vectors have played a crucial role in vaccine development. Vaccines such as Oxford-AstraZeneca and Johnson & Johnson COVID-19 vaccines, based on chimpanzee adenoviral vectors, have been globally deployed, contributing significantly to vaccination efforts.

Keywords: Nonreplicating, vector, vaccine, adjuvant, optimization

5.1 Introduction

In the field of vaccinology, nonreplicating viral vectors have emerged as promising tools for delivering vaccines. These vectors are engineered from viruses to carry antigenic material into cells without the ability to replicate, offering safety advantages over traditional vaccines. They include a variety of viruses like adenoviruses, lentiviruses, poxviruses, and adeno-associated viruses (AAVs), each with unique benefits for vaccine development [1]. The evolution of nonreplicating viral vectors is tightly intertwined with significant advancements in virology and genetic engineering. Beginning in the 1970s, the emergence of recombinant DNA technology, pioneered by scientists like Paul Berg, Herbert Boyer, and Stanley Cohen, enabled the manipulation of viral genomes, laying the groundwork for the development of custom-designed vectors [2]. Throughout the 1980s, researchers made substantial strides in this field, culminating in the creation of the first recombinant viral vectors. Adenoviruses, known for their well-characterized genome and broad host cell range, became prominent candidates for vector development. Scientists successfully engineered adenoviral vectors to transport foreign genes, marking a pivotal moment in gene therapy and vaccine research. In subsequent years, researchers focused on refining viral vector technology, particularly nonreplicating vectors [3]. Adenoviral vectors, along with platforms, like AAVs, lentiviruses, and poxviruses, underwent extensive optimization to improve safety, immunogenicity, and scalability. These efforts led to the approval of the world's first nonreplicating viral vector–based vaccine in the early 21st century, representing a significant advancement in combating infectious diseases [4]. One notable feature of these vectors is their ability to carry large amounts of genetic material, allowing for the delivery of multiple antigens in a single vaccine. This flexibility enables the creation of vaccines targeting complex pathogens or inducing broad immunity. Nonreplicating viral vectors possess a remarkable versatility that finds application in diverse fields such as vaccine development, gene therapy, and biomedical research.

Their unique characteristics offer numerous advantages over traditional methods, particularly in vaccine delivery [5]. These vectors are adept at eliciting robust immune responses, including both humoral and cellular immunity, making them highly effective in combating a broad spectrum of infectious diseases. Additionally, these vectors can be modified to enhance their potency and effectiveness, further improving their utility. The evolution of nonreplicating viral vectors has been driven by advancements in molecular biology, virology, and immunology. In the realm of vaccine development, nonreplicating viral vectors have been instrumental in creating vaccines against various viral and bacterial pathogens, ranging from HIV and influenza to Ebola and *Mycobacterium tuberculosis* [6]. Their flexibility allows for swift vaccine development in response to emerging infectious threats, as evidenced during the recent COVID-19 pandemic. Beyond infectious diseases, these vectors hold significant promise in gene therapy. By delivering therapeutic genes to target cells, they offer potential solutions for correcting genetic defects and treating inherited disorders. These advances have allowed for the precise engineering of vectors to optimize their performance and safety. Ongoing research continues to refine vector design and delivery strategies, promising even more effective vaccines in the future [7]. This chapter aims to provide a thorough overview of nonreplicating viral vectors for vaccine delivery. It discusses their mechanisms of action, the various vector platforms available, and the evidence supporting their efficacy and safety against infectious diseases. Challenges and limitations are also addressed, along with future research directions to enhance these technologies.

5.2 Nonreplicating Viral Vectors: Types and Characteristics

Nonreplicating viral vectors represent a sophisticated approach in genetic engineering, where viruses are altered to lose their ability to replicate within host cells while retaining their capacity to deliver genetic material. These vectors fall into two main categories: adenoviral and non-adenoviral vectors.

5.2.1 Adenoviral Vectors

Adenoviruses, known for their efficiency in infecting mammalian cells, are commonly utilized as vectors. Adenoviruses, members of the

Adenoviridae family, are renowned for their pivotal role in vaccine development. Through strategic genetic engineering, adenoviral vectors emerge as safe and potent vehicles for delivering vaccine payloads. These vectors are meticulously crafted, retaining infectivity while rendering themselves incapable of replication, thus ensuring safety [8]. In nonreplicating adenoviral vectors, essential viral genes for replication are removed or deactivated, ensuring the vector cannot self-replicate while still being able to deliver genes into target cells. Administered either topically to mucosal surfaces or via direct tissue injection, adenoviral vectors swiftly bind to cell surface receptors, prompting internalization through endocytosis. Once within the cell, they liberate their cargo into the cytoplasm, ultimately delivering it to the nucleus. There, the transgene is transcribed and translated, prompting the expression of the encoded antigen. This process elicits robust immune responses, essential for safeguarding against pathogens [9]. Adenoviral vectors boast several advantages, propelling their prominence in vaccine development. Their capacity to accommodate large transgenes facilitates the inclusion of multiple antigens or immunomodulatory molecules. Furthermore, they evoke durable immune responses, spanning both cellular and humoral immunity. Their scalability in manufacturing ensures high-titer production, while their safety profile alleviates concerns about genomic integration. Preexisting immunity poses a significant challenge, hindering vector efficacy due to neutralizing antibodies from prior adenovirus exposure. Mitigation strategies involve rare or nonhuman adenovirus serotypes or alternative vector platforms. Additionally, concerns regarding vector immunogenicity necessitate meticulous evaluation during vaccine formulation. Optimization of stability, storage, and delivery methods is crucial for ensuring vaccine efficacy [10].

5.2.2 Non-Adenoviral Vectors

Non-adenoviral vectors represent a diverse range of viral platforms and synthetic vectors utilized in vaccine development. Unlike adenoviral vectors, which employ adenoviruses for delivery, non-adenoviral vectors utilize alternative viral species or synthetic constructs derived from viruses. Notable examples include lentiviruses, alphaviruses, poxviruses, vesicular stomatitis viruses (VSVs), as well as synthetic vectors like nanoparticles and liposomes [11]. They are engineered to disable replication while retaining their ability to deliver genes. This versatility allows for tailored approaches in vaccine development, affecting target cell tropism and immunogenicity. These non-adenoviral vectors offer several advantages over their adenoviral counterparts. They typically induce weaker immune responses against the vector itself, reducing the risk of preexisting immunity that can affect vaccine efficacy. Additionally, they often boast superior safety profiles, minimizing adverse reactions or unintended consequences [12]. Their diverse nature allows tailored approaches to vaccine design, facilitating the incorporation of specific antigens, adjuvants, or targeting moieties to enhance effectiveness and immunogenicity. Non-adenoviral vectors have found applications in vaccine development against various infectious diseases, cancers, and medical conditions. Lentiviral vectors, for instance, have shown promise in gene therapy–based vaccines, while alphaviral vectors induce robust immune responses. Poxviral vectors, such as modified vaccinia Ankara (MVA), have been studied extensively for efficacy against diseases like HIV, malaria, and tuberculosis [13]. Synthetic vectors like lipid nanoparticles (LNPs) and virus-like particles (VLPs) offer versatile platforms for antigen delivery and immune modulation. However, non-adenoviral vectors face challenges. Integrating vectors like lentiviruses carry a risk of insertional mutagenesis or genomic integration, necessitating ongoing safety monitoring. Scalability and production feasibility pose challenges for large-scale vaccine manufacturing, requiring optimization of production processes and quality control measures. Regulatory considerations and public perception also influence the development and deployment of non-adenoviral vector vaccines, emphasizing the importance of transparent communication, rigorous evaluation, and adherence to ethical standards [14].

5.2.3 Key Characteristics of Nonreplicating Vectors

5.2.3.1 Immunogenicity

When it comes to nonreplicating viral vectors, their inherent ability to interact with various elements of the host's immune system is key to their immunogenicity. The level of antigenic protein expression by the viral vector within host cells plays a vital role in determining immunogenicity. Effective expression and presentation of antigens enhance the immune response. The viral vector's ability to target specific cell types or tissues influences immune response. Targeting antigen-presenting cells (APCs) like dendritic cells improves antigen presentation and immune activation. Nonreplicating viral vectors activate innate immune pathways upon entering host cells, leading to the production of pro-inflammatory molecules. This activation aids in recruiting and activating adaptive immune cells. Some nonreplicating viral vectors inherently possess adjuvant properties, which boost the immune response by aiding antigen presentation and enhancing T cell activation [15].

The immunogenicity of nonreplicating viral vectors arises from intricate interactions between the vector, host cells, and the immune system. Upon administration, viral vectors are recognized by pattern recognition receptors (PRRs) expressed on host cell surfaces or within endosomes. Activation of PRRs like Toll-like receptors (TLRs) and retinoic acid–inducible gene I (RIG-I)–like receptors (RLRs) initiates signaling cascades, leading to the production of type I interferons (IFNs) and proinflammatory molecules. Subsequent antigen expression within host cells leads to antigenic peptide presentation on major histocompatibility complex (MHC) molecules, facilitating recognition by T cells. This process activates antigen-specific $CD4^+$ T helper cells, which support B cells in antibody production, and $CD8^+$ cytotoxic T cells, responsible for eliminating infected cells. Moreover, nonreplicating viral vectors stimulate the production of neutralizing antibodies, which can directly impede viral entry or induce antibody-dependent cellular cytotoxicity (ADCC) [16].

5.2.3.2 Safety

By disabling replication, these vectors mitigate the risk of uncontrolled viral replication, enhancing safety for clinical use. These vectors are engineered to be incapable of replicating within host cells, thus greatly lowering the chance of inducing illness. By disabling key viral replication genes, they prevent spreading beyond the intended target cells. Unlike replicating vectors, nonreplicating ones typically express the desired genetic material temporarily. After delivering the payload, they are naturally eliminated from the body, reducing the likelihood of long-term side effects. Nonreplicating viral vectors undergo extensive safety assessments, including studies on distribution, tissue affinity, and potential immune reactions. This thorough evaluation ensures their safety and minimizes harm to vaccinated individuals [17]. Unlike replicating vectors, nonreplicating ones lack the ability to undergo genetic recombination, thus maintaining the stability of the vaccine construct and reducing the risk of generating unpredictable viral strains. Nonreplicating vectors are generally safer for use in people with compromised immune systems, as they pose minimal risk of uncontrolled viral replication and associated complications, which is crucial for those with underlying health conditions. Advances in genetic manipulation techniques allow for precise modifications to viral vector genomes, further enhancing safety. Techniques like codon optimization, insulator element incorporation, and the use of tissue-specific promoters can fine-tune vector behavior and minimize unintended effects [18].

5.2.3.3 *Stability*

Unlike live attenuated vaccines, nonreplicating vectors remain stable without genetic changes, facilitating storage and distribution. Physical stability is vital for preserving the structural integrity of viral vectors over time and under varying conditions. Maintaining the vector's form during storage and transit is essential to retain its infectivity and ability to trigger immune responses. Variables like temperature, pH, and freeze-thaw cycles can impact this stability. Scientists utilize methods like lyophilization and cryopreservation to bolster the physical resilience of these vectors, extending their shelf life. Genetic stability ensures that the vector's genome remains unchanged, safeguarding its functionality. These vectors are engineered to carry specific genetic payloads, like genes encoding antigens [19]. Consistent expression of these genes across production batches is crucial. Quality control measures such as sequencing and genome analysis are employed to monitor genetic stability throughout manufacturing. Immunological stability is pivotal for eliciting consistent and enduring immune responses postvaccination. Vectors must trigger robust immune reactions without adverse effects or immune evasion. Variables such as dosage, administration route, and host immune status impact the vaccine's ability to induce protective responses. Optimizing formulations and delivery methods maximizes vaccine immunogenicity and the longevity of protective immunity [20].

5.2.3.4 *Targeted Delivery*

Targeted delivery is a crucial aspect of utilizing nonreplicating viral vectors in vaccine development. It involves directing these vectors to specific cells or tissues within the body, enhancing immune responses while minimizing unintended effects. Scientists can engineer nonreplicating viral vectors to target specific cell types by altering the viral proteins. This modification redirects the vectors to desired cells while avoiding others, improving antigen delivery to key immune cells like dendritic cells and macrophages. By incorporating regulatory elements, such as cell-specific promoters, into viral vectors, researchers can control where and when the transgenes are expressed [21]. This precision allows for selective antigen presentation, enhancing vaccine efficacy and safety. The way viral vectors are administered affects where they go in the body. Different routes, like injection, nasal delivery, oral administration, or topical application, offer distinct advantages in targeting specific tissues or mucosal surfaces, influencing immune response quality and magnitude. Viral vectors can be engineered to adjust their immunogenicity, promoting desired immune responses while minimizing adverse reactions. This can involve incorporating immunomodulatory molecules or cytokines or using different viral envelopes, to fine-tune the immune response [22].

5.3 Engineering Nonreplicating Viral Vectors for Vaccine Design

Nonreplicating viral vectors represent a promising avenue in vaccine development, offering a safe and effective means to deliver antigenic material into target cells, thus eliciting robust immune responses against pathogens [23].

5.3.1 Capsid Modification

Capsid modification stands at the forefront of viral vector enhancement, aiming to tailor vectors for efficient vaccine delivery. This process involves altering capsid structures to achieve specific targeting and evade host immune responses, besides enhancing transduction efficiency. AAV2 is a promising candidate for gene therapy due to its favorable characteristics. However, its wide host range poses challenges in achieving tissue-specific gene transfer. This broad host range stems from the interaction between the AAV2 capsid and specific cellular receptors. To address this limitation, researchers have explored genetic modifications of the AAV2 capsid to alter its tropism. By introducing a targeting peptide called L14 into different regions of the AAV2 capsid, researchers aimed to redirect its binding to specific cellular receptors. Six AAV2 capsid mutants were generated, each carrying the L14 peptide in a different location identified through structural analysis. All generated mutants efficiently packaged genetic material. Importantly, three mutants successfully displayed the L14 peptide on their capsid surface. One of these mutants demonstrated the ability to infect cell lines resistant to wild-type AAV2, as these cells expressed the integrin receptor recognized by L14. These findings highlight the feasibility of modifying the AAV2 capsid with nonviral ligands, paving the way for the development of targeted AAV2 vectors for gene therapy applications in humans. Such targeted vectors hold promise for achieving precise gene delivery to specific tissues, potentially enhancing the efficacy and safety of gene therapy approaches [24].

Structural Optimization: Traditional techniques involve altering surface residues for receptor binding specificity. Advanced methods now utilize high-resolution structural analyses and computational modeling for precise engineering. This enables the design of variants with enhanced stability, reduced immunogenicity, and improved tissue targeting [25].

Biological Barriers: Overcoming biological barriers during vector delivery is crucial. Strategies like engineering stealthy capsid coatings with polymers can shield viral particles from the host immune system, enhancing circulation time. Additionally, developing variants capable of penetrating specific cellular barriers holds promise for neurological disorder therapies [26].

Evolutionary Algorithms: Directed evolution is pivotal, generating diverse capsid libraries subjected to selective pressures. Integration of machine learning accelerates the discovery of optimized capsid sequences [27].

5.3.2 Promoter Engineering

Promoter engineering is a powerful tool for controlling transgene expression dynamics and targeting specific cell types. Promoters play a pivotal role in regulating transgene expression within the infected cells. The choice of promoter depends on various factors, including the desired expression kinetics, tissue tropism, and immune response profile. Strong promoters, such as cytomegalovirus (CMV) or human elongation factor 1 alpha (EF1α), are commonly used to drive robust transgene expression. Tissue-specific promoters offer the advantage of targeting antigen expression to specific cell types or tissues, thereby enhancing vaccine efficacy while minimizing off-target effects. For example, selecting a promoter that is active in dendritic cells or APCs can promote efficient antigen presentation and immune activation [28].

Temporal Control: Inducible promoter systems regulate antigen presentation timing, enhancing vaccine safety and efficacy.

Tissue-Specific Targeting: Leveraging tissue-specific enhancers and regulatory elements restricts transgene expression to desired cell populations, optimizing immune responses.

Biosafety Considerations: Synthetic promoters prioritize biosafety, minimizing risks like insertional mutagenesis. Rational design and computational modeling identify sequences with optimal activity and minimal genotoxicity [29].

5.3.3 Transgene Optimization

Optimizing antigenic payload is crucial for eliciting robust immune responses.

Codon Optimization: Maximizing translational efficiency through species-specific codon preferences enhances antigen production and vaccine potency. Codon optimization is another essential aspect of transgene design. By aligning the codon usage of the transgene with the preferred codon usage of the vector host species, researchers can enhance translational efficiency and antigen expression levels. This optimization not only improves vaccine potency but also minimizes potential immune responses against non-native sequences [30].

Signal Peptide Modification: Rational modification enhances protein trafficking to antigen-presenting compartments, improving antigen processing and presentation efficiency.

Antigen Fusion Strategies: Fusion with immunostimulatory molecules amplifies immune responses, broadening protective immunity against complex pathogens [31].

5.3.4 Immune Evasion Strategies

Effective immune evasion is essential for sustained transgene expression.

Humoral Immune Responses: Nonreplicating viral vectors stimulate the production of antibodies tailored to the encoded antigens. These antibodies play a pivotal role in neutralizing the targeted pathogen, thereby thwarting infection. The effectiveness of this response depends on various factors, such as the levels of antigen expression, the structure of the antigen, and the tropism of the vector. To enhance the humoral immune response, researchers employ engineering strategies. These include incorporating adjuvants or immune modulators into the vaccine formulation. These additives serve as ADCC and complement activation [15].

Cellular Immune Responses: Apart from generating antibodies, nonreplicating viral vectors also activate cellular immunity. This involves the activation of cytotoxic T lymphocytes (CTLs) and T helper cells. CTLs identify and eliminate cells infected with the virus by recognizing the presented antigens, thus eradicating the infection and establishing long-lasting immunity. Developing robust cellular immunity is essential for combating intracellular pathogens and preventing disease relapse. To bolster this aspect of the immune response, researchers focus on optimizing pathways for antigen processing and presentation. Additionally, they explore methods to enhance antigen cross-presentation by APCs and manipulate co-stimulatory signals that are crucial for T cell activation [32].

Immune Checkpoint Inhibition: Inhibitors enhance immunogenicity by blocking inhibitory pathways, synergistically enhancing vaccine efficacy against infectious diseases and cancer. In recent years, immune checkpoint inhibitors (ICIs) have emerged as game-changers in the field of cancer treatment, leveraging the body's own immune defenses to combat tumor cells effectively. These inhibitors work by targeting specific molecules like programmed cell death protein 1 (PD-1), programmed death-ligand 1 (PD-L1), and cytotoxic T lymphocyte–associated protein 4 (CTLA-4), which normally act as brakes on immune responses. By blocking these inhibitory signals, ICIs unleash the immune system, leading to long-lasting responses in certain cancer patients. The success of ICIs in cancer has inspired researchers to explore their potential application in vaccine development. By integrating ICIs into nonreplicating viral vectors, scientists aim to enhance the immune response elicited by vaccines, particularly against infectious diseases where conventional vaccines may fall short [33].

Incorporating ICIs into viral vectors involves careful engineering to ensure both effectiveness and safety. One strategy involves fusing ICIs with viral proteins or antigenic fragments, ensuring their expression alongside vaccine antigens within infected cells. Alternatively, ICIs can be added as separate components, allowing for precise control over their expression levels. Additionally, the choice of viral vector and administration route plays a crucial role in determining the distribution and duration of ICI expression, thus impacting vaccine potency and safety. Numerous studies have demonstrated the feasibility of engineering viral vectors with ICIs for vaccine delivery [34]. For instance, adenoviral vectors encoding PD-L1 have been shown to boost T cell responses and enhance protection against viral infections in animal models. Similarly, vaccines based on AAVs expressing anti–CTLA-4 antibodies have induced robust immune responses against various pathogens, highlighting the versatility of this approach. Integrating ICIs into viral vectors can modulate various aspects of the immune response, influencing vaccine outcomes. By blocking inhibitory signals, ICIs enhance the activation and proliferation of antigen-specific T cells, improving their ability to eliminate pathogens [35]. Moreover, ICIs may influence the balance of regulatory T cells (T_{regs}) and effector T cells, shaping the overall strength and quality of the immune response. Furthermore, ICIs can stimulate neighboring immune cells, amplifying the overall response to vaccination. This bystander effect is particularly beneficial in scenarios where antigen presentation is limited or when targeting immune-privileged sites. However, excessive immune activation induced by ICIs may also trigger autoimmune reactions or immunopathology, emphasizing the need for careful dosing and monitoring in clinical settings [36].

5.4 Applications of Nonreplicating Viral Vectors in Vaccinology

The phase 3 clinical trial evaluated the safety, efficacy, and immunogenicity of a two-dose regimen of AZD1222 in preventing symptomatic and severe COVID-19. A total of 32,451 participants were randomized to receive either AZD1222 (n=21,635) or placebo (n=10,816). AZD1222 demonstrated a favorable safety profile with low rates of serious adverse events comparable to the placebo group. Local and systemic reactions were predominantly mild or moderate. The overall estimated efficacy of AZD1222 in preventing symptomatic and severe COVID-19 was 74.0%, with higher efficacy (83.5%) observed in individuals aged 65 years and older. Notably, no severe or critical symptomatic COVID-19 cases were reported in the fully vaccinated AZD1222 group, whereas eight cases occurred in the placebo group. This indicates a significant reduction in the risk of severe illness. Additionally, AZD1222 demonstrated efficacy in preventing SARS-CoV-2 infection, as evidenced by a 64.3% reduction in nucleocapsid antibody seroconversion compared to placebo. Furthermore, the vaccine induced a significant increase in spike protein binding and neutralizing antibody levels after both doses. These findings suggest that AZD1222 is a safe and effective vaccine against COVID-19, particularly in older adults, and elicits a robust immune response [37].

Researchers investigated the persistence and immune response dynamics of replication-defective adenovirus (Ad) vectors lacking the E1 gene, akin to those encountered in natural infections [38]. This study investigated the persistence and immunogenicity of adenoviral (Ad) vectors in mice. The vectors were found to persist in various tissues, including muscle, liver, and lymphatic tissues, particularly in T cells targeting the antigen encoded by the vector. The vector's genome remained active, leading to sustained production of transgene products and high levels of activated antigen-specific $CD8^+$ T cells and resting memory T cells. While persistent vaccines may present challenges for mass vaccination, this approach could potentially address the limitations of vaccines relying solely on T cell–mediated protection.

The study examined the kinetics of $CD8^+$ T cell responses induced by Ad vectors expressing a truncated Gag of HIV-1. BALB/c mice were vaccinated intramuscularly with AdC68 or AdHu5 vectors. Analysis of lymphocytes isolated from various tissues revealed high frequencies of IFN-γ–secreting $CD8^+$ T cells in spleens and peritoneal lavage, with lower frequencies in blood and lymph nodes. Interestingly, these frequencies remained stable or increased over time, suggesting a delayed development of central memory $CD8^+$ T cells. A booster immunization with a vaccinia virus recombinant expressing the same antigen further increased gag-specific $CD8^+$ T cells, and recall responses failed to contract in most compartments. To rule out the possibility that the transgene product was responsible for the lack of contraction, the study compared $CD8^+$ T cell responses induced by an AdHu5 vector expressing the glycoprotein of LCMV to those elicited by LCMV itself. Results showed that while the frequencies of $CD8^+$ T cells induced by the AdHu5 vector peaked later than those stimulated by LCMV, they remained stable throughout the experiment, whereas responses induced by LCMV rapidly declined [38].

A live attenuated measles vaccine (MV) offers potential as a dual pediatric vaccination approach, providing simultaneous protection against measles and human immunodeficiency virus type 1 (HIV-1). To investigate the ability of a recombinant MVSchw virus to elicit effective immune responses against HIV-1, we engineered the virus to express HIV-1 antigens. The study aimed to evaluate the induction of cytotoxic T cells (CTLs) and neutralizing antibodies targeting conserved HIV-1 epitopes. Our findings demonstrate that a recombinant MVSchw virus expressing an HIV-1–derived CTL polyepitope effectively stimulates HLA-A0201–restricted CTLs targeting multiple conserved HIV-1 epitopes in measles-susceptible mice humanized for HLA-A0201. Additionally, another recombinant MVSchw virus expressing an HIV-189.6 gp140 glycoprotein with deleted hypervariable V1, V2, and V3 loops (ΔV1V2V3gp140) elicits broadly neutralizing antibodies against primary HIV-1 isolates. These results suggest that the MVSchw pediatric vaccination vector is capable of inducing robust cellular and humoral immune responses specific to HIV-1 [39].

A study to investigate the immunogenicity of VSV expressing the structural proteins of hepatitis C virus (HCV), including core (C) and glycoproteins E1 and E2, using both replication-competent (VSV-C/E1/E2) and nonpropagating (VSVΔG-C/E1/E2) variants. Findings revealed that both VSV-C/E1/E2 and VSVΔG-C/E1/E2 efficiently expressed high levels of HCV C, E1, and E2 proteins, demonstrating authentic posttranslational processing. Moreover, the HCV E1-E2 glycoproteins produced by VSV formed noncovalently linked heterodimers and exhibited proper folding, as confirmed by sensitive antibody analysis. Intravenous or intraperitoneal immunization of BALB/c mice with either VSV-C/E1/E2 or VSVΔG-C/E1/E2 elicited significant and comparable antibody responses against HCV core or E2 proteins compared to control mice. Furthermore, both types of viruses induced HCV C-, E1-, or E2-specific $CD8^+$ T cell responses, as evidenced by enzyme-linked immunospot (ELISPOT) analysis. Mice immunized with VSVΔG-C/E1/E2 were also protected against tumor formation expressing HCV E2 (CT26-hghE2t) and showed specific $CD8^+$ T cell activity against E2. Additionally, when recombinant vaccinia virus (vvHCV.S) expressing HCV structural proteins was administered to mice immunized with VSV-C/E1/E2 or VSVΔG-C/E1/E2, viral replication was significantly reduced compared to control groups. These results demonstrate the potential of replication-defective VSV engineered to express authentic HCV glycoproteins. Such an approach holds promise for the development of effective vaccines and immunotherapies for HCV-related diseases [40].

5.5 Optimizing Nonreplicating Viral Vectors for Vaccine Delivery

5.5.1 Enhancing Transduction Efficiency

One of the primary challenges in using viral vectors for vaccine delivery is ensuring the effective transduction of target cells. Techniques to improve transduction efficiency include modifying the surface proteins of vectors to enhance binding to target cell receptors, refining vector production and purification processes, and employing specific ligands or promoters for cell-targeted delivery. By modifying the viral capsid, which encapsulates the viral genome, researchers can enhance vector stability, broaden tropism, and evade immune detection. Strategies such as rational design and directed evolution enable the creation of capsid variants with improved transduction properties and reduced immunogenicity [41]. Pseudotyping involves replacing native viral envelope proteins with those from other viruses to alter vector tropism and enhance transduction efficiency. For instance, incorporating fibers from different serotypes can expand the tropism of adenoviral vectors and bypass preexisting immunity. Fine-tuning the expression cassette encoding the transgene, including promoter strength, enhancer elements, and codon optimization, enhances transgene expression levels and duration. Integration of regulatory elements like microRNA target sites enables control of transgene expression and modulation of immune responses. Optimizing vector formulation, including buffer composition, particle size, and stabilizers, improves vector stability and bioavailability. Selecting appropriate routes of administration, such as intramuscular, intranasal, or intradermal delivery, enhances vector distribution and uptake by target cells [42].

5.5.2 Reducing Immunogenicity and Toxicity

Viral vectors, while nonreplicating, can trigger immune responses against their components, potentially compromising their effectiveness and safety. Strategies to mitigate these responses involve modifying vectors with heterologous envelope proteins to evade preexisting immunity, engineering vectors to minimize activation of the innate immune system, and optimizing dosing and administration routes. By enveloping viral vectors with biocompatible polymers like polyethylene glycol (PEG), we can obscure their surface characteristics, making them less recognizable to the immune system [43]. This "stealth coating" extends their presence in the bloodstream, improving vaccine delivery to target tissues and reducing immune responses. Co-administering immunomodulatory agents alongside viral vector vaccines helps manage inflammatory responses and lessen toxicity. Drugs like corticosteroids or immunosuppressants can mitigate adverse reactions and improve vaccine tolerability [44].

5.5.3 Improving Antigen Expression and Presentation

The level and duration of antigen expression are critical for eliciting robust immune responses. This can be achieved by selecting appropriate promoters and enhancers for transgene expression, engineering vectors to enhance protein stability and secretion, and incorporating immunostimulatory signals for improved antigen presentation and T cell activation. Researchers are exploring advanced techniques to augment vaccine efficacy through the integration of immune modulatory molecules within nonreplicating viral vectors. These vectors are engineered to express cytokines or co-stimulatory ligands, which play pivotal roles in enhancing antigen presentation and stimulating the immune response. By leveraging these molecules, APCs are stimulated, leading to enhanced T cell priming, ultimately resulting in a more robust and effective immune response against the target pathogen [45]. Another innovative approach involves the presentation of multivalent antigens on the surface of viral vectors. This strategy mimics the natural arrangement of antigens found on pathogens, thereby optimizing antigen presentation. Multivalent vaccines enable the cross-linking of antigen receptors on immune cells, amplifying the immune activation process. By presenting multiple copies of the antigen, these vaccines effectively enhance immune recognition and response, consequently improving vaccine efficacy. Adjuvants play a critical role in augmenting the immune response to vaccines by promoting antigen uptake and activation of APCs. Nonreplicating viral vectors can be engineered to deliver antigen-adjuvant combinations, thereby synergistically enhancing antigen presentation and eliciting robust immune responses. Through the strategic integration of adjuvants, vaccine formulations can achieve superior immunogenicity, leading to enhanced protection against the target pathogen [46]. Researchers are exploring innovative strategies to target specific subsets of APCs, such as dendritic cells or macrophages, by modifying the surface proteins of viral vectors. By directing viral vectors to these specialized APC subsets, antigen uptake and presentation can be optimized, leading to enhanced immune activation and vaccine efficacy. This targeted approach allows for precise modulation of the immune response, maximizing the effectiveness of the vaccine against the intended pathogen [47].

5.5.4 Addressing Preexisting Immunity

Preexisting immunity to viral vectors can hinder vaccine efficacy. Strategies to counter this include selecting vectors with low seroprevalence in target populations, engineering vectors to evade neutralizing antibodies, and using prime-boost vaccination regimens with different vector types. One promising avenue is customizing viral vectors to evade preexisting immunity while maintaining their antigen delivery efficiency. This can be accomplished by altering the surface proteins of the vector or introducing shielding molecules that obscure epitopes recognized by neutralizing antibodies. By reducing immune recognition and clearance of the vector, engineered vectors may improve vaccine uptake and antigen expression in target cells. Heterologous prime-boost strategies entail administering different vaccine vectors sequentially to induce robust and lasting immune responses [48]. By alternating between diverse vector platforms or delivery methods, researchers can circumvent vector-specific immunity and strengthen immune memory against target antigens. This tactic has demonstrated efficacy in overcoming vector neutralization and improving vaccine performance in both preclinical and clinical settings. Precision vaccine design involves selecting antigenic targets and vector platforms that are less affected by preexisting immunity. By focusing on conserved or novel antigenic epitopes and employing less immunogenic vector constructs, researchers can mitigate the impact of existing immunity on vaccine responses. Moreover, designing vaccines for mucosal delivery or alternative routes of administration can evade systemic immune responses and enhance vaccine effectiveness in individuals with preexisting immunity [48].

5.5.5 Targeting Vector Delivery to Secondary Lymphoid Organs

Efficient delivery of vaccine antigens to secondary lymphoid organs is essential for robust immune responses. Techniques involve engineering vectors for preferential homing to lymphoid tissues and optimizing administration routes for antigen transport to draining lymph nodes. Heterologous prime-boost strategies entail administering different vaccine vectors sequentially to induce robust and lasting immune responses. By alternating between diverse vector platforms or delivery methods, researchers can circumvent vector-specific immunity and strengthen immune memory against target antigens [49]. This tactic has demonstrated efficacy in overcoming vector neutralization and improving vaccine performance in both preclinical and clinical settings. Precision vaccine design involves selecting antigenic targets and vector platforms that are less affected by preexisting immunity. By focusing on conserved or novel antigenic epitopes and employing less immunogenic vector constructs, researchers can mitigate the impact of existing immunity on vaccine responses. Moreover, designing vaccines for mucosal delivery or alternative routes of administration can evade systemic immune responses and enhance vaccine effectiveness in individuals with preexisting immunity [50].

5.6 Challenges and Future Perspectives

Nonreplicating viral vectors have garnered attention for their potential in vaccine delivery, offering efficient antigen expression and strong immune responses. However, their development and implementation pose persistent challenges. Nonreplicating viral vectors face concerns regarding their immunogenicity and safety. Despite being engineered to be non-pathogenic, there remains a risk of immune reactions against the vector itself. Mitigating this challenge necessitates careful vector design to minimize immunogenicity while ensuring efficacy. Ensuring vector stability throughout manufacturing, storage, and delivery is a significant challenge. Nonreplicating viral vectors may degrade, impacting their potency and consistency. Developing robust manufacturing processes and storage conditions is vital to maintaining the reliability of these vectors for vaccine delivery. While nonreplicating viral vectors can trigger strong humoral immune responses, they may struggle to induce robust cellular immune responses, particularly cytotoxic T cell responses [51]. Enhancing the vector's ability to stimulate cellular immunity is crucial for defending against intracellular pathogens and providing long-lasting immunity. Preexisting immunity to the vector or its components can hinder vaccine efficacy. Many individuals may have prior exposure to similar viruses or vectors through infections or vaccinations, leading to immune responses that interfere with the desired vaccine response. Strategies to overcome preexisting immunity are essential for maximizing vaccine effectiveness. Advancements in vector engineering and synthetic biology are expected to drive the development of next-generation nonreplicating viral vectors with improved safety, immunogenicity, and stability. These vectors may incorporate novel modifications to evade host immune responses or enhance antigen expression, resulting in more potent vaccines. Tailored adjuvants and formulations can enhance the immunogenicity and efficacy of nonreplicating viral vectors. Adjuvants stimulating both humoral and cellular immune responses or modulating immune pathways could be integrated into vaccine formulations to enhance protective immunity. Targeted delivery of nonreplicating viral vectors to specific tissues or cells can enhance vaccine efficacy while minimizing off-target effects. Using tissue-specific promoters or engineering vector particles for cell-specific uptake could improve antigen presentation and immune activation at the desired site. Advances in personalized medicine and vaccine technology may enable the development of tailored vaccines based on individual immune profiles. Personalized nonreplicating viral vectors could elicit optimal immune responses in diverse populations, considering factors like age, genetics, and prior immune history [52].

Nonreplicating viral vectors offer a versatile platform for vaccine development against various infectious diseases, including viral, bacterial, and parasitic pathogens. Their ability to induce potent immune responses makes them valuable for expanding vaccine coverage and addressing unmet medical needs worldwide. Nonreplicating viral vectors could revolutionize pandemic preparedness by enabling rapid development and deployment of vaccines against emerging threats. Their scalability, flexibility, and established manufacturing processes make them suitable for responding to outbreaks and controlling infectious diseases. Developing nonreplicating viral vector vaccines could enhance vaccine accessibility in underserved regions and resource-limited settings. Their relatively simple production requirements and stability at ambient temperatures make them easier to distribute and administer in remote areas, promoting vaccine equity and global health security [53]. Nonreplicating viral vectors hold promise as platforms for long-term immunization strategies, offering durable protection against infectious diseases through booster vaccinations or multivalent formulations. Their ability to induce robust and sustained immune responses presents opportunities for developing vaccines with extended efficacy and durability. While nonreplicating viral vectors offer promise in vaccine delivery, addressing challenges like immunogenicity and vector stability is crucial for their success in public health and vaccination programs. Anticipated advancements in vector design, formulation, and delivery strategies present promising solutions to overcome these hurdles, maximizing the impact of nonreplicating viral vectors on global health. Harnessing these innovative vaccine platforms can enhance our ability to combat current and future infectious disease threats, ultimately benefiting populations worldwide [54].

5.7 Conclusion

Nonreplicating viral vectors have emerged as a transformative approach to vaccine delivery, offering significant advantages over traditional methods. Nonreplicating viral vectors utilize viral genetic material to deliver antigens into host cells without causing replication, ensuring safety while inducing strong immune responses. They have been widely used in developing vaccines for various diseases like HIV, influenza, Ebola, and, notably, COVID-19 due to their ability to present diverse antigens and evoke robust immune responses. These vectors possess inherent adjuvant properties, stimulating innate immune responses and enhancing antigen presentation, which, coupled with their ability to infect APCs, boosts vaccine efficacy. Compared to live attenuated vaccines, nonreplicating viral vectors offer a safer profile by preventing viral replication, thus reducing the risk of adverse events, especially crucial for immunocompromised individuals. Despite their benefits, challenges like preexisting immunity, vector immunogenicity, and stability persist, requiring concerted efforts to address and maximize their potential. Nonreplicating viral vectors signify a revolutionary approach to vaccine development, offering potent and versatile platforms for next-generation vaccines. Their success, exemplified by rapid COVID-19 vaccine development, highlights their potential in addressing global health challenges, not limited to pandemics but extending to diverse infectious agents. Moreover, their versatility extends beyond infectious diseases to areas like cancer immunotherapy, gene therapy, and therapeutic protein delivery, promising advancements in precision medicine.

References

1. Chavda, V.P., Bezbaruah, R., Athalye, M., *et al.*, Replicating Viral Vector-Based Vaccines for COVID-19: Potential Avenue in Vaccination Arena. *Viruses*, 14, 4, 759, 2022.
2. Berg, P. and Mertz, J.E., Personal Reflections on the Origins and Emergence of Recombinant DNA Technology. *Genetics*, 184, 1, 9–17, 2010.
3. Wang, D., Tai, P.W.L., Gao, G., Adeno-associated virus vector as a platform for gene therapy delivery. *Nat. Rev. Drug Discov.*, 18, 5, 358–378, 2019.
4. Trivedi, P.D., Byrne, B.J., Corti, M., Evolving Horizons: Adenovirus Vectors' Timeless Influence on Cancer, Gene Therapy and Vaccines. *Viruses*, 15, 12, 2378, 2023.
5. Mendonça, S.A., Lorincz, R., Boucher, P., Curiel, D.T., Adenoviral vector vaccine platforms in the SARS-CoV-2 pandemic. *npj Vaccines*, 6, 1, 97, 2021.
6. Fausther-Bovendo, H. and Kobinger, G.P., Pre-existing immunity against Ad vectors: Humoral, cellular, and innate response, what's important? *Hum. Vaccin. Immunother.*, 10, 10, 2875–2884, 2014.
7. Al Fayez, N., Nassar, M.S., Alshehri, A.A., *et al.*, Recent Advancement in mRNA Vaccine Development and Applications. *Pharmaceutics*, 15, 7, 1972, 2023.
8. Sakurai, F., Tachibana, M., Mizuguchi, H., Adenovirus vector-based vaccine for infectious diseases. *Drug Metab. Pharmacokinet.*, 42, 100432, 2022.
9. Tessarollo, N.G., Domingues, A.C.M., Antunes, F., *et al.*, Nonreplicating Adenoviral Vectors: Improving Tropism and Delivery of Cancer Gene Therapy. *Cancers*, 13, 8, 1863, 2021.
10. Chang, J., Adenovirus Vectors: Excellent Tools for Vaccine Development. *Immune Netw.*, 21, 1, e6, 2021.
11. Alhashimi, M., Elkashif, A., Sayedahmed, E.E., Mittal, S.K., Nonhuman Adenoviral Vector-Based Platforms and Their Utility in Designing Next Generation of Vaccines for Infectious Diseases. *Viruses*, 13, 8, 1493, 2021.
12. Wold, W. and Toth, K., Adenovirus Vectors for Gene Therapy, Vaccination and Cancer Gene Therapy. *Curr. Gene Ther.*, 13, 6, 421–433, 2014.
13. Schijns, V., Fernández-Tejada, A., Barjaktarović, Z., *et al.*, Modulation of immune responses using adjuvants to facilitate therapeutic vaccination. *Immunol. Rev.*, 296, 1, 169–190, 2020.
14. Yang, L., Gong, L., Wang, P., *et al.*, Recent Advances in Lipid Nanoparticles for Delivery of mRNA. *Pharmaceutics*, 14, 12, 2682, 2022.
15. Shirley, J.L., De Jong, Y.P., Terhorst, C., Herzog, R.W., Immune Responses to Viral Gene Therapy Vectors. *Mol. Ther.*, 28, 3, 709–722, 2020.
16. Arjomandnejad, M., Dasgupta, I., Flotte, T.R., Keeler, A.M., Immunogenicity of Recombinant Adeno-Associated Virus (AAV) Vectors for Gene Transfer. *BioDrugs*, 37, 3, 311–329, 2023.

17. De Haan, P., Van Diemen, F.R., Toscano, M.G., Viral gene delivery vectors: the next generation medicines for immune-related diseases. *Hum. Vaccin. Immunother.*, 17, 1, 14–21, 2021.
18. Trovato, M., Sartorius, R., D'Apice, L., Manco, R., De Berardinis, P., Viral Emerging Diseases: Challenges in Developing Vaccination Strategies. *Front. Immunol.*, 11, 2130, 2020.
19. Crommelin, D.J.A., Volkin, D.B., Hoogendoorn, K.H., Lubiniecki, A.S., Jiskoot, W., The Science is There: Key Considerations for Stabilizing Viral Vector-Based Covid-19 Vaccines. *J. Pharm. Sci.*, 110, 2, 627–634, 2021.
20. Chavda, V.P., Soni, S., Vora, L.K., Soni, S., Khadela, A., Ajabiya, J., mRNA-Based Vaccines and Therapeutics for COVID-19 and Future Pandemics. *Vaccines*, 10, 12, 2150, 2022.
21. Robert-Guroff, M., Replicating and non-replicating viral vectors for vaccine development. *Curr. Opin. Biotechnol.*, 18, 6, 546–556, 2007.
22. Bezbaruah, R., Chavda, V.P., Nongrang, L., *et al.*, Nanoparticle-Based Delivery Systems for Vaccines. *Vaccines*, 10, 11, 1946, 2022.
23. Kutzler, M.A. and Weiner, D.B., DNA vaccines: ready for prime time? *Nat. Rev. Genet.*, 9, 10, 776–788, 2008.
24. Girod, A., Ried, M., Wobus, C., *et al.*, Genetic capsid modifications allow efficient re-targeting of adeno-associated virus type 2. *Nat. Med.*, 5, 9, 1052–1056, 1999.
25. Yang, Q., Mamounas, M., Yu, G., *et al.*, Development of Novel Cell Surface CD34-Targeted Recombinant Adenoassociated Virus Vectors for Gene Therapy. *Hum. Gene Ther.*, 9, 13, 1929–1937, 1998.
26. Suk, J.S., Xu, Q., Kim, N., Hanes, J., Ensign, L.M., PEGylation as a strategy for improving nanoparticle-based drug and gene delivery. *Adv. Drug Delivery Rev.*, 99, 28–51, 2016.
27. Ghauri, M.S. and Ou, L., AAV Engineering for Improving Tropism to the Central Nervous System. *Biology*, 12, 2, 186, 2023.
28. Smirnova, O.G. and Kochetov, A.V., Choice of the Promoter for Tissue and Developmental Stage-Specific Gene Expression [Internet], in: *Biolistic DNA Delivery in Plants*, S. Rustgi and H. Luo (Eds.), pp. 69–106, Springer US, New York, NY, 2020, [cited 2024 May 9]. Available from: http://link.springer.com/10.1007/978-1-0716-0356-7_4.
29. Devkota, P. and Wuchty, S., Promoter/enhancer-based controllability of regulatory networks. *Sci. Rep.*, 12, 1, 3528, 2022.
30. Paremskaia, A.I., Kogan, A.A., Murashkina, A., *et al.*, Codon-optimization in gene therapy: promises, prospects and challenges. *Front. Bioeng. Biotechnol.*, 12, 1371596, 2024.
31. Lee, W. and Suresh, M., Vaccine adjuvants to engage the cross-presentation pathway. *Front. Immunol.*, 13, 940047, 2022.
32. Raskov, H., Orhan, A., Christensen, J.P., Gögenur, I., Cytotoxic CD8+ T cells in cancer and cancer immunotherapy. *Br. J. Cancer*, 124, 2, 359–367, 2021.

33. Batista-Duharte, A., Hassouneh, F., Alvarez-Heredia, P., Pera, A., Solana, R., Immune Checkpoint Inhibitors for Vaccine Improvements: Current Status and New Approaches. *Pharmaceutics*, 14, 8, 1721, 2022.
34. Lin, D., Shen, Y., Liang, T., Oncolytic virotherapy: basic principles, recent advances and future directions. *Signal Transduct. Target. Ther.*, 8, 1, 156, 2023.
35. Koger-Pease, C., Perera, D.J., Ndao, M., Recent Advances in the Development of Adenovirus-Vectored Vaccines for Parasitic Infections. *Pharmaceuticals*, 16, 3, 334, 2023.
36. González-Navajas, J.M., Fan, D.D., Yang, S., *et al.*, The Impact of Tregs on the Anticancer Immunity and the Efficacy of Immune Checkpoint Inhibitor Therapies. *Front. Immunol.*, 12, 625783, 2021.
37. Falsey, A.R., Sobieszczyk, M.E., Hirsch, I., *et al.*, Phase 3 Safety and Efficacy of AZD1222 (ChAdOx1 nCoV-19) Covid-19 Vaccine. *N. Engl. J. Med.*, 385, 25, 2348–2360, 2021.
38. Tatsis, N., Fitzgerald, J.C., Reyes-Sandoval, A., *et al.*, Adenoviral vectors persist in vivo and maintain activated CD8+ T cells: implications for their use as vaccines. *Blood*, 110, 6, 1916–1923, 2007.
39. Lorin, C., Delebecque, F., Labrousse, V., *et al.*, A recombinant live attenuated measles vaccine vector primes effective HLA-A0201-restricted cytotoxic T lymphocytes and broadly neutralizing antibodies against HIV-1 conserved epitopes. *Vaccine*, 23, 36, 4463–4472, 2005.
40. Majid, A.M., Ezelle, H., Shah, S., Barber, G.N., Evaluating Replication-Defective Vesicular Stomatitis Virus as a Vaccine Vehicle. *J. Virol.*, 80, 14, 6993–7008, 2006.
41. Bulcha, J.T., Wang, Y., Ma, H., Tai, P.W.L., Gao, G., Viral vector platforms within the gene therapy landscape. *Signal Transduct. Target. Ther.*, 6, 1, 53, 2021.
42. Cronin, J., Zhang, X.-Y., Reiser, J., Altering the Tropism of Lentiviral Vectors through Pseudotyping. *Curr. Gene Ther.*, 5, 4, 387–398, 2005.
43. Zeng, J., Jaijyan, D.K., Yang, S., Pei, S., Tang, Q., Zhu, H., Exploring the Potential of Cytomegalovirus-Based Vectors: A Review. *Viruses*, 15, 10, 2043, 2023.
44. Jan, N., Madni, A., Khan, S., *et al.*, Biomimetic cell membrane-coated poly(lactic-*co*-glycolic acid) nanoparticles for biomedical applications. *Bioeng. Transl. Med.*, 8, 2, e10441, 2023.
45. Williams, J., Vector Design for Improved DNA Vaccine Efficacy, Safety and Production. *Vaccines*, 1, 3, 225–249, 2013.
46. Caradonna, T.M. and Schmidt, A.G., Protein engineering strategies for rational immunogen design. *npj Vaccines*, 6, 1, 154, 2021.
47. Melgoza-González, E.A., Bustamante-Córdova, L., Hernández, J., Recent advances in antigen targeting to antigen-presenting cells in veterinary medicine. *Front. Immunol.*, 14, 1080238, 2023.

48. Wang, W.-C., Sayedahmed, E.E., Mittal, S.K., Significance of Preexisting Vector Immunity and Activation of Innate Responses for Adenoviral Vector-Based Therapy. *Viruses*, 14, 12, 2727, 2022.
49. Ding, Y., Li, Z., Jaklenec, A., Hu, Q., Vaccine delivery systems toward lymph nodes. *Adv. Drug Deliv. Rev.*, 179, 113914, 2021.
50. Schijns, V., Majhen, D., Van Der Ley, P., *et al.*, Rational Vaccine Design in Times of Emerging Diseases: The Critical Choices of Immunological Correlates of Protection, Vaccine Antigen and Immunomodulation. *Pharmaceutics*, 13, 4, 501, 2021.
51. Naim, H.Y., Applications and challenges of multivalent recombinant vaccines. *Hum. Vaccin. Immunother.*, 9, 3, 457–461, 2013.
52. Van Schaik, E.J., Fratzke, A.P., Gregory, A.E., Dumaine, J.E., Samuel, J.E., Vaccine development: obligate intracellular bacteria new tools, old pathogens: the current state of vaccines against obligate intracellular bacteria. *Front. Cell. Infect. Microbiol.*, 14, 1282183, 2024.
53. Deng, S., Liang, H., Chen, P., *et al.*, Viral Vector Vaccine Development and Application during the COVID-19 Pandemic. *Microorganisms*, 10, 7, 1450, 2022.
54. Vrba, S.M., Kirk, N.M., Brisse, M.E., Liang, Y., Ly, H., Development and Applications of Viral Vectored Vaccines to Combat Zoonotic and Emerging Public Health Threats. *Vaccines*, 8, 4, 680, 2020.

6

Genetically Modified Viral Vectors for Vaccine Delivery

Deepshi Arora[1], Yugam Taneja[2], Diksha Gulati[1], Manish Kumar[3], Anil Pareek[4] and Rupesh K. Gautam[5*]

[1]Guru Gobind Singh College of Pharmacy, Yamunanagar, Haryana, India
[2]Nutrascience, Sidcul, Haridwar, India
[3]Department of Pharmaceutics, ISF College of Pharmacy, Moga, Punjab, India
[4]Lachoo Memorial College of Science and Technology (Autonomous), Jodhpur, Rajasthan, India
[5]Indore Institute of Pharmacy, IIST Campus, Indore, Madhya Pradesh, India

Abstract

Viral vectors that have been genetically altered are ushering in a revolutionary era in vaccine research. These vectors, which are generated from harmless viruses and are designed to transmit certain genetic material, have amazing potential for overcoming immunization difficulties. They can deliver genetic instructions that code for antigens with adaptability and precision, allowing for increased immune responses and the promise of more potent and precisely targeted vaccines for a variety of diseases. To realize the full potential of this technology, prudent development and cautious regulation are essential. It is crucial to strike a careful balance between scientific advancement and ethical considerations, including informed consent and equal access. It is morally necessary to make sure that everyone can benefit from this ground-breaking technology, regardless of their location or any social, economic, or environmental restrictions. This chapter examines the vital significance of moral behavior and the requirement for thorough control in the area of vaccines using genetically engineered viral vectors. It places a focus on the moral issues that must be addressed to protect individual rights and autonomy, such as informed consent and data privacy. Additionally, it emphasizes the importance of maintaining fair access, ensuring that the advantages of this ground-breaking technology are accessible to a variety of global populations. Future developments in this field's study and technology could drastically alter the

**Corresponding author*: drrupeshgautam@gmail.com

Vivek P. Chavda and Vasso Apostolopoulos (eds.) Viral Vectors for Vaccine Delivery, (149–178) © 2025 Scrivener Publishing LLC

practice of preventative medicine. In the future, vaccines will not only be effective and safe but also personalized for specific individuals, increasing social resistance to health emergencies and enhancing global health outcomes. A future where preventative medicine is an unwavering pillar of hope, preserving humanity's health, and promoting a healthier, more just world, is foreshadowed by the revolutionary potential of genetically modified viral vector vaccines.

Keywords: Viral vectors, antigens, genetically modified techniques, novel vaccine platforms, adenovirus, immune, clinical, immunotherapy

6.1 Introduction

Modern biotechnology and medicine have greatly advanced thanks to genetically modified viral vectors, which serve as adaptable tools that are carefully, precisely, and purposefully made. These vectors are produced from viruses that have undergone careful genetic modification to serve as effective carriers of particular genetic material into target cells [1]. To ensure

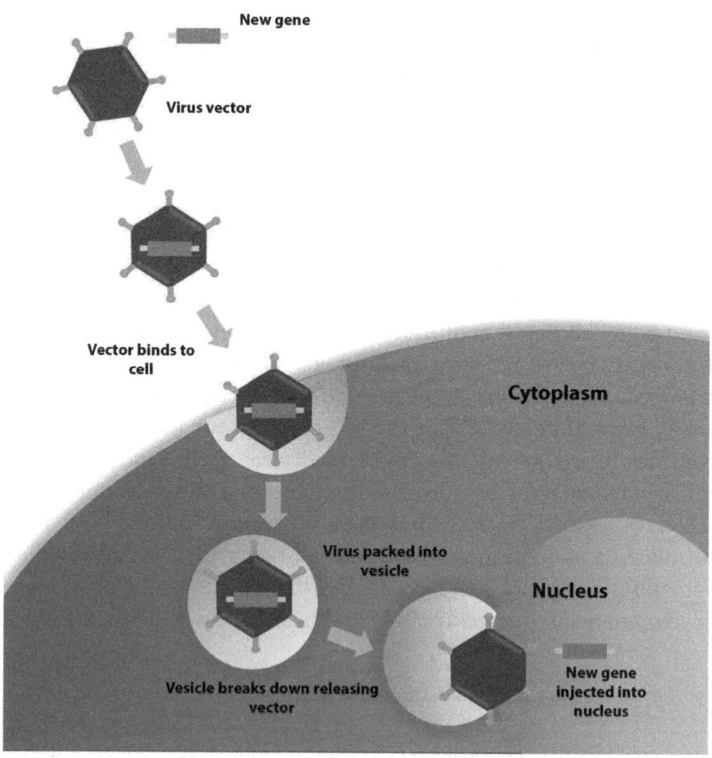

Figure 6.1 Delivery of inserted gene into the host cell.

security, effectiveness, and selectivity in the delivery of desired genetic cargo, this altering method incorporates intentional genetic engineering.

Viruses are clever biological agents that, in their natural state, are known for their capacity to infect host cells by introducing their genetic material—typically DNA or RNA—into the cellular machinery of the host [2]. This innate property of viruses has made them desirable candidates for gene delivery applications, providing a basis for the development of

Table 6.1 Summary of different types of viral vectors along with their descriptions, advantages, and disadvantages.

Type of viral vector	Description	Advantages	Limitations
Adenoviruses	Non-enveloped, double-stranded DNA viruses with a broad host range. They efficiently deliver genes to dividing and nondividing cells.	- Efficient gene delivery to a wide range of cells. - High transduction efficiency and transient gene expression. - Suitable for *in vitro* and *in vivo* gene transfer.	- Immune responses may reduce efficacy for subsequent administrations. - Limited duration of transgene expression. - Preexisting immunity in the population may limit effectiveness.
Lentiviruses	A subgroup of retroviruses with a single-stranded RNA genome. They integrate their genetic material into the host genome, allowing long-term transgene expression in both dividing and nondividing cells.	- Stable, long-term transgene expression due to integration into the host genome. - Suitable for both dividing and nondividing cells. - Low immunogenicity and reduced risk of inflammatory responses.	- More complex production and purification processes compared to other viral vectors. - Integration may cause insertional mutagenesis or disrupt endogenous genes.

(*Continued*)

Table 6.1 Summary of different types of viral vectors along with their descriptions, advantages, and disadvantages. (*Continued*)

Type of viral vector	Description	Advantages	Limitations
Vesicular stomatitis viruses	Negative-sense, single-stranded RNA viruses that have been modified to serve as viral vectors. They are replication-defective.	- High transduction efficiency and rapid expression of transgenes. - Effective gene delivery to various cell types. - Relatively simple to engineer and produce.	- Preexisting immunity in the population against VSV may limit effectiveness. - Potential for induction of immune responses.
Other viral vectors	Various other viral vectors like retroviruses, adeno-associated viruses (AAV), herpes simplex viruses (HSV), etc. Each has unique characteristics, advantages, and limitations.	- Vary based on specific vector types.	- Advantages and limitations depend on the specific vector type.

genetically altered viral vectors. Specific genetic components are altered, added, or removed by carefully manipulating the viral genome, allowing for customized changes that maximize its utility for gene therapy, research, and vaccine production [3].

The genetic alterations made to these viral vectors are purposefully planned with safety as their priority. Important viral genes associated with virulence or unchecked replication are often silenced or deleted entirely [4]. As a result, there is no chance that the resulting viral vector can spread disease to the host. Various genetic sequences, sometimes known as transgenes, are simultaneously inserted into the viral genome. These transgenes convey the desired genetic payload, which may include vaccine-inducing pathogen antigens or therapeutic genes for gene therapy [4].

The effective and precise delivery of the inserted genetic material into the target cells is the main goal of genetically modified viral vectors. The natural infection process that the original virus undertook is mirrored by this delivery method [5]. Researchers may, however, direct the vector to carry out advantageous acts without harming by altering the genetic makeup. As a result, the genetically altered viral vector maintains its capacity to enter host cells, enabling efficient and precise delivery of the inserted genetic material (Figure 6.1).

The summary of different types of viral vectors along with their descriptions, advantages, and disadvantages is shown in Table 6.1.

6.2 Genetic Modification of Viral Vectors

A. Selection of Antigen Genes:

Designing viral vectors for gene delivery requires careful consideration of the antigen genes to be chosen, especially in the context of vaccine development. Antigen genes produce proteins that the immune system can recognize and react to. Several factors affect the choice of antigen genes [6]:

- **Pathogen-Specific Antigens:** These antigens are crucial for infection, replication, or the development of disease in the target pathogen (viral, bacterial, or parasitic). They serve as prime targets for immune responses and possible vaccine candidates because they include surface proteins, poisons, or virulence factors as examples [7].
- **Conservation and Variation:** Favored antigens are those that show a high level of conservation across different strains or serotypes of the pathogen. The vaccine's ability to properly target a wide range of strains is ensured by conservation, which increases its coverage and overall efficacy [8]. However, to address strain-specific immunity or immune evasion mechanisms, consideration of varied antigens is crucial.
- **Immunogenicity:** Emphasis is placed on antigens with the capacity to elicit a strong and focused immunological response, such as the generation of antibodies or stimulation of T cell responses. The antigen's structural characteristics, expression levels, and cellular localization inside the host are all factors that affect immunogenicity, and they all work together to produce a strong immune response [9].

- **Safety Profile:** To avoid negative consequences or autoimmune reactions, it is essential to choose antigens with a good safety profile [10]. To ensure the overall safety and acceptability of the vaccination to recipients, vaccine design prioritizes antigens that are well-tolerated by the host and do not cause adverse reactions.

B. Methods for Gene Insertion:

To ensure effective expression and presentation of the antigen to the host immune system, genetic engineering techniques are used to insert target antigen genes into viral vectors. Typical techniques include the following:

- **Restriction Enzyme Digestion and Ligation:** The viral vector genome and antigen gene are properly cut by restriction enzymes at predetermined locations. In order to create a vaccine, genetic engineering requires a critical step, after which the components are fused to create a recombinant genome.
- **Polymerase Chain Reaction (PCR)–Based Cloning:** By amplifying antigen genes and introducing certain DNA sequences, such as restriction sites, PCR makes it simple to clone antigen genes into viral vector genomes. By creating a large number of copies of the antigen gene and including the appropriate changes for quick integration, this approach speeds up the process [12].
- **Homologous Recombination:** Antigen genes are added to a plasmid that has parts that are identical to the viral vector genome. An exact technique in genetic engineering allows for the seamless insertion of the antigen gene into the vector by recombination between the vector genome and the plasmid [13].
- **Transposon-Mediated Integration:** The antigen gene is incorporated at specified target places within the viral vector genome using transposons, mobile DNA elements [14]. This method enables targeted insertion, increasing the antigen gene's precision and efficiency of integration into the vector.
- **Cas9 Editing:** By directing the insertion of the antigen gene into a specific location within the viral vector genome, Cas9 technology provides accurate gene editing [15].

This cutting-edge method offers precision and control, ensuring that the antigen gene is exactly positioned for the best possible vaccine production.

6.3 Applications of Genetically Modified Viral Vectors

Historic Use in Vaccine Development

Vectors from genetically altered viruses are essential for creating vaccines. In earlier methods, vaccinations were made by attenuating or inactivating wild-type viruses. These techniques raised questions about safety, though. A new era opened up with the advent of genetic engineering, allowing the creation of more secure and potent vaccinations using viral vectors. Viral vectors are safe to use thanks to genetic alterations that make them effective carriers of vital genetic material needed to trigger a strong immune response without the hazards associated with live, attenuated viruses. This development transformed vaccine development, resulting in the development of vaccinations with improved safety and effectiveness characteristics [16].

Current Applications:

- **Viral Vector Vaccines:** Inserting genes that encode antigens from different pathogens, such as viruses and bacteria, into the viral vectors genome constitutes a genetic alteration of viral vectors. Once included, the viral vector functions as an effective delivery system, controlling how these antigens are expressed within the host organism [17]. The host's immune system responds vigorously to this tactical deployment, producing antibodies and activating immune cells as a result. As a result, the person develops immunity against the target infection, serving as the foundation for the creation of vaccines. The development of COVID-19 vaccines using adenoviral vectors, which produce the spike protein antigen of the SARS-CoV-2 virus and trigger a protective immunological response in the recipient, is a prime example of this technology in action.
- **Multivalent Vaccines:** The amazing capacity of viral vectors to contain and deliver several antigen genes is a property that offers great promise for the development of multivalent

vaccinations. These vaccines, which can simultaneously target different strains or serotypes of the disease, are especially important for preventing quickly changing viruses like influenza. This strategy greatly expands the scope of the vaccine's protection, ensuring that the immune system is prepared to detect and neutralize a wide range of virus types. Multivalent viral vector vaccines pave the path for more thorough and adaptive immunization regimens, ultimately strengthening human defenses against ever-evolving infectious dangers [18]. They do this by tackling the difficulty of antigenic variation typical of viruses like influenza.

Emerging Infectious Diseases and Vaccine Development

Infectious diseases that are just now emerging are a hazard to global health. To lessen their impact and rate of transmission, rapid vaccine development is important. Genetically modified viral vectors offer a productive and flexible platform for the development of vaccines against recently emerging infectious diseases.

Applications:

- **Rapid Response Vaccines:** Viral vectors that have been genetically altered provide a flexible foundation for quickly responding to newly developing infectious illnesses [19]. By employing viral vectors, the genetic engineering procedure can be sped up when a new pathogen is discovered to express antigens from the novel threat. The expedited creation of vaccinations specifically crafted to fight the particular virus is made possible by this quick adaptability. One significant instance is the speedy creation of the Ebola and Zika vaccines, where genetic alterations allowed for the quick introduction of viral vector–based immunizations to aid in outbreak containment [20].
- **Pandemic Preparedness:** Because preexisting viral vector systems are flexible, we are prepared to respond quickly in the event of pandemics. Scientists can quickly integrate genes encoding antigens of a recently discovered pathogen by using well-established viral vector frameworks [21]. Our ability to act quickly to emerging infectious illnesses on a worldwide scale is made possible by our agility, which also

permits the rapid development of vaccines. The adaptability of viral vectors makes it possible to develop vaccines that are effective against a variety of new infections, ensuring pandemic preparedness and enhancing our ability to control the spread of infectious threats.

Cancer Immunotherapy

The goal of cancer immunotherapy is to activate the immune system to combat cancer cells. By facilitating the delivery of therapeutic genes or the modification of immune cells, genetically modified viral vectors emerge as powerful partners in this endeavor [22]. These vectors can be modified to carry genes that boost antitumor responses, causing the immune system to be more effective at identifying and combating cancer cells. They can also be used to change immune cells, such as T cells, giving them chimeric antigen receptors (CARs) to improve their capacity to target malignancy. The combination of immunotherapy and genetic modification has great promise for improving cancer treatment methods [23].

Applications:

- **Tumor Antigen Delivery:** Genetically modified viral vectors can be precisely tailored to express tumor antigens, which are proteins unique to cancer cells. By engineering these vectors to carry and deliver tumor antigens, they effectively stimulate the immune system to recognize these abnormal proteins as threats [24]. Consequently, the immune response is galvanized to selectively target and attack cancer cells while sparing healthy ones. This targeted approach holds immense potential in cancer immunotherapy, offering a way to train the immune system to identify and combat the specific markers present in cancer cells.
- **Immune Cell Modification:** Viral vectors are instrumental in modifying immune cells, particularly T cells, to express CARs [25]. CAR-T cell therapy involves genetically altering the patient's T cells to express these receptors, which are designed to specifically recognize and bind to cancer cells. By leveraging viral vectors for the precise integration of CARs into T cells, the immune system's ability to identify and eradicate cancer is significantly enhanced [26]. This innovative approach marks a paradigm shift in cancer treatment,

empowering the immune system to mount a potent and targeted response against malignancies.

Gene Therapy Applications

The goal of gene therapy, a cutting-edge medical strategy, is to introduce, correct, or replace genes within a patient's cells to treat or prevent disease [27]. By acting as precise delivery systems for genes, genetically engineered viral vectors are essential in this sector. These vectors, designed to carry therapeutic genes in specific cells with exceptional accuracy, are safe and effective carriers. The repair of genetic flaws at their root is made possible by this focused gene delivery [28]. The combination of gene therapy with genetically altered viral vectors has the potential to completely transform how a variety of genetic illnesses and diseases are treated [29].

Applications:

- **Gene Replacement Therapy:** Through gene replacement therapy, viral vectors have expanded the possibilities for treating genetic illnesses [30]. Viral vectors can transmit functional copies of these genes to affected cells in diseases where faulty genes are the source of the illness, such as cystic fibrosis or muscular dystrophy. By adding the proper genetic material, the cellular machinery can now generate the necessary proteins, reducing or even reversing the consequences of the disease. By directly treating the genetic root cause and reestablishing normal cellular function, this strategy holds enormous promise for offering effective treatment for a variety of genetic diseases [31].
- **Gene Editing:** Viral vectors that have been genetically altered are essential for developing gene-editing methods like CRISPR-Cas9. These instruments enable targeted mutation or editing of genes within a patient's cells, and they are accurately supplied through viral vectors [32]. We can fix mutations, eliminate detrimental genetic components, or even add helpful genetic alterations by directing these molecular scissors (CRISPR-Cas9) to particular gene sequences. By accurately modifying the genetic code, gene editing has the potential to treat hereditary illnesses at their root, ushering in a new era of therapeutic possibilities with the potential to revolutionize medicine [33].

6.4 Administration of Vaccines

A. Routes of Administration

There are several ways to give vaccines, and each is selected based on the vaccine's characteristics and the desired immunological response:

- **Intramuscular (IM) Injection:** Using this technique, the vaccine is injected into a muscle, usually the deltoid in the upper arm. A strong immunological response is made possible by the IM route's delayed and continuous delivery of the vaccine into the bloodstream. It is a typical and efficient method of administering several vaccines, including those that guard against influenza, measles, and hepatitis [34].
- **Subcutaneous (SC) Injection:** Under the skin, subcutaneous injections are given, typically in the fat of the upper arm. This method is appropriate for some vaccination types since it allows for a delayed absorption of the vaccine. It is frequently used to ensure a powerful immunological response and simple administration of vaccines against rabies and measles.
- **Intradermal (ID) Injection:** With intradermal injections, the vaccine is injected into the skin's dermis layer. This short injection can improve the immunological response while requiring a lesser dose of the vaccine [35]. With the help of the skin's abundant immune cell population, it is employed for particular vaccines like the Bacillus Calmette-Guérin (BCG) vaccine for tuberculosis, which allows for an effective response.
- **Oral Administration:** Common oral vaccines include those for polio and rotavirus, effectively inducing immunity through the gastrointestinal tract. Oral vaccines are delivered through the mouth, frequently as drops or tablets [36]. This administration method provides ease of use, making it particularly useful for mass vaccination programs [37]. It offers the potential for increased compliance, especially in children and those averse to injections.
- **Nasal Administration:** The vaccination is given via the nasal passages using sprays or droplets during nasal administration. Intranasal vaccinations are appropriate for this route, particularly for respiratory illnesses like influenza [38].

Targeting mucosal immune responses in the respiratory system, a crucial region for infections offers a noninvasive and practical approach.

- **Intravenous (IV) Injection:** Intravenous injections deliver the vaccine directly into a vein, allowing rapid and complete distribution of the vaccine throughout the body [39]. This route is reserved for specific vaccines and situations, often in a clinical setting where precise dosing and immediate systemic distribution of the vaccine are required for diseases like yellow fever or certain travel vaccines.

B. Vaccine Delivery Mechanisms

Needle and Syringe: This time-honored approach to vaccination administration has shown to be effective and popular. It is appropriate for a variety of injection methods, including intramuscular (IM), subcutaneous (SC), and intradermal (ID), and it enables accurate dosage management. Despite being successful, the use of needles may be unsettling for some people.
Jet Injectors: Without using needles, jet injectors use high pressure on a small skin incision to administer immunizations [40, 41]. For those who have a needle phobia, this technology provides a needle-free alternative that may be extremely helpful. Jet injectors can also speed up the procedure, improving the effectiveness of large immunization efforts.
Microneedle Patches: The vaccine is delivered through the skin using small, painless needles found in microneedle patches. They provide a practical and possibly self-administrable substitute for conventional injections [42]. Microneedles are particularly helpful for vaccination, especially in situations where self-administration or more straightforward immunization techniques are desirable since their lack of pain improves patient acceptance.

C. Clinical Trials and Regulatory Approvals

Clinical Trials:

Phase 1 Clinical Trial: The vaccine is first administered to a small group of healthy volunteers to evaluate its safety, dose, and capacity to elicit an immunological response [43]. Participants are continuously watched by researchers for any negative effects, and dosages are changed as necessary.
Phase 2 Clinical Trial: This phase involves a bigger group and attempts to assess safety and effectiveness further. It offers information on

recommended dosages, lists typical adverse effects, and starts to compile statistics on the vaccine's efficacy [44].
Phase 3 Clinical Trial: This level involves a much larger group—often thousands of people. Its main objectives are to verify the vaccine's effectiveness, carefully monitor side effects, and gather further safety information. For regulatory approval, it offers critical proof.
Phase 4 Clinical Trial: Following regulatory approval, this phase encompasses post-marketing surveillance [45]. To maintain the vaccine's safety and efficacy, it wants to monitor its long-term impacts and performance in the general population on a larger scale.

Regulatory Approvals:

Preclinical Testing: Vaccines are rigorously tested on animals and in laboratories before being used in human trials to determinc their safety, effectiveness, and prospective effectiveness. The decision to proceed with clinical trials is based on the vital information provided at this point [46].
Investigational New Drug (IND) Application: A preclinical test application, or IND, is a submission to a regulatory body like the FDA that contains specific data from the preclinical testing. It asks permission to begin human clinical trials and provides proof of the vaccine's security and possible advantages [47].
New Drug Application (NDA): NDA requires the submission of extensive data on the vaccine's manufacture, quality control, safety, and efficacy. It is a formal request made to regulatory bodies asking for permission to commercialize and distribute the vaccine [48].
Regulatory Review and Approval: This process entails a thorough evaluation by regulatory agencies like the FDA or EMA to ascertain whether the vaccine satisfies the requirements for market authorization in terms of safety, efficacy, and quality. Safe public health is ensured through a thorough evaluation [49].

6.5 Immune Response and Protection

A. Mechanism of Immune Response:

Innate Immune Response: Innate immunity provides instant, all-encompassing defense against viruses and other infections. Examples of components include skin as a physical barrier, macrophages and dendritic cells as cells, and cytokines and interferons as chemicals. Pathogen-associated molecular patterns (PAMPs), which are common characteristics of viruses, are recognized by innate immune cells when they come into contact with them [50].

Adaptive Immune Response: It takes time for the particular adaptive immune response to emerge. Equal parts of cellular and humoral responses are involved. B cells produce antiviral antibodies and are involved in the humoral response [51]. T cells, which are part of the cellular response, recognize contaminated cells and assist in their destruction ($CD4^+$ helper T cells and $CD8^+$ cytotoxic T cells).

Antigen Presentation: Dendritic cells, in particular, are specialized antigen-presenting cells (APCs), which present antigens produced by the virus to T lymphocytes. The activation of T cells and the beginning of the adaptive immune response—a crucial line of defense against infection—are sparked by this interaction, which serves as a catalyst [52].

Memory Cells: The immune system creates memory B cells and memory T cells, which are specialist memory cells, after coming into touch with a virus through infection or immunizations. These cells retain a "memory" of the different antigens the virus exposed [53]. Memory B cells are ready to produce antibodies right away if the same antigen reappears, allowing for a speedier and more efficient antibody response. Memory T cells, on the other hand, can immediately recognize and attack contaminated cells, effectively halting the virus's ability to spread throughout the body. The immunological memory supports long-lasting protection against specific pathogens.

B. Immune Memory and Long-Term Protection:

Memory B Cells: When exposed to the virus again, memory B cells can quickly develop into plasma cells that generate antibodies, resulting in a quick and effective immune response [54].

Memory T Cells: Memory long-term immunity depends on T cells. They can identify and target infected cells, stopping the virus's internal spread [55].

Long-Term Immunity: Memory cells provide long-term protection that lessens the intensity and duration of subsequent infections.

C. Effectiveness of Genetically Modified Viral Vector Vaccines:

Viral Vector Vaccines: Viral vector vaccines that have undergone genetic modification use a benign virus called the viral vector as a secure and reliable delivery method [56]. This vector carries genes that code for particular antigens from the target virus. Once injected, the vector quickly and effectively delivers this substance into cells, triggering an immune response that kills the intended virus. The immune system is efficiently prepared to fight off the actual virus by simulating the natural infection process.

Immune Response Induction: The viral vector's genes give instructions to cells on how to make antigens specific to the target virus [57]. As a result, the immune system detects these antigens as foreign and launches a potent defense. This comprises the activation of T cells and the synthesis of antibodies by B cells, which cooperate to neutralize the danger and create an immunological memory [58].

Long-Term Protection: The ability to provide enduring protection against the target virus is a strength of genetically modified viral vector vaccines. For the development of long-lasting immunity, the dual-pronged immune response involving both antibodies and T cells is essential [59]. When exposed to the antigens again, memory B cells quickly produce antibodies because they "remember" them. Memory T cells locate and eliminate contaminated cells to stop the spread of viruses inside the body. The risk and severity of recurrent infections are considerably decreased by this long-lasting immunity.

Enhanced Immune Memory: The vector-based strategy promotes the development of memory cells by inducing a strong immunological response [60]. This improved immunological memory aids in long-lasting defense against the target pathogen. The memory B cells and memory T cells produced continuously patrol the body, prepared to perform a quick and effective response when the virus is encountered again. This characteristic increases immunity's longevity, possibly outlasting the protection offered by several other vaccination kinds.

6.6 Case Studies

Adenoviruses for COVID-19: Johnson & Johnson (Janssen) and AstraZeneca (Vaxzevria) deploy genetically modified adenoviruses in their COVID-19 vaccines to combat the SARS-CoV-2 virus. The genetic information for the spike protein of the SARS-CoV-2 virus is transmitted via a modified adenovirus vector. The introduction of this genetic material into cells via the vector results in the production of the spike protein. Because the immune system perceives the protein as being foreign, it reacts violently [61]. This response prepares the body to combat the virus on its own if it reappears. These vaccinations have greatly aided global immunization initiatives and have been efficient in avoiding COVID-19.

Vesicular Stomatitis Viruses for Ebola: In their COVID-19 vaccines, Johnson & Johnson (Janssen) and AstraZeneca (Vaxzevria) use genetically modified adenoviruses to combat the SARS-CoV-2 virus. The genetic information for the spike protein produced by the SARS-CoV-2 virus has been added to the adenovirus vector [62]. The vector carries this genetic material into cells, resulting in the production of the spike protein. The immune system reacts powerfully because it perceives the protein as being foreign. The body is prepared to battle the virus on its own if it reappears as a result of this reaction. These vaccines have been successful in preventing COVID-19, and they have made a substantial contribution to global vaccination campaigns.

Various Viral Vectors for HIV, Malaria, etc.: In the fight against challenging diseases like HIV and malaria, many viral vectors are being studied for their potential to deliver specific antigens and induce targeted immune responses. Experimental vaccines against HIV and malaria transmit genetic material encoding antigens linked to these diseases via viral vectors [63]. When given, these immunizations cause the immune system to recognize the associated pathogens and mount an assault against them. Despite the fact that these vaccinations are still at the experimental stage, this approach shows promise in revolutionizing preventive measures against HIV, malaria, and other dangerous diseases, providing hope for more successful immunization in the future. Table 6.2 shows a comparison of genetically modified viral vector vaccines.

Table 6.2 Comparison of genetically modified viral vector vaccines.

Vaccine	Disease targeted	Genetic material encoded	Safety profile	Efficacy	Potential for personalization
Johnson & Johnson COVID-19	COVID-19	SARS-CoV-2 spike protein	Well-established	High efficacy	Potential for customization
AstraZeneca COVID-19	COVID-19	SARS-CoV-2 spike protein	Well-established	High efficacy	Potential for customization
Ervebo	Ebola	Ebola virus glycoprotein	Proven	High efficacy	Potential for customization
Potential Future Vaccines	Various (e.g., cancer and genetic disorder)	Disease-specific antigens	Ongoing research	Varied efficacy	Promising potential

6.7 Challenges and Future Directions

A. Safety Concerns and Risk Mitigation:

Adverse Events: A major worry is the safety profile of any intervention, including viral vector–based therapy [64]. Viral vector–related adverse events might range from minor side effects like discomfort at the injection site to more serious allergic reactions. Before any medicine is approved, extensive preclinical and clinical testing is done to reduce these risks. This includes lengthy safety evaluations in lab settings and subsequent human subject studies [65]. A functioning pharmacovigilance system is in place to keep track of unfavorable outcomes after approval. Maintaining the public's trust and promptly addressing any emergent safety concerns need prompt and proper responses to unfavorable situations.
Integration and Genomic Stability: The possibility for viral vector DNA to be incorporated into the host genome is a worry in gene therapy that uses viral vectors. Such integration might impair the function of the host gene normally and have long-term consequences, such as oncogenesis. Vector design strategies concentrate on minimizing integration events to reduce this danger [66]. It is now possible to create non-integrating vectors, which do not integrate their genetic material into the host genome. These vectors guarantee the desired genetic modifications while preventing unwanted genomic changes. As a result, there is a considerably lower chance of upsetting normal genomic stability, which is consistent with the safety objectives of gene therapy and viral vector applications.

B. Regulatory Considerations:

Approval and Standardization: For genetically engineered viral vector vaccines to be approved, clear regulatory requirements must be established. These regulations ought to include a thorough assessment of production consistency, effectiveness, and safety. A standardized method guarantees that all vaccinations go through a thorough and uniform evaluation procedure, giving regulators and the public a basis for comparison and assurance [67]. It also increases trust in the security and effectiveness of these novel vaccines. To speed up the deployment of these vaccinations on a larger scale and facilitate their timely access to populations across numerous countries, it is essential to achieve global standardization in approval processes.
Adaptability and Flexibility: The rules governing vaccines made with genetically engineered viral vectors ought to be flexible and adaptable.

Genetic engineering and viral vector technology are fields that are developing quickly [68]. Regulations ought to be adaptable enough to take into account new developments in science and our understanding of viral vectors. This adaptability fosters ongoing innovation and permits prompt responses to newly developing infectious illnesses. Regulations that are timely adjusted ensure that cutting-edge research and technical advancements can be promptly turned into safe and effective vaccinations, which ultimately benefit public health and efforts to manage diseases globally [69].

C. Advances in Vector Design and Technology:

Enhanced Specificity and Efficiency: The goal of improvements in viral vector design is to target particular cells or tissues with greater precision [70]. These vectors can successfully carry therapeutic payloads, such as genetic material or vaccinations, to the intended target by focusing on certain cellular receptors or surface indicators. This increased specificity reduces off-target effects and lowers the possibility of unwanted repercussions in cells that are not the target. This improvement greatly strengthens the vaccine's therapeutic or preventative effects and ensures a more effective and focused distribution of the appropriate therapeutic ingredients [71].

Non-Integrating Vectors: Safety problems related to the potential genomic integration of viral vector components are addressed by the creation of non-integrating viral vectors. Concerns about mutagenesis and oncogenesis are raised by the possibility that integrating vectors could alter the DNA of host cells [72]. These safety concerns are allayed by the fact that non-integrating vectors do not integrate into the host DNA. Non-integrating vectors decrease the possibility of long-term genetic changes while preserving payload delivery efficacy, ensuring a safer profile for the treatment strategy. This development is especially important for long-term applications, such as gene treatments, where preventing irreversible genetic modifications is essential for patient safety and the overall effectiveness of the therapeutic process [73].

D. Potential for Personalized Vaccines:

Individualized Immunization: Future advancements in viral vector technology may result in a ground-breaking strategy—personalized vaccines created to address a person's particular genetic makeup and medical issues. Scientists can modify viral vector–based vaccinations to optimize immune responses by examining a person's genetic makeup and health information [74]. This customization enables targeted antigen selection, resulting in a more potent and focused immune response. We may be able to unlock improved vaccine efficacy and responsiveness by utilizing customized viral vectors, which might result in a new era of personalized medicine in the field of immunization [75].

Cancer Immunotherapies: With the introduction of personalized viral vector vaccines for cancer immunotherapies, the boundaries of cancer treatment are being rewritten. Based on the distinct tumor profile of each patient, these vaccines are designed to target certain tumor antigens [76]. The immune system is stimulated to recognize and target cancer cells with unparalleled specificity by using viral vectors to transfer genetic material encoding tumor-specific antigens. The body's inherent defenses against cancer can be strengthened by using this personalized strategy, which could result in more effective and precise cancer therapies. A key step forward in the fight against cancer is the customization of the vaccine to a patient's tumor profile, demonstrating the potential of viral vectors in personalized oncological therapies [78].

E. Ethical and Societal Implications:

Equitable Access: To reduce global health inequities, equitable access to genetically engineered viral vector vaccines is essential. To do this, it is necessary to ensure the equitable distribution and accessibility of these cutting-edge vaccines, particularly in low-income nations where healthcare resources could be few [79]. To promote technology transfer, reasonable pricing, and assist regional manufacturing capacity, we should encourage cooperation between governments, international organizations, and pharmaceutical corporations. By pooling resources and expertise to ensure equitable vaccination allocation, programs like COVAX also play a crucial role in ensuring equitable access and, eventually, addressing health inequities on a global scale [80].

Informed Consent and Transparency: Informed consent and openness are pillars of the ethical framework governing vaccinations using genetically engineered viral vectors. Before agreeing to get these vaccines, people must be thoroughly educated about their nature, potential risks, and advantages [81]. The importance of open and transparent communication of the associated genetic modifications, potential side effects, and overall safety profiles cannot be overstated. To build trust and understanding, governments, healthcare practitioners, and researchers must communicate openly with the general population. To ensure that vaccination decisions are well-informed, this entails spreading information through a variety of channels, such as understandable instructional materials and public forums [82].

Privacy and Data Security: When using individual genetic data for the creation of personalized vaccinations, privacy protection and strong data security measures are crucial. To preserve public confidence and safeguard people's right to privacy, sensitive genetic data must be protected from unauthorized access or misuse [83]. It is crucial to strike the correct balance between using this important information for scientific research and making sure that all data are strictly anonymized and encrypted. It is crucial to put in place strict regulatory frameworks that specify how genetic data should be gathered, maintained, and disseminated while giving individuals control over their data. Such actions will support privacy while simultaneously promoting involvement in genetic research for the greater good [84].

6.8 Conclusion

A. Summary of Key Points:

Mechanism of Immune Response: Innate immunity provides immediate, nonspecific defense mechanisms against pathogens, while adaptive immunity is a targeted and specific response that involves B cells, which produce antibodies, and T cells, which orchestrate targeted attacks on infected or abnormal cells. This response culminates in the formation of memory cells, which provide long-term protection by recognizing and swiping away foreign substances.

Genetically Modified Viral Vector Vaccines: To transmit genetic material encoding antigens of a target pathogen, genetically modified viral vector vaccines, such as the COVID-19 vaccines made by Johnson & Johnson and AstraZeneca and the Ebola vaccine Ervebo, use weak or nonpathogenic viruses as carriers (viral vectors). When the host cells display these antigens, a powerful immune response is triggered against the targeted illness. HIV and malaria vaccines are being investigated for promising applications, demonstrating the adaptability and potential of this technology in combating several difficult diseases.

Efficacy, Safety, and Impact: Genetically modified viral vector vaccines, such as the COVID-19 vaccines produced by Johnson & Johnson and AstraZeneca and the Ebola vaccine Ervebo, use weak or nonpathogenic viruses as carriers (viral vectors) to convey genetic material encoding antigens of a target pathogen. A potent immune response is generated against the targeted sickness when the host cells exhibit these antigens. The versatility and potential of this technology in battling several challenging diseases are illustrated by the investigation of HIV and malaria vaccines for prospective applications.

Challenges and Future Directions: The development of vaccines using genetically engineered viral vectors is shaped by several important problems and prospects. It is crucial to address safety issues and stringent regulatory requirements to make sure the vaccinations adhere to high safety standards. Vector design and technology advancements are crucial for these vaccines' effectiveness and specificity to be maximized. Additionally, there is significant promise in researching genetically tailored vaccines. To respect ethical norms while maximizing the potential of this technology for improvements to public health, ethical concerns including informed consent, data protection, and equitable distribution also need to be carefully considered. These factors influence how viral vector–based vaccines may develop in the future.

B. The Role of Genetically Modified Viral Vectors in the Future of Vaccine Development:

By addressing immunization issues, genetically engineered viral vectors demonstrate potential in the creation of vaccines. The promise for more effective and targeted vaccinations against a variety of diseases is fostered by their adaptability and accuracy in delivering genetic material encoding antigens, which promotes increased immune responses.

Efficiency and Specificity: The invention of genetically altered viral vectors is a shining example of how to develop vaccines with more precision and efficacy. Vector design advancements allow for the exact targeting of particular cells and tissues throughout the body. Vaccines can be administered precisely by modifying these vectors to recognize and bind to specific cellular receptors or surface indicators. Ensuring that the desired immune response is elicited in the proper cells and minimizing off-target effects improves vaccine effectiveness by lowering the possibility of unexpected reactions in areas that are not targeted. In the end, this precision paves the door for extremely potent and specifically tailored vaccinations, boosting the immunization sector.

Customization and Personalization: Genetically altered viral vectors provide a promising avenue for individualized and customized vaccines, signaling a paradigm shift in healthcare. These vectors can be modified to accommodate a person's particular genetic profile and medical needs.

Vaccines can be precisely adjusted to each person's unique genetic information to elicit the best immune responses. This novel strategy has the potential to transform healthcare by offering a level of personalization that ensures each person's utmost safety and effectiveness. A new era in healthcare where vaccinations are specially created to match each patient's unique needs and characteristics is the personalized vaccine era, which is soon to arrive.

Broad Application Spectrum: Genetically engineered viral vectors' adaptability and versatility broaden their range of potential uses beyond infectious illnesses. These vectors are an effective tool for creating vaccines against a variety of illnesses, such as genetic abnormalities and cancer immunotherapies. Viral vectors can trigger tailored immune responses against cancer cells or rectify genetic defects by integrating the genetic material encoding certain antigens linked to these disorders. This adaptability demonstrates the enormous potential of genetically altered viral vectors to treat a wide range of health issues, from infectious diseases to complicated genetic disorders, ushering in a new era of therapeutic interventions and developments in contemporary medicine.

C. Closing Thoughts on the Significance of This Technology:

In the field of vaccination, genetically altered viral vectors have become a ground-breaking technique that holds great promise for addressing persistent health issues. These vectors exhibit amazing versatility since they were created from nonpathogenic viruses and modified to convey certain genetic material. Their adaptability comes from their capacity to transmit genetic instructions that encode antigens, imitate diseases, and elicit specific immune reactions. This adaptability is essential for successfully treating a variety of illnesses, such as infectious disorders like COVID-19, as demonstrated by the vaccines developed by Johnson & Johnson and AstraZeneca, among other illnesses.

Vaccines using genetically engineered viral vectors are known for their effectiveness and safety. Their safety profiles are ensured by extensive study and rigorous testing, making them appropriate for widespread use. Furthermore, their ability to trigger powerful immune responses makes them effective weapons against disease. Their efficiency is significantly increased by the potential to produce long-lasting defense by producing memory cells.

Looking ahead, the potential for a healthcare revolution with customized vaccines is provided by genetically engineered viral vectors. Personalized vaccinations can be created to optimize immune responses by utilizing unique genetic and health characteristics. This portends a time when vaccines will be made specifically for each person, maximizing their capacity for prevention.

However, careful regulation and prudent development are essential. To ensure that the advantages of new technology reach all populations and leave no one behind, it is essential to strike a balance between advancement and ethical considerations, informed consent, and fair access. In the end, the ongoing development of research and technology in this area promises to transform the practice of preventive medicine, possibly resulting in a world with more efficient, safe, and customized vaccines that significantly improve societal resilience to health crises and global health outcomes.

References

1. Travieso, T., Li, J., Mahesh, S., Mello, J.D., Blasi, M., The use of viral vectors in vaccine development. *npj Vaccines*, 7, 1, 75, 2022 Jul 4.
2. Rampersad, S. and Tennant, P., Replication and expression strategies of viruses. *Viruses*, 55, 2018.
3. Kim, J., Eygeris, Y., Gupta, M., Sahay, G., Self-assembled mRNA vaccines. *Adv. Drug Deliv. Rev.*, 170, 83–112, 2021 Mar 1.
4. Dwivedi, S., Purohit, P., Vasudeva, A., Kumar, M., Agrawal, R., Sheikh, N.A., Misra, R., Kishore, S., Misra, S., Gene therapy and gene editing in healthcare, in: *Biotechnology in Healthcare,* pp. 147–175, Academic Press, United States, 2022 Jan 1.
5. Sasso, E., D'Alise, A.M., Zambrano, N., Scarselli, E., Folgori, A., Nicosia, A., New viral vectors for infectious diseases and cancer. *Semin. Immunol.*, 50, 101430, 2020 Aug 1, Academic Press.
6. Merten, O. W., and Gaillet, B., Viral vectors for gene therapy and gene modification approaches. *Biochem. Eng. J.*, 108, 98–115, 2016 Apr 15.
7. Ali, A., Waris, A., Khan, M.A., Asim, M., Khan, A.U., Khan, S., Zeb, J., Recent advancement, immune responses, and mechanism of action of various vaccines against intracellular bacterial infections. *Life Sci.*, 28, 121332, 2022 Dec.
8. Graves, C.J., Ros, V.I., Stevenson, B., Sniegowski, P.D., Brisson, D., Natural selection promotes antigenic evolvability. *PLoS Pathog.*, 9, 11, e1003766, 2013 Nov 14.
9. Nooraei, S., Bahrulolum, H., Hoseini, Z.S., Katalani, C., Hajizade, A., Easton, A.J., Ahmadian, G., Virus-like particles: Preparation, immunogenicity and their roles as nano vaccines and drug nanocarriers. *J. Nanobiotechnol.*, 19, 1, 1–27, 2021 Dec.
10. Riley, R.S., June, C.H., Langer, R., Mitchell, M.J., Delivery technologies for cancer immunotherapy. *Nat. Rev. Drug Discov.*, 18, 3, 175–96, 2019 Mar.
11. Mackett, M.I., Smith, G.L., Moss, B.E., General method for production and selection of infectious vaccinia virus recombinants expressing foreign genes. *J. Virol.*, 49, 3, 857–64, 1984 Mar.

12. Mardanova, E.S., Blokhina, E.A., Tsybalova, L.M., Peyret, H., Lomonossoff, G.P., Ravin, N.V., Efficient transient expression of recombinant proteins in plants by the novel pEff vector based on the genome of potato virus X. *Front. Plant Sci.*, 8, 247, 2017 Feb 28.
13. Yee, J.K., Miyanohara, A., LaPorte, P., Bouic, K., Burns, J.C., Friedmann, T., A general method for the generation of high-titer, pantropic retroviral vectors: highly efficient infection of primary hepatocytes. *Proc. Natl. Acad. Sci.*, 91, 20, 9564–8, 1994 Sep 27.
14. Moretti, A., Ponzo, M., Nicolette, C.A., Tcherepanova, I.Y., Biondi, A., Magnani, C.F., The past, present, and future of non-viral CAR T cells. *Front. Immunol.*, 13, 867013, 2022 Jun 9.
15. Fajrial, A.K., He, Q.Q., Wirusanti, N.I., Slansky, J.E., Ding, X., A review of emerging physical transfection methods for CRISPR/Cas9-mediated gene editing. *Theranostics*, 10, 12, 5532, 2020.
16. Liu, M.A., DNA vaccines: a historical perspective and view to the future. *Immunol. Rev.*, 239, 1, 62–84, 2011 Jan.
17. Afrough, B., Dowall, S., and Hewson, R., Emerging viruses and current strategies for vaccine intervention. *Clin. Exp. Immunol.*, 196, 2, 157–166, 2019.
18. Harris, C.L., Pouw, R.B., Kavanagh, D., Sun, R., Ricklin, D., Developments in anti-complement therapy; from disease to clinical trial. *Mol. Immunol.*, 102, 89–119, 2018 Oct 1.
19. Mastellos, D. C., Hajishengallis, G., and Lambris, J. D., A guide to complement biology, pathology and therapeutic opportunity. *Nat. Rev. Immunol.*, 24, 2, 118–141, 2024 Feb.
20. Bloom, K., van den Berg, F., Arbuthnot, P., Self-amplifying RNA vaccines for infectious diseases. *Gene Ther.*, 28, 3-4, 117–29, 2021 Apr.
21. Gebre, M.S., Brito, L.A., Tostanoski, L.H., Edwards, D.K., Carfi, A., Barouch, D.H., Novel approaches for vaccine development. *Cell*, 184, 6, 1589–603, 2021 Mar 18.
22. Kinloch, N., Addressing and leveraging within-and between-host HIV genetic diversity towards ending the HIV pandemic.
23. Keshavarz, A., Salehi, A., Khosravi, S., Shariati, Y., Nasrabadi, N., Kahrizi, M.S., Maghsoodi, S., Mardi, A., Azizi, R., Jamali, S., Fotovat, F., Recent findings on chimeric antigen receptor (CAR)-engineered immune cell therapy in solid tumours and haematological malignancies. *Stem Cell Res. Ther.*, 13, 1, 1–22, 2022 Dec.
24. Choi, Y., and Chang, J., Viral vectors for vaccine applications. Clinical and experimental vaccine research, 2, 2, 97–105, 2013.
25. Labbé, R.P., Vessillier, S., Rafiq, Q.A., Lentiviral vectors for T cell engineering: clinical applications, bioprocessing and future perspectives. *Viruses*, 13, 8, 1528, 2021 Aug 2.
26. Dana, H., Chalbatani, G.M., Jalali, S.A., Mirzaei, H.R., Grupp, S.A., Suarez, E.R., Rapôso, C., Webster, T.J., CAR-T cells: Early successes in blood cancer

and challenges in solid tumours. *Acta Pharm. Sin. B*, 11, 5, 1129–47, 2021 May 1.
27. Haidar, Z.S., Introductory Chapter: Unraveling the Complexities of DNA Replication, Epigenetics, and Gene Therapy Applications, in: *DNA Replication-Epigenetic Mechanisms and Gene Therapy Applications*, IntechOpen, United Kingdom, London, 2023 Sep 6.
28. Yin, H., Kanasty, R.L., Eltoukhy, A.A., Vegas, A.J., Dorkin, J.R., Anderson, D.G., Non-viral vectors for gene-based therapy. *Nat. Rev. Genet.*, 15, 8, 541–55, 2014 Aug.
29. Chandrasekaran, S.N., Ceulemans, H., Boyd, J.D., Carpenter, A.E., Image-based profiling for drug discovery: due for a machine-learning upgrade? *Nat. Rev. Drug Discov.*, 20, 2, 145–59, 2021 Feb.
30. Li, H., Yang, Y., Hong, W., Huang, M., Wu, M., Zhao, X., Applications of genome editing technology in the targeted therapy of human diseases: mechanisms, advances and prospects. *Signal transduct. target. ther.*, 5, 1, 1, 2020 Jan 3.
31. van Haasteren, J., Li, J., Scheideler, O.J., Murthy, N., Schaffer, D.V., The delivery challenge: fulfilling the promise of therapeutic genome editing. *Nat. Biotechnol.*, 38, 7, 845–55, 2020 Jul.
32. Zhang, H., Qin, C., An, C., Zheng, X., Wen, S., Chen, W., Liu, X., Lv, Z., Yang, P., Xu, W., Gao, W., Application of the CRISPR/Cas9-based gene editing technique in basic research, diagnosis, and therapy of cancer. *Mol. Cancer*, 20, 1–22, 2021 Dec.
33. Li, T., Yang, Y., Qi, H., Cui, W., Zhang, L., Fu, X., He, X., Liu, M., Li, P.F., Yu, T., CRISPR/Cas9 therapeutics: progress and prospects. *Signal Transduct. Target. Ther.*, 8, 1, 36, 2023 Jan 16.
34. Khoshandam, M., Soltaninejad, H., Mousazadeh, M., Hamidieh, A.A., Hosseinkhani, S., Clinical applications of the CRISPR/Cas9 genome-editing system: Delivery options and challenges in precision medicine. *Genes Dis.*, 11, 1, 268–82, 2023 Mar 25.
35. Zhao, Z., Li, C., Tong, F., Deng, J., Huang, G., and Sang, Y., Review of applications of CRISPR-Cas9 gene-editing technology in cancer research. *Biol. Proced. Online*, 23, 1–13, 2021.
36. Ramirez, J.E., Sharpe, L.A., Peppas, N.A., Current state and challenges in developing oral vaccines. *Adv. Drug Deliv. Rev.*, 114, 116–31, 2017 May 15.
37. Homayun, B., Lin, X., Choi, H.J., Challenges and recent progress in oral drug delivery systems for biopharmaceuticals. *Pharmaceutics*, 11, 3, 129, 2019 Mar 19.
38. Wilk, M.M., and Mills, K.H., CD4 TRM cells following infection and immunization: implications for more effective vaccine design. *Front. Immunol.*, 9, 1860, 2018 Aug 10.
39. Chaudhary, N., Weissman, D., Whitehead, K.A., mRNA vaccines for infectious diseases: principles, delivery and clinical translation. *Nat. Rev. Drug Discov.*, 20, 11, 817–38, 2021 Nov.

40. Bik, L., van Doorn, M.B., Boeijink, N., Wennekers, M., Meesters, A.A., Bloemen, P., Haedersdal, M., Wolkerstorfer, A., Clinical endpoints of needle-free jet injector treatment: An in-depth understanding of immediate skin responses. *Lasers Surg. Med.*, 54, 5, 693–701, 2022 Jul.
41. Fenton, O.S., Olafson, K.N., Pillai, P.S., Mitchell, M.J., Langer, R., Advances in biomaterials for drug delivery. *Adv. Mater.*, 30, 29, 1705328, 2018 Jul.
42. Monin, L., Laing, A.G., Muñoz-Ruiz, M., McKenzie, D.R., Del Barrio, I.D., Alaguthurai, T., Domingo-Vila, C., Hayday, T.S., Graham, C., Seow, J., Abdul-Jawad, S., Safety and immunogenicity of one versus two doses of the COVID-19 vaccine BNT162b2 for patients with cancer: interim analysis of a prospective observational study. *Lancet Oncol.*, 22, 6, 765–78, 2021 Jun 1.
43. Battistoni, C., Giraldo Nohra, C., Barbero, S., A systemic design method to approach future complex scenarios and research towards sustainability: A holistic diagnosis tool. *Sustainability*, 11, 16, 4458, 2019 Aug 17.
44. Artaud, C., Kara, L., Launay, O., Vaccine development: from preclinical studies to phase 1/2 clinical trials, in: *Malaria Control and Elimination*, pp. 165–76, 2019.
45. Rao, A.K., Petersen, B.W., Whitehill, F., Razeq, J.H., Isaacs, S.N., Merchlinsky, M.J., Campos-Outcalt, D., Morgan, R.L., Damon, I., Sánchez, P.J., Bell, B.P., Use of JYNNEOS (smallpox and monkeypox vaccine, live, nonreplicating) for preexposure vaccination of persons at risk for occupational exposure to orthopoxviruses: recommendations of the Advisory Committee on Immunization Practices—United States, 2022. *Morb. Mortal Wkly. Rep.*, 71, 22, 734, 2022 Jun 6.
46. Simpson, S., Chakrabarti, A., Robinson, D., Chirgwin, K., Lumpkin, M., Navigating facilitated regulatory pathways during a disease X pandemic. *npj Vaccines*, 5, 1, 101, 2020 Oct 23.
47. Zhuang, X. and Lu, C., PBPK modelling and simulation in drug research and development. *Acta Pharm. Sin. B*, 6, 5, 430–40, 2016 Sep 1.
48. Baylor, N.W., Role of the national regulatory authority for vaccines. *Int. J. Health Gov.*, 22, 3, 128–37, 2017 Sep 4.
49. Johnson, R. A., White, R. C., and Disbrow, G. L., Advancing development of medical countermeasures: incorporating COVID-19 lessons learned into future pandemic preparedness planning. *Hum. Vaccin. Immunother.*, 18, 6, 2129930, 2022.
50. Chen, X., Liu, S., Goraya, M.U., Maarouf, M., Huang, S., Chen, J.L., Host immune response to influenza A virus infection. *Front. Immunol.*, 9, 320, 2018 Mar 5.
51. Daniels, B.P., Holman, D.W., Cruz-Orengo, L., Jujjavarapu, H., Durrant, D.M., Klein, R.S., Viral pathogen-associated molecular patterns regulate blood-brain barrier integrity via competing innate cytokine signals. *MBio*, 5, 5, 10–128, 2014 Oct 31.

52. Zabel, F., Kündig, T.M., Bachmann, M.F., Virus-induced humoral immunity: on how B cell responses are initiated. *Curr. Opin. Virol.*, 3, 3, 357–62, 2013 Jun 1.
53. Eiz-Vesper, B., and Schmetzer, H. M., Antigen-presenting cells: potential of proven und new players in immune therapies. *Transfus. Med. Hemother.*, 47, 6, 429–431, 2020 Dec, 3.
54. Akkaya, M., Kwak, K., Pierce, S.K., B cell memory: building two walls of protection against pathogens. *Nat. Rev. Immunol.*, 20, 4, 229–38, 2020 Apr.
55. Walsh, S.R., Simovic, B., Chen, L., Bastin, D., Nguyen, A., Stephenson, K., Mandur, T.S., Bramson, J.L., Lichty, B.D., Wan, Y., Endogenous T cells prevent tumour immune escape following adoptive T cell therapy. *J. Clin. Invest.*, 129, 12, 5400–10, 2019 Dec 2.
56. Sayed, N., Allawadhi, P., Khurana, A., Singh, V., Navik, U., Pasumarthi, S.K., Khurana, I., Banothu, A.K., Weiskirchen, R., Bharani, K.K., Gene therapy: Comprehensive overview and therapeutic applications. *Life Sci.*, 294, 120375, 2022 Apr 1.
57. Corrado, M. and Pearce, E.L., Targeting memory T cell metabolism to improve immunity. *J. Clin. Invest.*, 132, 1, 2022 Jan 4.
58. Murray, A.A., Plant Virus Nanoparticle *in Situ* Cancer Immunotherapies, Case Western Reserve University, 2018.
59. Lee, K.L., High Aspect Ratio Viral Nanoparticles for Cancer Therapy, Case Western Reserve University, 2016.
60. Upreti, S. and Samant, M., A review on immunological responses to SARS-CoV-2 and various COVID-19 vaccine regimens. *Pharm. Res.*, 39, 9, 2119–34, 2022 Sep.
61. Hadj Hassine, I., Covid-19 vaccines and variants of concern: a review. *Rev. Med. Virol.*, 32, 4, e2313, 2022 Jul.
62. Rijkers, G.T., Weterings, N., Obregon-Henao, A., Lepolder, M., Dutt, T.S., van Overveld, F.J., Henao-Tamayo, M., Antigen presentation of mRNA-based and virus-vectored SARS-CoV-2 vaccines. *Vaccines*, 9, 8, 848, 2021 Aug 3.
63. Ghattas, M., Dwivedi, G., Lavertu, M. and Alameh, M.G., Vaccine technologies and platforms for infectious diseases: Current progress, challenges, and opportunities. *Vaccines*, 9, 12, 1490, 2021.
64. Bezeljak, U., Cancer gene therapy goes viral: viral vector platforms come of age. *Radiol. Oncol.*, 56, 1, 1–3, 2022 Feb 11.
65. Subramanian, M., Wojtusciszyn, A., Favre, L., Boughorbel, S., Shan, J., Letaief, K.B., Pitteloud, N., Chouchane, L., Precision medicine in the era of artificial intelligence: implications in chronic disease management. *J. Transl. Med.*, 18, 1, 1–2, 2020 Dec.
66. Amer, M.H., Gene therapy for cancer: present status and future perspective. *Mol. Cell. Ther.*, 2, 1, 1–9, 2014 Dec.
67. Lawrence, R.S., Durch, J.S., Stratton, K.R. (Eds.), *Vaccines for the 21st century: a tool for decisionmaking*, National Academies Press (US), 2000.

68. Hajebi, S., Yousefiasl, S., Rahimmanesh, I., Dahim, A., Ahmadi, S., Kadumudi, F.B., Rahgozar, N., Amani, S., Kumar, A., Kamrani, E., Rabiee, M., Genetically Engineered Viral Vectors and Organic-Based Non-Viral Nanocarriers for Drug Delivery Applications. *Adv. Healthcare Mater.*, 11, 20, 2201583, 2022 Oct.
69. Kim, E., Lim, E.K., Park, G., Park, C., Lim, J.W., Lee, H., Na, W., Yeom, M., Kim, J., Song, D., Haam, S., Advanced Nanomaterials for Preparedness Against (Re-) Emerging Viral Diseases. *Adv. Mater.*, 33, 47, 2005927, 2021 Nov.
70. Maeder, M. L., and Gersbach, C. A., Genome-editing technologies for gene and cell therapy. *Molecular Therapy*, 24, 3, 430–446, 2016.
71. Hollingsworth, R.E. and Jansen, K., Turning the corner on therapeutic cancer vaccines. *npj Vaccines*, 4, 1, 7, 2019 Feb 8.
72. Pauwels, K., Gijsbers, R., Toelen, J., Schambach, A., Willard-Gallo, K., Verheust, C., Debyser, Z., Herman, P., State-of-the-art lentiviral vectors for research use: risk assessment and biosafety recommendations. *Curr. Gene Ther.*, 9, 6, 459–74, 2009 Dec 1.
73. Li, Y., Tenchov, R., Smoot, J., Liu, C., Watkins, S., Zhou, Q., A comprehensive review of the global efforts on COVID-19 vaccine development. *ACS Cent. Sci.*, 7, 4, 512–33, 2021 Mar 29.
74. Poland, G.A., Ovsyannikova, I.G., Kennedy, R.B., Personalized vaccinology: a review. *Vaccine*, 36, 36, 5350–7, 2018 Aug 28.
75. Bisgin, A., Sanlioglu, A.D., Eksi, Y.E., Griffith, T.S., Sanlioglu, S., Current update on severe acute respiratory syndrome coronavirus 2 vaccine development with a special emphasis on gene therapy viral vector design and construction for vaccination. *Hum. Gene Ther.*, 32, 11-12, 541–62, 2021 Jun 1.
76. Jain, K.K. and Jain, K.K., Personalized immuno-oncology, in: *Textbook of Personalized Medicine*, 479–508, 2021.
77. Kazdin, A.E., Innovations in psychosocial interventions and their delivery: Leveraging cutting-edge science to improve the world's mental health, Oxford University Press, Oxford, 2018 Mar 5.
78. Peacocke, E.F., Heupink, L.F., Frønsdal, K., Dahl, E.H., Chola, L., Global access to COVID-19 vaccines: a scoping review of factors that may influence equitable access for low and middle-income countries. *BMJ Open*, 11, 9, e049505, 2021 Sep 1.
79. Doody, O. and Noonan, M., Nursing research ethics, guidance and application in practice. *Br. J. Nurs.*, 25, 14, 803–7, 2016 Jul 28.
80. Ahmad Rizal, A.R., Nordin, S.M., Ahmad, W.F., Ahmad Khiri, M.J., Hussin, S.H., How does social media influence people to get vaccinated? The elaboration likelihood model of a person's attitude and intention to get COVID-19 vaccines. *Int. J. Environ. Res. Public Health*, 19, 4, 2378, 2022 Feb 18.
81. Sahin, U. and Türeci, O., Personalized vaccines for cancer immunotherapy. *Science*, 359, 6382, 1355–60, 2018 Mar 23.

82. Vicini, P., Fields, O., Lai, E., Litwack, E.D., Martin, A.M., Morgan, T.M., Pacanowski, M.A., Papaluca, M., Perez, O.D., Ringel, M.S., Robson, M., Precision medicine in the age of big data: the present and future role of large-scale unbiased sequencing in drug discovery and development. *Clin. Pharmacol. Ther.*, 99, 2, 198–207, 2016 Feb.
83. Chen, J., Yi, C., Okegbile, S.D., Cai, J., Shen, X.S., Networking Architecture and Key Supporting Technologies for Human Digital Twin in Personalized Healthcare: A Comprehensive Survey. *IEEE Commun. Surv. Tutor.*, 26, 1, 706–46, 2023 Sep 4.
84. Sleigh, J. and Vayena, E., Public engagement with health data governance: the role of visuality. *Humanit. Soc. Sci. Commun.*, 8, 1, 1–2, 2021 Jun 18.

7

DNA- and RNA-Based Viral Vectors

Devesh U. Kapoor[1], Bhumi Bhatt[2], Dipansu Sahu[3], Rajiv R. Kakkar[4], Sonam M. Gandhi[5] and Rupesh K. Gautam[6]*

[1]*Dr. Dayaram Patel Pharmacy College, Bardoli, Gujarat, India*
[2]*S.S. Agarwal Institute of Pharmacy, Navsari, Gujarat, India*
[3]*Shree Naranjibhai Lalbhai Patel College of Pharmacy, Umrakh, Bardoli, Gujarat, India*
[4]*School of Pharmacy, Raffles University, Neemrana, Alwar, Rajasthan, India*
[5]*Shree Dhanvantary Pharmacy College, Kim, Gujarat, India*
[6]*Indore Institute of Pharmacy, IIST Campus, Indore, Madhya Pradesh, India*

Abstract

Vaccine delivery is an innovative and promising method for treating genetic and acquired diseases. One of the key challenges in gene therapy is delivering therapeutic genes to the intended cells effectively. Among the various types of viral vectors, DNA- and RNA-based vectors have attracted considerable interest due to their distinctive properties and potential. This book chapter aims to provide a comprehensive overview of DNA- and RNA-based viral vectors in the context of gene therapy. It begins by elucidating the fundamental principles of viral vector design and construction, focusing on the key features that make DNA- and RNA-based vectors attractive for gene delivery applications. The chapter extensively examines RNA-based viral vectors, encompassing retroviruses, lentiviruses, and adeno-associated viruses (AAVs). These vectors possess distinct advantages, such as prolonged expression of the therapeutic gene, effective delivery to non-dividing cells, and limited immune responses. The chapter also discusses recent progress and novel approaches utilized to improve the safety, effectiveness, and targeting abilities of DNA- and RNA-based viral vectors. Furthermore, the chapter addresses the obstacles and constraints related to DNA- and RNA-based viral vectors. These include issues such as immune system reactions, potential genetic mutations caused by vector integration, and limitations in vector packaging. This book chapter offers a thorough examination of DNA- and RNA-based viral

**Corresponding author*: drrupesgautam@gmail.com

Vivek P. Chavda and Vasso Apostolopoulos (eds.) Viral Vectors for Vaccine Delivery, (179–220) © 2025 Scrivener Publishing LLC

vectors, providing insights into their design, applications, and potential advancements in the field of vaccine delivery.

***Keywords*:** Adenoviral vectors, gene therapy, viral vectors, RNA-based virus, lentiviral vectors

7.1 Introduction to Viral Vectors

7.1.1 Definition and Overview

The genetic material of a virus penetrates the cell membrane and into the nucleus of a host cell, allowing it to express and duplicate its own genetic material before spreading to other cells [1]. The virus must therefore be genetically altered to replace a pathogenic gene's function with the therapeutic gene while keeping its nonpathogenic structures. Presently, gene therapy trials predominantly rely on viral vectors due to their exceptional *in vivo* transfection efficiency. However, these vectors do come with certain limitations, including the risk of acute immune responses, potential carcinogenic effects, high costs for production also restricted carrying ability for genetic materials [2].

7.1.2 Importance in Vaccine Delivery and Vaccination

Both gene therapy and immunization depend on viral vectors, which provide a potent method of introducing vaccine antigens into cells [3]. By providing a secure and efficient way of transferring vaccine antigens into target cells, vectors have transformed the area of biomedicine. To achieve effective gene delivery targeted antigen presentation, adaptability, and modifiability, as well as to generate a robust immune response, viral vectors play a crucial role in vaccine therapy and immunization [4].

7.2 Basics of Deoxyribonucleic Acid (DNA) and Ribonucleic Acid (RNA) Viruses

Viruses can be divided into two main groups depending on the structure of genetic makeup: DNA and RNA viruses. DNA viruses hold double-stranded DNA (dsDNA) as their genetic makeup. By the using mechanism of the host cell, they duplicate their genetic material and convert DNA into RNA, which acts as a blueprint for the synthesis of proteins. Some well-known DNA viruses include herpesviruses (e.g., herpes simplex virus), papillomaviruses (e.g., human papillomavirus), adenoviruses, and poxviruses (e.g., variola virus—responsible for smallpox). These DNA viruses can induce a variety of diseases, ranging from minor infections like cold sores (herpes simplex) to severe illnesses like smallpox (variola virus) [5]. RNA viruses are numerous and diverse, with examples including Influenza viruses (orthomyxoviruses), human immunodeficiency virus (HIV), measles, and also coronavirus [6].

7.2.1 Structure and Replication of DNA Viruses

The majority of DNA viruses possess a singular linear dsDNA genome. The polyoma and papillomaviruses are, among the papovaviruses, and their circular DNA genomes have a size of between 5.1- and 7.8-kilobase (kb) pairs. The dsDNA molecule plays a dual role as a template for both mRNA synthesis and self-transcription. The capsid of papovaviruses is made up of either three or two structural proteins, in addition to encoding five to six nonstructural proteins. These nonstructural proteins serve essential functions in transcribing the virus, replicating DNA, and transforming cells. Within the virion, there exist two to four distinct structural protein species, each originating in a distinct way from the same gene product. The adeno-associated virus (AAV) cannot generate progeny virions independently; instead, it relies on the presence of helping viruses (adenovirus or herpesvirus) to facilitate replication and virion production. The circovirus family harbors the smallest autonomously replicating viruses, characterized by their circular single-stranded DNA, which spans a compact size of only 1.7 to 2.3 kb. The 17-nm-long, isometric capsid is composed of just two protein species.

7.2.2 Structure and Replication of RNA Viruses

RNA viruses, containing 70% of all viruses, exhibit remarkable diversity in their genome structures. Due to the error ratio of enzymes engaged in RNA replication, these viruses typically exhibit significantly higher mutation amounts compared to DNA viruses [7]. Mutation amounts on the order of 10^4 result in the constant generation of diverse virus variants that demonstrate remarkable adaptableness to infecting new hosts. The viral genome may be dispersed throughout one or more discrete segments (segmented genomes) or it may be single-stranded (ss) or double-stranded (ds) strands of RNA. Furthermore, within a single-stranded genome, the messenger RNA (mRNA) strand can exist as either the sense strand, also known as the plus strand, or the antisense strand which is also known as the minus strand. The antisense strand is complementary to the sense strand but lacks the ability to directly translate into proteins. Sense viral RNA, due to its capability to function as mRNA, can initiate the translation of the virus's encoded proteins and replicate independently if introduced into cells. In contrast, antisense RNA lacks a role in translation and cannot autonomously generate viral components [8].

7.2.3 Characteristics Relevant to Vector Development

Vectors utilized in molecular biology and genetic engineering possess distinct characteristics that make them highly suitable for specific purposes. Figure 7.1 illustrates the characteristics essential for vector development in the context of vaccine delivery.

7.2.3.1 Plasmids

It is dsDNA molecules and circular which can autonomously multiply in host cells. They frequently have a replication origin that enables the plasmid to replicate within the host in a somewhat independent manner [9]. Bacteria and some eukaryotes, like yeast, have plasmids. They are frequently used for cloning and are simple to work with in the lab. A "multiple cloning site" on plasmids used as cloning vectors may allow fragments of DNA to be incorporated. They can also be used as transcription or expression vectors to produce proteins [10].

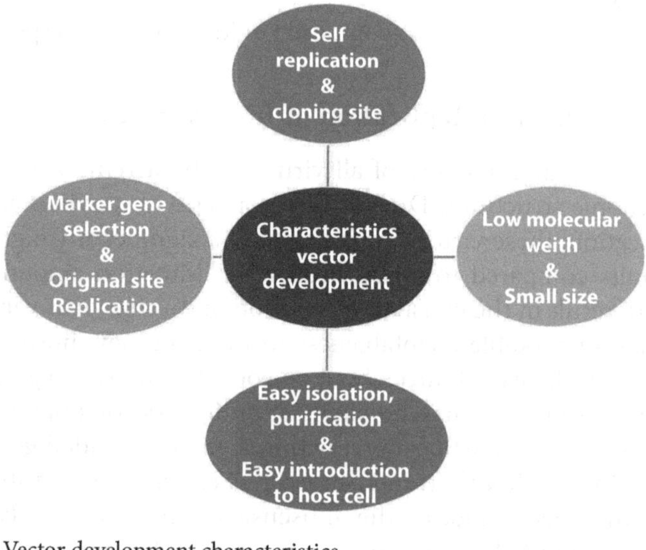

Figure 7.1 Vector development characteristics.

7.2.3.2 *Viral Vectors*

These modified viral vectors, adapted for vaccine delivery, have undergone genetic engineering to serve as carriers for foreign DNA or RNA in host cells. Despite their noninfectious nature, they retain viral promoters and transgenic sequences, enabling the host cell to produce the transgene efficiently [11, 12]. These vectors have the capacity for sustained expression and are proficient at delivering genetic material to various cell types. However, for broad-scale delivery, they may require helper viruses or packaging systems. After incorporating the transgene, viral vectors like retroviruses may leave specific genetic imprints within the host genome [13].

7.2.3.3 *Artificial Chromosomes*

Large DNA fragments are carried by artificial chromosomes, which are constructed chromosome-like structures. It can be classified into yeast artificial chromosomes (YACs), bacterial artificial chromosomes (BACs), or human artificial chromosomes (HACs). DNA pieces up to hundreds of thousands of nucleotides long can fit inside YACs and BACs. To support consistent replication and segregation during cell division, they comprise crucial elements such as a centromere, telomeric end sequences, and replication origins [14].

7.3 DNA-Based Viral Vectors

DNA viruses' viral genomes can be either single- or double-stranded. In relation to their utility as a means of gene transfer, the adenovirus, AAV, and herpes simplex virus are the most common DNA viruses. These viruses possess exceptional attributes for packaging vaccines, achieving widespread target cell infection, and facilitating efficient viral infection for vaccine delivery. As a result, they are extensively employed to develop vector systems for vaccine delivery applications [15].

7.3.1 Adenoviral Vectors

Adenoviruses, which do not have an envelope and contain dsDNA of about 35 kb, were first identified in 1953 [16]. There are 49 distinct serotypes that can be again divided into A to F subclasses according to their capabilities of haemagglutination. Types 2 (Ad2) and 5 (Ad5) of adenoviruses, which is a type of the C subgroup, have been studied the most thoroughly. It shows that adenovirus serotypes are not linked to severe disease in people and hence appropriate for *in vivo* uses, they were employed for creating the initial adenoviral vectors [17]. Modifications in the adenoviral genome will remove early gene 1 which is E1A that will be replication-incompetent vectors, thereby creating ample room for the insertion of genes. This is necessary as the E1A gene plays a vital role in virus replication. To make more room for gene insertion, these first-generation adenoviral vectors also partially delete the E1B and E3 genes in addition to the E1A gene. These adenoviral vectors' packing capacity ranges from 7 to 8 kb, which may not be their maximum insertion capacity. Helper cells are required for the production of infectious viral particles because they supply the necessary E1A protein in trans for effective viral encapsulation. This function is carried out for the creation of recombinant viral stocks by the broadly useful human kidney cell line 293, which has the E1A gene stably inserted [18, 19].

The inverted terminal repeats (ITR), the transgene, and the psi packaging sequences were the only viral coding areas left in more recent faulty adenovirus vectors, which have been referred to as being "gutted" or "gutless." Both the full-length dystrophin gene and the cystic fibrosis transmembrane conductance regulator (CFTR) gene were successfully expressed using such adenoviral vectors [20]. Such vectors have the benefit of being less immunogenic and producing high viral titers in the 293 cell line. Adenoviruses that are replication-competent are also employed for gene therapy approaches, particularly for cancer gene therapy, in addition to the adenoviral vector systems that are replication incompetent that were stated earlier. They make use of the cytopathic effect of viral replication in the targeted cells, where the E1A protein actively facilitates the lysis of tumor cells. Figure 7.2 illustrates the different DNA-based viral vectors.

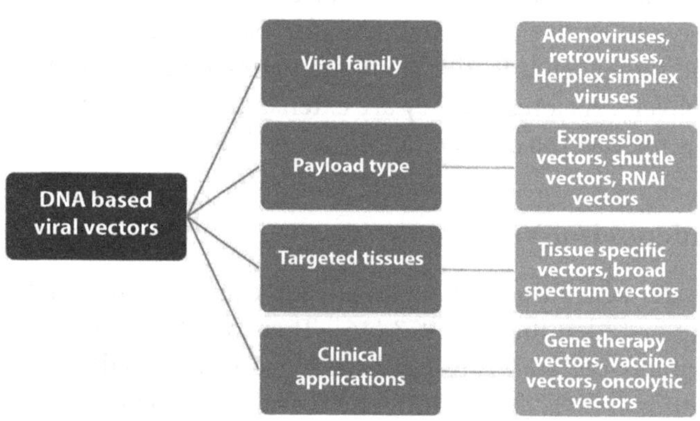

Figure 7.2 DNA-based viral vectors.

Usually, after adenoviral infection, the adenoviral E1B protein prevents cells from lysing as a result of E1A-mediated and p53-dependent apoptosis. Therefore, a mutation in the E1B gene would result in a virus that is unable to replicate itself in a useful manner in healthy cells that have active p53. However, such a virus will reproduce in cells deficient in active p53. Because p53 is frequently damaged in tumor cells, the adenovirus targets these cells for destruction. As a result, the E1B-defective virus can grow and propagate to neighboring tumor cells in tumor tissues while normal cells are unaffected. Such replication-competent adenoviruses have also been paired with HSV-tk suicide gene expression in other experiments to more effectively eradicate tumors. The benefits of adenoviral vectors with lower immunogenicity and long-lasting, high-level production of therapeutic genes are currently being combined using a variety of ways [21]. The fusion of adenovirus and retrovirus in chimeric vector systems combines adenoviral vectors' effectiveness in infecting target cells both *in vitro* and *in vivo* with the stable integration ability of retroviruses into the host genome, thereby establishing a connection with sustained long-term expression [22, 23].

7.3.1.1 Advantages and Limitations of Adenoviral Vectors

Adenoviral vectors offer several advantages in gene delivery and gene therapy applications:

1. High virus titers: Adenovirus vectors can be easily formed to achieve high titers (up to 10^{10} pfu/ml) in cell culture, allowing for efficient transduction of target cells and maximizing the therapeutic effect [24].
2. High-level gene expression: Adenoviral vectors are capable of driving strong and sustained gene expression in transduced cells. This is mainly advantageous for applications that require the robust and long-standing appearance of the therapeutic gene [24, 25].
3. Large insert capacity: Adenoviral vectors can accommodate relatively large DNA inserts, up to 7 to 8 kb, making them suitable for delivering larger genes or multiple therapeutic genes as part of a single vector construct [24, 25].
4. Broad cell tropism: Since adenoviral vectors may infect both proliferating and nonproliferating cells, their spectrum of potential uses is greater. Many other viral vectors, such as retroviruses, can only transduce actively dividing cells, limiting their usefulness in certain tissues and cell types [24].

5. Low risk of genomic integration: Adenoviral vectors, unlike retroviruses, do not incorporate their genetic material. This reduces the risk of mutagenesis, a potential concern in gene therapy approaches [24].
6. Rapid and transient gene expression: Gene expression caused by an adenoviral vector is often brief, which is useful when long-term expression is undesirable. This characteristic allows for a controlled and predictable duration of therapeutic gene expression [24].
7. Immunogenicity and immunomodulatory effects: These viral vectors can stimulate an immune response, which can be beneficial in certain gene therapy applications where immune activation is desired, such as in cancer immunotherapy [24, 25].
8. High *in vivo* transduction efficacy: The *in vivo* transduction effectiveness of adenoviral vectors has been found to be relatively high, making them a promising tool for *in vivo* delivery of genes in animals and maybe in human clinical trials.

It is crucial to recognize that adenoviral vectors have limitations and safety issues, including the probability of triggering immune responses in the host and the presence of previous immunity in certain individuals due to previous exposure to adenoviruses. These factors require careful evaluation and consideration when applying gene therapy to specific situations [24].

7.3.1.2 Adenoviral Vectors Applications in Vaccination

Due to their special qualities, adenoviral vectors are mostly used in both gene therapy and immunization. These vectors are recognized on adenoviruses, which are viruses that commonly cause respiratory illnesses in individuals. However, they have been engineered to be replication-deficient, meaning that they cannot replicate and cause disease. This makes them suitable for use as delivery vehicles for therapeutic genes or vaccine antigens. Here is how they are used in vaccination:

a. Viral Vector Vaccines: In viral vector vaccines, the adenoviral vector is engineered to carry genetic material encoding the antigen of interest from a pathogen (like a virus or bacterium). When administered, the vector delivers the antigen to host cells, triggering an immune response. The immune system recognizes the antigen as foreign, prominent to the activate T and B cells, thereby conferring immunity against the target pathogen [26].

b. Prime-Boost Strategies: Adenoviral vectors can be used in prime-boost vaccination strategies. In this approach, an adenoviral vector vaccine is given as the initial "prime," followed by a different type of vaccine (often a protein-based or mRNA vaccine) as a "boost." This strategy enhances and prolongs the immune response, leading to increased protection [27].
c. Speed of Development: In comparison to other conventional vaccine techniques, adenoviral vectors may be created and manufactured quite quickly. This makes them valuable tools during disease outbreaks and pandemics when rapid response is crucial.

It is worth noting that adenoviral vectors have also faced challenges in some applications. Preexistent immunity to natural adenoviruses in the number of people can limit the effectiveness of these vectors, especially for vaccines. Investigators are continuously working to address these tasks and develop the safety and efficiency of adenoviral vector–based therapies and vaccines [28].

7.3.2 Lentiviral Vectors

A lentivirus known as HIV causes AIDS. AIDS is known to be brought on by HIV. For the growth of lentiviral vector systems, this type of retrovirus offers several characteristics that are interesting. One of these characteristics is HIV's capacity to infect and integrate into cells that are not dividing, a capability that MLV-based vectors do not have [29, 30]. Lentiviruses are able to target the nucleus without the need for mitosis, which accounts for their capacity. HIV integration occurs without cellular mitosis thanks to a subset of virus-encoded proteins called vpr and p17 [31]. HIV integrates into many target cell types using various viral protein sets. A comprehensive genetic overhaul of the viral genome is important to ensure safe gene transfer and to expand the host range beyond the virus's "natural" target cells, such as $CD4^+$ cells. This is essential to utilize HIV in a manner similar to retroviral vector systems. In recent years, HIV-based vectors have been developed and tested for their biological safety and effectiveness in gene transfer in order to rule out the possibility of reinfecting the patient with pathogenic HIV-1 that is capable of replication. In order to achieve this, transient expression methods have been developed for the creation of recombinant lentivirus particles. In these systems, the transgenes are carried by the lentiviral vector, which has two distinct plasmids carrying the viral packaging genes [32]. It was shown that distinguished macrophages and neurons can both be successfully infected *in vitro* and *in vivo* by galactosidase or luciferase reporter gene transfer utilizing HIV-1–derived vectors. The new worries about potential cell growth dysregulation, mutagenesis, and recombination that have a significant influence on the prospective therapeutic use of these vectors are supported by the intricacy of the HIV genome and regulation mechanisms of viral replication. Therefore, before using human gene therapy can be considered, significant research on the biosafety of lentiviral vectors is required [33, 34].

7.3.2.1 Advantages and Limitations of Lentiviral Vectors

7.3.2.1.1 Infect Proliferating and Nonproliferating Cells

Both proliferating and nonproliferating cells can be effectively infected by lentiviral vectors. This is mainly important for gene therapy applications, as many target cells in the human body, such as neurons, are post-mitotic and do not divide. The spectrum of target tissues that can be efficiently treated expands thanks to the capacity to transduce nonproliferating cells [35].

7.3.2.1.2 Stable Gene Expression

The expression of the transgene is steady and long-lasting thanks to lentiviral vectors, which incorporate their genetic material into the genome of the host cell. This is in contrast to some other viral vectors like adenoviral vectors, which do not integrate and often result in transient gene expression [36].

7.3.2.1.3 Large Insert Capacity

Given their relatively high carrying capacity, lentiviral vectors can contain genetic material up to 10 kb in size. This feature is advantageous when delivering larger genes or multiple genes together as part of a therapeutic approach [37].

7.3.2.1.4 Pseudotyping Flexibility

Lentiviral vectors can be pseudotyped with various envelope proteins. Pseudotyping enhances their ability to target specific tissues [38].

7.3.2.1.5 Low Immunogenicity

As compared to other viral vectors, this viral vector has a low immunogenicity profile. This is advantageous for reducing potential immunological reactions that can restrict the efficacy of gene therapy therapies [39].

7.3.2.1.6 Versatile Applications

Lentiviral vectors are frequently utilized in many different types of studies, including fundamental studies, investigations into the function of genes, and gene therapy. They are useful tools for figuring out how genes work and creating fresh treatment plans because of their ability to transport and stably express genes in a variety of cell types.

However, it is worth noting that while lentiviral vectors have many advantages, there are also some challenges and safety considerations associated with their use. These include concerns about potential insertional mutagenesis, immune responses to viral proteins, and the need for stringent biosafety measures when working with lentiviral vectors. Therefore, their use should be carefully evaluated and carried out in compliance with appropriate safety guidelines and regulations [40].

7.3.2.2 Lentiviral Vectors Applications in Vaccination

Lentiviral vectors have demonstrated considerable promise in vaccine applications. Here are some of the key applications of lentiviral vectors in these fields:

Viral Vector Vaccines: Lentiviral vectors can be strategically engineered to transport genes encoding specific pathogen–derived antigens, enabling the production of these antigenic proteins. Utilizing these viral vector platforms for vaccine delivery offers a remarkable advantage in eliciting robust and enduring immune responses against the targeted pathogen [4].

Cancer Vaccines:

Lentiviral vectors have been investigated as a platform for cancer vaccines. They can be used to deliver tumor-specific antigens or immunomodulatory genes to stimulate the immune system's recognition and attack against cancer cells [41].

Therapeutic Antibodies:

Therapeutic antibody genes have been delivered using lentiviral vectors. These gene-modified antibodies can provide prolonged expression of specific antibodies, potentially offering passive immunity against infectious agents or cancer cells [42].

It is important to highlight that while lentiviral vectors offer numerous advantages, there are still challenges to overcome, such as safety concerns related to potential insertional mutagenesis and immune responses. Researchers and clinicians continue to develop and refine lentiviral vector technologies, optimizing their safety and efficacy profiles to unlock their full potential in gene therapy and vaccination applications [43].

7.3.3 Adeno-Associated Viral Vectors

The AAV is a single-stranded DNA–dependent virus that is a member of the parvovirus family. AAV infection can affect a number of cell types. Despite the fact that the majority of people are AAV seropositive, viral infection has not been linked to any pathology [44]. Two genes in the AAV, rep and cap, code for polypeptides necessary for AAV replication and encapsidation. A fruitful AAV infection also requires the adenoviral E1B and E4 proteins. The second AAV DNA strand is synthesized with the help of the adenoviral E4 protein [45]. The adoption of recombinant AAV (rAAV) vectors for human gene therapy is currently hampered by the challenge of completely eliminating helper viruses. Adenovirus superinfection is necessary for the production of rAAV particles, which makes it challenging to find high-quality viral stocks. Recently, high-titer packing cell lines were created, making it easier to get higher-quality rAAV supplies and eliminating the possibility of replication-competent AAV [46]. By substituting adenovirus with adenovirus helper plasmids, more recent rAAV production approaches get over the issues with adenovirus-dependent rAAV creation [47].

7.3.3.1 Advantages and Limitations of AAV

AAV vectors have gained important attention in gene therapy and other gene delivery applications due to several advantageous characteristics. Here are the main advantages of using AAV vectors:

1. **Infect Proliferating and Nonproliferating Cells**
In contrast to certain other viral vectors that can only target proliferating cells, AAV vectors can infect both actively proliferating and nonproliferating cells, which is a considerable advantage. This feature allows AAV vectors to effectively target various cell types in different tissues and organs [24].

2. Broad Cell Tropism:
AAV vectors exhibit a broad range of cell tropism, meaning that they can target a number of cell types across different tissues. This versatility is valuable in gene therapy applications, where targeting specific cell types is crucial for treating various genetic disorders and diseases [48].

3. Potential for Targeted Integration:
AAV vectors may be specifically incorporated into the genome of the host cell. This feature allows lasting gene expression and stable inheritance of the therapeutic gene, increasing the effectiveness of gene therapy treatments [49].

4. Low Immunogenicity:
AAV vectors generally provoke a weak immune response in the host matched to any other viral vectors. This lower immunogenicity reduces the risk of adverse effects and allows for repeated administration of the vector if necessary [50].

5. Nonpathogenic:
The AAV is a nonpathogenic virus. The parent virus does not cause any known diseases in humans, making AAV vectors a safer choice for gene therapy and gene delivery applications [51].

6. Long-Term Gene Expression:
These vectors can lead to long-lasting gene expression in the target cells, providing sustained therapeutic effects. This is especially beneficial for treating chronic conditions and genetic disorders that require continuous gene expression [52].

7. Compatibility with Different Delivery Methods: AAV vectors can be delivered through various administration routes, including intravenous, intramuscular, intrathecal, and local injections. This flexibility allows for a wide range of applications and potential therapeutic targets [53]. Adeno-associated viral vectors have several limitations, including a restricted capacity for transgenes (4 kb), challenges in generating high virus titers, and a dependency on adenovirus or herpesvirus for AAV replication [54].

7.3.3.2 AAV Applications in Gene Therapy and Vaccination

AAV vectors have demonstrated considerable promise in a number of gene therapy and vaccination-related applications. Here are a few of their main uses:

1. **Gene Therapy:** Gene therapy employs AAV vectors frequently to treat a variety of inherited diseases and genetic problems. By introducing functional genes in place of damaged or absent ones, they can deliver therapeutic genes to targeted cells and tissues. AAV-mediated gene therapy has been successful in treating conditions such as inherited retinal disorders (e.g., Leber congenital amaurosis) and certain types of muscular dystrophy [55].

2. **Central Nervous System Disorders:** AAV vectors can effectively target cells in the CNS by bridging the blood-brain barrier. They are especially useful for treating neurodegenerative conditions like Parkinson's and Alzheimer's diseases because of this feature. Therapeutic genes have been delivered to neurons using AAV vectors in an effort to improve or restore their functionality [56].

3. **Hemophilia Treatment:** Hemophilia, a bleeding illness brought on by the absence of particular clotting factors, has been studied as a possible candidate for gene therapy using AAV vectors. AAV vectors can deliver the missing clotting factor gene to liver cells, leading to the production of the deficient protein and reducing bleeding episodes in patients [57].

4. **Cancer Gene Therapy:** AAV vectors can be contrived to carry genes that promote tumor suppression or stimulate the immune system to target cancer cells. These vectors are being explored as potential tools for cancer gene therapy, either as standalone treatments or in combination with other therapies [58].

5. **Vaccination:** AAV vectors have emerged as promising platforms for vaccine development. They can be engineered to carry and deliver specific antigens from pathogens, triggering an immune response without causing disease. AAV-based vaccines have been studied for various infectious diseases, including HIV, influenza, and Zika virus [59].

6. **Gene Editing:** AAV vectors can also deliver gene-editing tools, such as CRISPR-Cas9, to target specific genes and modify their sequences. This approach holds the potential for correcting disease-causing mutations and treating genetic disorders at the DNA level [60].

7. **Immunotherapy:** AAV vectors can be engineered to express specific proteins that activate or modify the immune system. This property has led to their exploration of cancer immunotherapy, where immune-stimulating chemicals can be delivered using AAV-based vectors to improve the body's capacity to identify and destroy cancer cells [61].

7.3.4 Other DNA-Based Viral Vectors

7.3.4.1 Baculoviral Vectors

Baculoviral vectors are gene-delivery tools derived from baculoviruses, a family of insect viruses. These viruses are suitable for use in gene transfer applications because they have a sizable circular dsDNA genome and are not pathogenic to humans or the majority of vertebrates [62]. Baculoviral vectors have become valuable tools in various biotechnological and biomedical applications, including gene expression studies, protein production, gene therapy, and vaccine development. Some key features and applications of baculoviral vectors: Baculoviral vectors are widely used to express recombinant proteins in insect cells and other host systems. Large amounts of protein production in infected cells can be attained by introducing the desired gene under the control of a potent viral promoter into the baculovirus genome. Complex and challenging-to-express proteins can now be produced using this technique for both research and commercial uses. Additionally, it helps with protein production [63].

7.3.4.2 Herpes Simplex Virus Vectors

HSV-1 is a DNA virus possessing a linear double-stranded genome spanning 150 kb, which contains the genetic information for approximately 70 to 80 genes. This genome structure accounts for the HSV-1's great packaging capability for the insertion of foreign genes of 30 to 50 kb. The virus can infect both proliferating and nonproliferating cells and has a wide variety of target cell types. At the moment, HSV-1 vectors that are genetically altered to lack these specific ICP genes result in decreased toxicity [64]. The virus only expresses itself briefly in infected cell populations because it does not participate in the host genome. HSV is of interest primarily because of its high ability for insertion of foreign DNA and natural preference for neuronal cells, which can be used for either cancer gene therapies for neurogenic tumors or correcting gene therapies [65]. This vector contains the replication and packaging signals from the HSV origin, and it needs to be superinfected with the HSV helper virus to spread [66].

7.3.4.3 Poxviral Vectors

Viruses from the Poxviridae family, including the vaccinia virus, avipoxviruses also known as canarypox virus, and countless others, are frequently utilized. These viruses' great insertion capability for several foreign genes is a benefit. Greater than 25 kbp of foreign DNA can be successfully included in the viral genome. Distinct from the methods employed in other vector systems, the introduction of transgene sequences into recombinant vaccinia viral vectors (rVV) [67]. Since poxviruses employ their own transcriptional machinery to proliferate in the cytoplasm, viral promoters are necessary for the expression of foreign genes [68]. Recombinant poxviruses have garnered attention for their capability to stimulate both cell-mediated and humoral immune reactions. It holds promise in vaccination strategies aimed at expressing crucial proteins for eliciting immune responses against diseases and cancer. The T cell responses triggered by poxviruses make them particularly valuable for use as live cancer vaccines. To treat prostate cancer, colorectal cancer, breast cancer, and lung cancer, numerous clinical trials are currently being conducted to examine the anti-cancer effectiveness of poxviruses [69]. According to a study, people who get the rVV vaccine have memory cytotoxic T cells that are specific to the human papillomavirus. Further research is needed to increase the safety of poxvirus vectors and lower the possibility of cytopathic effects due to their complicated structure and biology [70].

7.4 RNA-Based Viral Vectors

7.4.1 Retroviral Vectors

Retroviral vectors are a class of viral vectors commonly employed in gene therapy and genetic engineering. They originate from retroviruses, a group of RNA viruses capable of performing reverse transcription, a process that converts their RNA genetic material into DNA upon infecting host cells. This distinct characteristic of retroviruses renders them highly advantageous for delivering therapeutic genes into specific target cells during medical treatments [71]. The core elements of the retroviral vector include the packaging system, which contains crucial genes from the retrovirus essential for generating new viral particles. These essential genes typically consist of gag, pol, and env (group-specific antigen, polymerase, and envelope, respectively). In the context of gene therapy, these viral genes are often substituted with the therapeutic gene of interest [72]. Another component is long terminal repeats (LTR), found at both ends of the retroviral genome, which play a pivotal role in the viral life cycle by facilitating the integration of viral DNA into the host cell genome and initiating viral gene expression [73]. Furthermore, the therapeutic gene, also known as the transgene, is the specific DNA sequence incorporated into the retroviral vector, intended for delivery into the target cells. This genetic material may consist of a functional copy of a mutated gene, a gene encoding a therapeutic protein, or a gene designed to rectify a genetic abnormality [74].

The process of utilizing retroviral vectors in gene therapy typically involves two main steps:

1. Transduction: The retroviral vector is specifically modified to carry the therapeutic gene of interest. It is then introduced into the target cells, either within the body (*in vivo*) or outside the body (*ex vivo*). During transduction, the viral vector integrates its DNA, including the therapeutic gene, into the host cell's genetic material [75].

2. Expression: After integrating into the host cell's genome, the therapeutic gene becomes active and undergoes transcription and translation processes. This leads to the production of the desired therapeutic protein or RNA molecule, enabling the corrected or functional gene to carry out its intended effect [76].

Retroviral vectors have proven to be highly efficient in transferring genes into actively dividing cells. Nevertheless, their effectiveness is limited in nondividing cells since they rely on cell division for successful integration into the host genome. Moreover, there are concerns regarding insertional mutagenesis, where the viral integration could potentially interfere with or activate genes, underscoring the critical need for thorough safety evaluations in clinical use.

Although retroviral vectors face challenges, they still hold significant value in gene therapy, particularly for specific applications that align with therapeutic objectives. Ongoing research and innovation in vector design and safety protocols aim to enhance their effectiveness and mitigate potential risks, making them more reliable and safer tools for gene therapy.

7.4.1.1 Advantages and Limitations

Retroviral vectors demonstrate exceptional efficiency in transferring therapeutic genes into target cells, especially those undergoing division. As a result, they are well-suited for specific applications that demand high transduction rates. Persistent transgene expression is a notable advantage of retroviral vectors. After integration into the host cell's genetic material, the therapeutic gene remains active for an extended duration, ensuring lasting therapeutic outcomes. Stable integration is a key advantage of retroviral vectors, as they can become a permanent part of the host cell's genetic material. This allows for consistent and heritable expression of the therapeutic gene as the host cell undergoes division and replication. Retroviruses exhibit reduced immunogenicity in comparison to certain other types of viral vectors, leading to a decreased likelihood of eliciting a robust immune response in the host.

Retroviral vectors possess the advantage of accommodating larger gene inserts in comparison to certain other viral vectors. This feature enables the delivery of larger therapeutic genes in gene therapy applications [77].

Retroviral vectors rely on the active division of target cells for successful integration into the host genome. As a result, their efficacy is restricted in nondividing cells like neurons and muscle cells. The incorporation of retroviral DNA into the host genome carries the risk of disturbing or activating host genes, possibly resulting in unintended effects or the development of tumors. While retroviral vectors offer a relatively larger gene capacity compared to certain vectors, they still face constraints in delivering very large genes or multiple genes due to size limitations. This can pose challenges in accommodating extensive genetic information within the vector for therapeutic purposes. The manufacture of retroviral vectors for clinical applications can be a complex and time-consuming process. It demands specialized facilities and expertise to produce replication-defective vectors of high quality. Although retroviruses generally provoke a low immune response, the host's immune system can still react to the viral particles, leading to a decrease in their presence within the body over time. Targeting specific tissues with retroviral vectors is a complex task due to their reliance on the envelope protein for tropism, which may not always enable accurate and precise targeting. This difficulty in achieving tissue-specific delivery poses a challenge in utilizing retroviral vectors for highly targeted gene therapy applications [78].

7.4.2 Lentiviral Vectors

Lentiviral vectors are specialized viral vectors derived from lentiviruses, which are a subgroup of retroviruses. These vectors are extensively employed in gene delivery and gene therapy applications due to their distinctive characteristics, particularly their remarkable capacity to effectively integrate their genetic payload into the DNA of the target cell.

Lentiviral vectors possess a wide range of cell tropism, allowing them to infect both actively dividing cells and nondividing cells effectively. This characteristic makes lentiviral vectors a suitable choice for targeting diverse cell types, including stem cells and fully differentiated cells [79].

Once integrated into the host cell's genome, lentiviral vectors ensure enduring transgene expression, resulting in sustained and long-lasting gene expression within the targeted cells. This stable transgene expression is a key feature that contributes to the effectiveness of lentiviral vectors in gene therapy applications.

Lentiviral vectors possess a notable advantage in accommodating substantial genetic material, enabling the efficient delivery of extensive gene sequences, full-length genes, or multiple therapeutic elements. This feature makes them valuable tools in gene therapy and genetic research applications.

Lentiviral vectors offer flexibility in regulating transgene expression by incorporating different regulatory elements, such as promoters, enhancers, and response elements. These elements enable the control of transgene activity and responsiveness to specific cellular signals and conditions. Lentiviral vectors possess the ability to adopt the characteristics of other viruses by incorporating their envelope proteins. This feature enables the vectors to modify their host cell targeting and immune response evasion properties [80].

Lentiviral vectors are designed to be non-replicative, ensuring that they cannot cause viral infections. Furthermore, modern vector design has significantly reduced the risk of insertional mutagenesis, addressing potential genotoxicity concerns. These safety features make lentiviral vectors a safer and more reliable tool for gene delivery and therapeutic applications.

Lentiviral vectors have demonstrated their utility in diverse research areas, encompassing fundamental biology investigations, disease modeling, and drug discovery. Additionally, researchers are actively exploring their potential as a gene therapy tool for the treatment of genetic disorders and specific acquired diseases. These versatile vectors continue to pave the way for advancements in both scientific research and therapeutic applications.

7.4.2.1 Advantages and Limitations

Lentiviral vectors are highly favored in gene delivery and gene therapy applications due to their numerous valuable benefits and advantages. Their versatility, efficiency, long-term gene expression, and potential for treating various genetic disorders make them a popular and widely adopted choice in the field of gene therapy and research [81].

Lentiviral vectors exhibit a broad cell tropism, enabling them to infect a diverse array of cell types, including both actively dividing and nondividing cells. This characteristic makes them highly versatile in targeting different tissues and cell types within various organs of the body.

Lentiviral vectors, upon integration into the host cell's genetic material, enable stable and enduring transgene expression. This extended duration of expression proves advantageous for therapeutic interventions that demand continuous production of therapeutic proteins or RNA molecules [82].

Lentiviral vectors possess a notable advantage in their capacity to carry substantial genetic material, enabling the delivery of complex genes and multiple therapeutic agents within a single vector. This feature provides flexibility and versatility in gene delivery applications, making them an ideal choice for various genetic engineering and gene therapy approaches.

Lentiviral vectors have undergone specific engineering to minimize their immunogenicity, which reduces the likelihood of inducing strong immune responses upon administration. This modification enhances their safety profile, making them suitable for repeated treatments in various therapeutic applications [83].

Lentiviral vectors excel in gene delivery due to their remarkable transduction efficiency. This means they can efficiently introduce genes into specific target cells, making them a valuable tool in successful gene therapy and gene editing applications. Lentiviral vectors have the ability to integrate their genetic material into the DNA of the host cell. This integration ensures that the transgene is stably maintained and passed on to daughter cells after cell division, resulting in long-term and heritable expression of the inserted gene. Lentiviral vectors offer the versatility of both *in vivo* and *ex vivo* approaches for gene delivery. In the *in vivo* method, the vectors are directly administered to the target tissues within the living organism. On the other hand, in *ex vivo* gene therapy, cells are modified outside the body and then reintroduced into the patient. This flexibility allows for tailored and effective gene delivery strategies, making lentiviral vectors a valuable tool in gene therapy research and clinical applications. Extensive strides have been taken to enhance the safety of lentiviral vectors, focusing on reducing the chances of insertional mutagenesis and mitigating any possible negative consequences. Lentiviral vectors show the potential to address diverse medical conditions, including genetic disorders, hereditary diseases, and acquired illnesses. They offer promising therapeutic options, especially in cases where traditional treatments have limitations or are less effective [84].

Lentiviral vectors play a crucial role as valuable tools in scientific research, providing opportunities to investigate gene function, regulation, and disease mechanisms. They also aid in the development of novel therapies. Due to their versatility and effectiveness, lentiviral vectors are extensively utilized in preclinical research and hold immense potential in therapeutic applications, solidifying their prominent position in the field of gene delivery and gene therapy [85].

Lentiviral vectors have different applications in gene therapy, which are mentioned in Table 7.1 [86].

Lentiviral vectors hold great potential in vaccine development because of their efficient delivery of antigen genes and their ability to trigger strong and effective immune responses. The different applications of lentiviral vectors are mentioned in Figure 7.3.

Table 7.1 Different applications of lentiviral vectors in gene therapy.

S. no	Application	Description
01.	Monogenic disorders	Lentiviral vectors have the capability to transport intact and functional copies of faulty genes associated with monogenic genetic disorders. This allows them to potentially correct the genetic defects responsible for these specific inherited conditions.
02.	Cancer therapies	Lentiviral vectors have the capability to modify immune cells or transport therapeutic genes to specifically target and address cancer cells, presenting a potential approach for cancer treatment.
03.	Inherited diseases	Lentiviral vectors hold the potential to provide a curative approach for inherited diseases by transporting corrected genes to the affected tissues.
04.	Hematopoietic disorders	Lentiviral vectors have the capability to modify hematopoietic stem cells, enabling the treatment of a wide range of blood-related disorders.
05.	Neurological diseases	Lentiviral vectors show great potential for delivering therapeutic genes to the central nervous system, offering a promising approach for treating neurological diseases.
06.	Viral vector vaccines	Lentiviral vectors have the potential to be utilized as a foundation for creating viral vector vaccines aimed at combating infectious diseases.

(*Continued*)

Table 7.1 Different applications of lentiviral vectors in gene therapy. (*Continued*)

S. no	Application	Description
07.	Gene editing	Lentiviral vectors have the capability to transport gene editing tools, such as CRISPR/Cas9, allowing for precise modifications of targeted gene sequences.
08.	Immunotherapy	Lentiviral vectors are employed to modify immune cells for adoptive cell therapies, enabling them to effectively target cancerous cells or combat viral infections.
09.	Tissue repair	Lentiviral vectors have the capability to transport therapeutic genes that facilitate tissue regeneration and repair, offering potential treatments for a range of tissue-related disorders.
10.	Metabolic disorders	Lentiviral vectors hold promise for addressing metabolic disorders by potentially correcting deficiencies in metabolic enzymes.

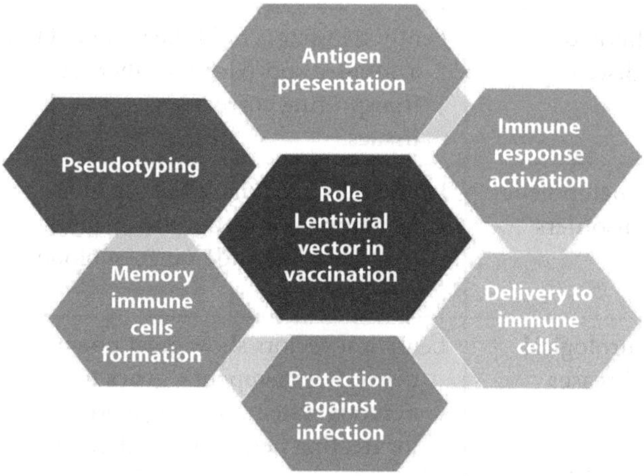

Figure 7.3 Application of lentiviral vector in vaccination.

7.4.3 Alphaviral Vectors

Alphaviral vectors are viral vectors that originate from alphaviruses, which are a class of single-stranded RNA viruses with a positive-sense genome. These vectors have garnered significant interest as a potential solution for gene delivery and vaccine development due to their distinct attributes and beneficial properties. Alphaviral vectors demonstrate high transduction efficiency, enabling them to efficiently deliver genes to the desired target cells. Additionally, alphaviruses have limited replication in host cells, contributing to their safety profile and minimizing the potential for uncontrolled viral dissemination [87].

Alphaviral vectors possess a wide tissue tropism, enabling them to infect diverse cell types and tissues. This versatility makes them well-suited for various therapeutic applications. Furthermore, alphaviral vectors usually lead to transient gene expression, which is beneficial for scenarios that demand short-term or time-specific production of proteins. Alphaviral vectors are advantageous as they usually do not integrate into the host genome, reducing the likelihood of causing genetic mutations or long-term alterations. Additionally, these vectors can trigger the host's innate immune response, enhancing their immunogenicity and making them attractive candidates for vaccine development. Alphaviral vectors hold promise as live attenuated vaccines that can confer immunity without causing severe illness. Moreover, these vectors offer the advantage of straightforward production in significant quantities using conventional laboratory techniques, making them well-suited for large-scale manufacturing in clinical settings [88].

Despite the advantages offered by alphaviral vectors, they do come with certain challenges. For instance, their cargo capacity is limited, which can be problematic when attempting to deliver large genetic material. Additionally, there may be preexisting immunity in the human population to specific alphaviruses, posing a hurdle for their widespread use. However, researchers are actively working to overcome these limitations and unlock the full potential of alphaviral vectors for gene therapy and vaccine development, making them a promising option in the realm of viral vectors [89].

7.4.3.1 Advantages and Limitations

The alpha viral vectors have several benefits, which are mentioned in Table 7.2 [90].

Although alphaviral vectors offer several benefits, they also come with certain limitations that require attention and resolution to fully harness their potential in gene therapy and vaccine development. Alphaviral vectors

Table 7.2 Numerous advantages of alpha viral vectors.

S. no.	Benefits	Description
01.	High transduction efficiency	Alphaviral vectors demonstrate high transduction efficiency, enabling them to efficiently deliver genes into desired target cells.
02.	Transient replication	Alphaviruses exhibit restricted replication within host cells, which improves their safety profile and decreases the likelihood of uncontrolled viral dissemination.
03.	Broad tissue tropism	Alphaviral vectors possess the ability to effectively infect diverse cell types and tissues, rendering them well-suited for a wide array of therapeutic applications.
04.	Transient gene expression	Alphaviral vectors are advantageous for applications requiring short-term or time-specific protein production since they facilitate transient gene expression. This means that the genetic material delivered by the vectors is only active for a limited duration, providing flexibility and control over protein production timelines.
05.	Minimal integration into host genome	Alphaviral vectors have the ability to stimulate the host's innate immune response, which enhances their immunogenicity and makes them promising candidates for vaccine development.
06.	Innate immune activation	Alphaviral vectors have the ability to trigger the host's innate immune response, enhancing their immunogenicity and making them attractive candidates for vaccine development.
07.	Potential for live attenuated vaccines	Certain alphaviruses can be genetically modified to serve as live attenuated vaccines, inducing immune responses and conferring protection against the targeted pathogen without causing severe illness.
08.	Ease of production	Alphaviral vectors can be efficiently produced in large quantities using standard laboratory techniques, making them well-suited for large-scale manufacturing in clinical applications.

possess a small cargo capacity, which limits the amount of genetic material they can deliver. This constraint may impede the delivery of larger genes or multiple therapeutic elements using a single vector. Preexisting immunity in certain individuals, either from previous exposure or vaccinations to specific alphaviruses, can diminish the effectiveness of alphaviral vectors in these individuals. This immune response may impact the vectors' ability to elicit the desired therapeutic effect. Alphaviral vectors typically result in the temporary production of the desired protein as they mediate transient gene expression. In therapeutic applications where sustained expression is needed, this limitation may require multiple vector administrations. Immunogenicity is a concern with alphaviral vectors as they can activate the host's innate immune system, potentially causing inflammation and immune reactions. This aspect of their nature may affect the safety and effectiveness of the vectors in practical applications. Attaining accurate targeting and delivery to specific tissues or cell types presents a significant challenge for alphaviral vectors, thereby restricting their utility in certain diseases. While replication-defective alphaviral vectors are generally considered safe, there are safety concerns associated with replication-competent alphaviruses. These concerns arise from the potential risk of uncontrolled viral replication and increased virulence, which need to be carefully addressed in their use for gene therapy and vaccine development. Integration into the host genome is a concern with alphaviral vectors, as although they usually show restricted integration, any integration events have the potential to lead to insertional mutagenesis. In the *in vivo* environment, alphaviral vectors might undergo degradation or elimination by the host's immune system or other factors, which can affect their stability and effectiveness.

7.4.4 Other RNA-Based Viral Vectors

RNA-based viral vectors are captivating vehicles used in genetic engineering and vaccine development. One intriguing example is the vesicular stomatitis virus (VSV) vector. Scientists have tinkered with VSV to carry and deliver packages of genetic material, allowing us to insert desired genes into specific cells. This has shown exciting potential in creating vaccines. Imagine the VSV acting like a delivery truck loaded with harmless snippets of pathogens that teach our immune system to respond effectively without making us sick.

Another remarkable player in this field is the measles virus vector. Yes, the same virus that causes measles has been repurposed for good. It is like giving the virus a new job—delivering important RNA cargo into cells. This could be a game-changer in cancer treatment. Think of it as a precision-guided missile. Scientists can program the modified measles virus to specifically target and eliminate cancer cells, leaving healthy cells unharmed. This clever tactic taps into the virus's natural ability to infiltrate our bodies. Lentiviruses, including HIV, have also joined the RNA-based viral vector party. They have been enlisted in gene therapy, acting like microscopic couriers. Their mission is to carry therapeutic genes and drop them off exactly where they are needed in our bodies. This has the potential to treat genetic disorders and other illnesses rooted in our genes. By tweaking the lentiviral RNA, researchers make sure these tiny carriers integrate with our genetic material, offering a potential long-term fix for various health challenges. All in all, these RNA-based viral vectors are at the forefront of modern biology and medicine. They are like versatile tools, aiding us in uncovering the secrets of genetics, crafting innovative treatments, and even combating infectious diseases. The ongoing research in this realm is like an adventure that keeps opening new doors, showing us exciting possibilities for the future of biotechnology and healthcare.

7.4.4.1 Sendai Virus Vectors

Sendai virus (SeV), also referred to as murine parainfluenza virus type 1, stands out as an RNA-based viral vector with valuable applications in genetic studies and biotechnology. It has garnered attention for its efficient delivery of genetic material into specific cells, avoiding the integration into the host's genetic material. Scientists have capitalized on SeV's distinctive characteristics to create vectors tailored for diverse purposes. These vectors can transport RNA payloads, such as therapeutic agents or genes of interest, into various cell types. Importantly, SeV vectors come with the advantage of not posing a risk of modifying the host's DNA, ensuring safety for specific applications [91].

A particularly promising domain for SeV vectors is the realm of induced pluripotent stem cell (iPSC) production. These specialized cells can be reprogrammed to adopt different roles, offering great potential for disease modeling and regenerative medicine. By effectively introducing reprogramming factors into somatic cells, SeV vectors streamline iPSC generation. This technique addresses challenges associated with alternative methods and opens avenues for personalized medicine and innovative cellular therapies [92].

7.4.4.2 *Vesicular Stomatitis Virus Vectors*

VSV vectors have emerged as a potent tool in the realm of genetic engineering and biotechnology. These RNA-based viral vectors have been tailored to efficiently deliver genetic material into specific target cells. Their proficient and secure transportation of RNA payloads enhances their applicability across various fields. In the context of vaccine development, VSV vectors can be personalized to express antigens sourced from diverse pathogens. This strategic customization provokes a robust immune response, potentially offering remedies for infectious diseases. Moreover, VSV vectors exhibit encouraging potential in oncolytic virotherapy, enabling them to be designed for the precise infection and eradication of cancer cells. The exceptional ability of VSV vectors to exploit cellular pathways, combined with their wide host range, underscores their significance in driving genetic comprehension and pioneering innovative medical strategies. As ongoing research unveils fresh possibilities, the versatile potential of VSV vectors continues to captivate scientists across diverse scientific arenas [93].

7.5 Vector Engineering and Modifications

Vector engineering and modifications form a vibrant and evolving domain within genetic research and biotechnology, with a primary focus on customizing viral vectors to amplify their efficiency, safety, and specificity for a multitude of applications. These engineered vectors act as conveyors, transporting genetic material into intended cells and assuming pivotal roles in gene therapy, vaccine innovation, and other groundbreaking methodologies. Researchers adeptly manipulate the genetic composition of viral vectors, often employing methodologies like genetic recombination and gene editing to refine their performance. Such alterations encompass adjustments in the viral envelope, optimization of gene expression promoters, and introduction of precise targeting sequences [94].

Through these meticulous refinements, scientists can bolster vector durability, augment cellular intake, and precisely direct the cargo to designated cell types, thus elevating the overall success of the intended genetic manipulation. Within the scope of gene therapy, vector engineering becomes instrumental in ensuring the accurate delivery of therapeutic genes to rectify genetic disorders. By meticulously adapting viral vectors to adeptly infiltrate designated tissues and cells, researchers open avenues for enduring solutions to inherited ailments. Similarly, in the realm of vaccine development, tailored vectors can be devised to express pathogen-derived antigens, inciting potent immune responses sans inducing illness. This strategic groundwork forms the bedrock for effective immunization strategies. The realm of vector engineering and modifications also extends its reach to oncolytic virotherapy, where vectors are meticulously customized to selectively infect and dismantle cancerous cells [95].

This holds substantial promise as a precisely targeted and potentially less invasive approach to combat cancer. Concurrently, as we delve into the intricacies of diverse ailments, these bespoke vectors contribute to unraveling the convoluted web of molecular pathways and biological processes. Fundamentally, vector engineering and modifications constitute a dynamic and continuously evolving arena that empowers researchers to fully harness the potential harbored by viral vectors. This ongoing stream of innovation and adaptation reshapes our capacities and deepens our comprehension of genetic manipulation, ultimately contributing to the advancement of genetics, medicine, and biotechnology. This incessant progress stands to enhance human health and further the bounds of scientific exploration [96].

7.5.1 Enhancing Vector Safety

Advancing the safety of viral vectors is a critical goal in the field of genetic engineering and biotechnology. This essential effort involves a multifaceted strategy to minimize potential risks associated with using these vectors in various applications like gene therapy and vaccine development. Researchers employ diverse approaches to enhance vector safety. This starts with careful vector design and adjustments. By tailoring viral components, such as eliminating replication genes or adding control mechanisms, scientists can reduce the chances of uncontrolled viral replication and potential harm. Thorough testing and analysis are also key to improving vector safety. Comprehensive preclinical assessments help understand how vectors behave and potential toxicities, providing insights to refine their design and performance. Refining delivery methods and targeting precision are crucial as well [97].

Optimizing how vectors are introduced into cells or tissues helps decrease unintended effects and maximizes therapeutic impact. Innovations in delivery techniques, tissue-specific triggers, and viral trafficking mechanisms contribute to this endeavor. Integrating fail-safe mechanisms adds an extra layer of security. By incorporating features or switches that can stop vector activity, researchers can have better control and mitigate possible adverse outcomes. Regular monitoring of treated individuals is important for assessing long-term safety. Continuous surveillance aids in the early detection of unexpected effects, allowing prompt adjustments if needed. In essence, elevating vector safety involves careful design, rigorous testing, precise targeting, fail-safe measures, and consistent posttreatment monitoring. These combined efforts aim to maximize the benefits of viral vectors while minimizing potential risks, creating a safer and more effective landscape for scientific progress [98].

7.5.2 Improving Vector Targeting and Tropism

Advancing the precision of vector targeting and tropism is a focal point in the realm of genetic engineering and biotechnology. This crucial objective aims to refine how viral vectors efficiently engage specific cells or tissues, optimizing their potential for various applications.

Researchers employ a range of strategies to enhance vector targeting and tropism. Customized adjustments to the viral envelope or surface proteins enable vectors to exhibit a preference for particular cell types, ensuring a more tailored and effective delivery. This approach reduces the chance of unintended interactions and potential side effects. Further refining vector targeting involves implementing advanced delivery techniques [99].

Utilizing nanoparticle-based systems, tissue-specific promoters, and engineered viral trafficking pathways contributes to the accuracy of vector delivery, increasing the likelihood of successful therapeutic outcomes. Equally important is optimizing vector tropism for specific applications. By engineering vectors to zero in on specific tissues, like tumor cells in cancer treatment, researchers can magnify therapeutic impact while sparing healthy cells. This approach holds promise for boosting treatment effectiveness and minimizing unintended consequences. The intricate interplay between vector adjustments and delivery methods is paramount. Combining tailored viral modifications with refined delivery strategies ensures vectors effectively reach their intended destination while sidestepping unintended effects. In essence, elevating vector targeting and tropism is a nuanced endeavor that blends tailored modifications, sophisticated delivery methods, and a deep understanding of cellular interactions. This collaborative effort aims to unlock the complete potential of viral vectors, creating a more precise and efficient platform for genetic engineering and biotechnological applications [100].

7.5.3 Regulatory Considerations and Quality Control

Managing regulatory aspects and maintaining robust quality control procedures are critical components in the realm of genetic engineering and biotechnology. These crucial elements are essential to ensure the safety, effectiveness, and ethical integrity of applications involving viral vectors, such as gene therapy and vaccine development. Regulatory compliance involves adhering to established guidelines and protocols set by relevant governing bodies [101].

A comprehensive understanding of and adherence to these regulations is vital to ensure the responsible and safe utilization of viral vectors in medical and research contexts. Equally important are measures to control and assure quality. Stringent testing protocols are utilized to assess the safety, purity, and potency of viral vector preparations. This involves meticulous evaluation of vector integrity, genetic stability, and the absence of contaminants to prevent potential harm. Additionally, thorough documentation practices are crucial for maintaining traceability and accountability throughout vector development and production. Precise records detailing vector design, manufacturing steps, and testing outcomes are indispensable for transparency, regulatory audits, and quality assurance. Post-administration monitoring of vector performance is another pivotal aspect. Analyzing the vector's behavior within the host and its interaction with target cells offers vital insights into therapeutic effectiveness and potential side effects. This ongoing evaluation aids in refining vector design and application strategies. Collaboration among regulatory experts, scientists, and manufacturing professionals is essential to seamlessly integrate regulatory considerations and quality control measures. A multidisciplinary approach ensures that all facets of vector design, production, and application adhere to the highest standards of safety and efficacy [102].

7.6 Preclinical and Clinical Applications

Preclinical applications constitute a crucial phase preceding human trials in the realm of scientific research and medical development. This stage involves rigorous experimentation and testing, often spanning several years, where researchers assess the safety, efficacy, and feasibility of potential interventions. Through the use of cell cultures, animal models, and *in vitro* experiments, preclinical studies aim to uncover potential benefits and risks associated with a new drug, treatment, or medical device. Key considerations include evaluating dose-response relationships and potential toxicity, all of which contribute to informed decision-making regarding whether to proceed to clinical trials. While not requiring regulatory approval, preclinical findings play a pivotal role in shaping the direction of subsequent research [103].

On the other hand, clinical applications encompass studies involving human subjects, marking a critical transition from the preclinical phase. Clinical trials are designed to rigorously evaluate the safety, efficacy, dosing, and potential adverse effects of interventions in a controlled and ethical manner. Human volunteers and patients participate in these trials, which are often conducted in multiple phases to progressively gather more comprehensive data. Patient responses to treatments, along with safety evaluations and observed outcomes, play a central role in guiding drug and device approval decisions. Ethical guidelines and regulatory approvals are stringent prerequisites for conducting clinical trials, ensuring patient well-being and adherence to established standards [104].

7.6.1 Gene Therapy Applications

Gene therapy is an innovative technique that aims to treat or prevent genetic and acquired disorders by modifying genes. It holds great promise in addressing various medical conditions, such as inherited genetic diseases, cancer, and viral infections, among others. This cutting-edge approach opens up new possibilities for personalized and targeted treatments, potentially transforming the landscape of modern medicine.

7.6.1.1 Inherited Disorders

Inherited disorders refer to a group of medical conditions that are passed down from parents to their children through their genetic material. These disorders arise due to mutations or changes in specific genes, which can affect various aspects of health and development. Examples of inherited disorders include cystic fibrosis, where mutations in the CFTR gene lead to respiratory and digestive problems, and sickle cell anemia, caused by mutations in the HBB gene, resulting in abnormal red blood cells. Other inherited disorders encompass conditions like hemophilia, where blood clotting is impaired due to genetic mutations, and Huntington's disease, which involves progressive neurological degeneration due to genetic changes in the HTT gene. These inherited disorders underscore the significance of genetic inheritance in shaping an individual's health and highlight the ongoing efforts in medical research and genetic counseling to better understand, diagnose, and manage these conditions [105].

7.6.1.2 Neurological Disorders

Neurological disorders encompass a broad spectrum of medical conditions that affect the nervous system, which includes the brain, spinal cord, and peripheral nerves. These disorders arise from a complex interplay of genetic, environmental, and lifestyle factors, often leading to disruptions in the normal functioning of the nervous system. Conditions like Alzheimer's disease, characterized by cognitive decline and memory impairment, and Parkinson's disease, which involves motor symptoms such as tremors and stiffness, are well-known examples of neurological disorders. Genetic mutations, protein misfolding, and neuronal degeneration play roles in these disorders [106]. Other neurological disorders include multiple sclerosis, where the immune system attacks the protective covering of nerve fibers, and amyotrophic lateral sclerosis (ALS), a progressive degeneration of motor neurons that control muscle movement. The study and treatment of neurological disorders are complex and challenging due to the intricate nature of the nervous system. Ongoing research aims to better understand the underlying mechanisms, develop targeted therapies, and improve the quality of life for individuals affected by these conditions. Early diagnosis, advancements in medical technology, and innovative treatment approaches, including gene therapies and neurodegenerative techniques, offer hope for managing and potentially mitigating the impact of neurological disorders [107].

7.6.2 Vaccination Applications

Vaccination is a pivotal aspect of immunization, serving as a vital tool in preventing and managing infectious diseases. By administering vaccines containing weakened or inactive disease-causing agents, the immune system is primed to develop antibodies, providing protection without causing illness. This essential practice contributes significantly to public health, reducing the prevalence of various infectious diseases and safeguarding communities worldwide. Table 7.3 describes the different applications of vaccination [108].

7.6.2.1 Viral Vector–Based Vaccines

Viral vector–based vaccines represent a ground-breaking approach to immunization that harnesses the power of viruses to stimulate a protective immune response. These innovative vaccines use harmless viruses, often modified to be non-replicating or weakened, as vehicles to deliver specific

Table 7.3 Applications of vaccination.

Vaccination applications	Description
Infectious disease prevention	Prevents a wide range of infectious diseases, from common childhood illnesses to severe threats.
Emerging infectious diseases	Rapidly develops vaccines during outbreaks of new or emerging infectious diseases.
Cancer prevention	Targets infections linked to increased cancer risk, like the HPV vaccine for cervical cancer.
Travel and global health	Protects travelers from region-specific infections and contributes to global health initiatives
Herd immunity	Creates collective immunity in a population to reduce outbreak risks, benefitting vulnerable groups.
Allergy and autoimmune research	Explores vaccination strategies to address allergies and autoimmune diseases.
Maternal and neonatal health	Provides protection to both pregnant women and newborns against certain infections.
Biodefense and bioterrorism preparedness	Serves as a crucial component of biodefense strategies and preparedness.

genetic material into human cells. This genetic material encodes antigens from a target pathogen, prompting the immune system to recognize and mount a defense against the antigen without causing the disease itself [109].

The viral vectors used in these vaccines act as carriers, effectively introducing the antigen-producing genetic instructions to cells. This prompts the cells to generate the antigen, which is then presented to the immune system. The immune system responds by producing antibodies and activating immune cells, such as T cells, to remember and fight the pathogen if encountered in the future. Viral vector–based vaccines offer several advantages, including their ability to induce strong and long-lasting immune responses. They can also be engineered to carry antigens from multiple pathogens, potentially enabling the development of combination vaccines. Notable examples include the Oxford-AstraZeneca vaccine for COVID-19, which employs a chimpanzee adenovirus vector, and the Johnson & Johnson COVID-19 vaccine, which uses a human adenovirus vector. These vaccines have demonstrated their potential in combatting a range of infectious diseases and are also being explored for their potential in other fields, such as cancer immunotherapy. While they offer exciting prospects, ongoing research continues to refine their design, safety, and effectiveness, contributing to the advancement of modern vaccine development and the prevention of a variety of illnesses [110].

7.6.2.2 Genetic Vaccines

Genetic vaccines, a cutting-edge innovation in the field of immunization, represent a novel approach to triggering immune responses against infectious diseases. Unlike traditional vaccines that use weakened or inactivated pathogens, genetic vaccines leverage the power of genetic material to stimulate immunity. In genetic vaccines, a small piece of genetic material, often DNA or mRNA, is introduced into the body. This genetic material carries instructions to produce a specific antigen from the target pathogen. Once inside the body's cells, these instructions prompt the cells to generate the antigen, which is then recognized by the immune system as foreign. The immune system responds by producing antibodies and activating immune cells, preparing the body to mount a defense if it encounters the actual pathogen [111]. One remarkable aspect of genetic vaccines is their ability to mimic natural infection without causing the disease itself. This stimulates a robust immune response that offers protection. Genetic vaccines have shown promising results in various applications, including infectious diseases like COVID-19, influenza, and Zika virus. They offer advantages such as rapid development, versatility, and potential for broad-spectrum protection. For instance, during the COVID-19 pandemic, mRNA-based vaccines from Pfizer-BioNTech and Moderna were developed and authorized for emergency use in record time. While genetic vaccines hold immense potential, ongoing research continues to refine their design, delivery methods, and long-term safety. The rapid advancements in this field not only transform vaccine development but also pave the way for innovative approaches to prevent and control a wide range of diseases.

7.7 Conclusion

In summary, DNA and RNA viral vectors have revolutionized gene therapy and biotechnology. These innovative vectors hold immense potential for treating genetic disorders, cancer, and infectious diseases, and ongoing research will be critical to harnessing their power for personalized medicine and improved healthcare. In the ever-evolving realm of gene therapy, DNA and RNA viral vectors offer transformative possibilities, ushering in a new era of medical breakthroughs. Continuous research, advancements in technology, and rigorous safety evaluations will play a pivotal role in unleashing the complete capabilities of DNA and RNA viral vectors and ensuring their secure and successful implementation in medical treatments. Looking ahead, the prospects for DNA and RNA viral vectors are incredibly bright, paving the way for an exciting era of precision medicine and personalized therapies.

References

1. Chowdhury, E.H., *Nanotherapeutics: From Laboratory to Clinic*, CRC press, Boca Raton, Florida, 2016, ISBN 1-4987-0752-1.
2. Smith, A.E., Viral Vectors in Gene Therapy. *Annu. Rev. Microbiol.*, *49*, 807–838, 1995.
3. Louz, D., Bergmans, H.E., Loos, B.P., Hoeben, R.C., Cross-species Transfer of Viruses: Implications for the Use of Viral Vectors in Biomedical Research, Gene Therapy and as Live-virus Vaccines. *J. Gene Medicine Cross-disciplinary J. Res. Sci. Gene Transfer Clin. Appl.*, *7*, 1263–1274, 2005.
4. Ura, T., Okuda, K., Shimada, M., Developments in Viral Vector-Based Vaccines. *Vaccines*, *2*, 624–641, 2014.
5. Robinson, H.L. and Pertmer, T.M., DNA Vaccines for Viral Infections: Basic Studies and Applications, 2000.
6. Holland, J.J.D., De La Torre, J., Steinhauer, D., RNA Virus Populations as Quasispecies. *Genet. Diversity RNA Viruses*, 176, 1–20, 1992.
7. Gelderblom, H.R., Structure and Classification of Viruses, in: *Medical Microbiology*, 4th edition, 1996.
8. Gajdusek, D.C., Unconventional Viruses and the Origin and Disappearance of Kuru. *Science*, *197*, 943–960, 1977.
9. Shareck, J., Choi, Y., Lee, B., Miguez, C.B., Cloning Vectors Based on Cryptic Plasmids Isolated from Lactic Acid Bacteria: Their Characteristics and Potential Applications in Biotechnology. *Crit. Rev. Biotechnol.*, *24*, 155–208, 2004.
10. Mairhofer, J. and Lara, A.R., Advances in Host and Vector Development for the Production of Plasmid DNA Vaccines. *Cancer Vaccines Methods Protoc.*, 1139, 505–541, 2014.
11. Rodrigues, T., Carrondo, M.J., Alves, P.M., Cruz, P.E., Purification of Retroviral Vectors for Clinical Application: Biological Implications and Technological Challenges. *J. Biotechnol.*, *127*, 520–541, 2007.

12. Vuppu, S., Mishra, T., Gholap, A.D., Balar, P.C., Gogoi, N.R., Chavda, V.P., Expression System and Purification Process for the Vaccine Production, in: *Advanced Vaccination Technologies for Infectious and Chronic Diseases*, pp. 131–151, Elsevier, 2024, ISBN 978-0-443-18564-9.
13. Lentz, T.B., Gray, S.J., Samulski, R.J., Viral Vectors for Gene Delivery to the Central Nervous System. *Neurobiol. Dis.*, *48*, 179–188, 2012.
14. Monaco, A.P. and Larin, Z., YACs, BACs, PACs and MACs: Artificial Chromosomes as Research Tools. *Trends Biotechnol.*, *12*, 280–286, 1994.
15. Flotte, T. and Carter, B., Adeno-Associated Virus Vectors for Gene Therapy. *Gene Ther.*, *2*, 357–362, 1995.
16. Enders, J.F., Bell, J.A., Dingle, J.H., Francis Jr., T., Hilleman, M.R., Huebner, R.J., Payne, A.-M., "Adenoviruses": Group Name Proposed for New Respiratory-Tract Viruses. *Science*, *124*, 119–120, 1956.
17. Walther, W. and Stein, U., Viral Vectors for Gene Transfer: A Review of Their Use in the Treatment of Human Diseases. *Drugs*, *60*, 249–271, 2000.
18. Graham, F.L., Smiley, J., Russell, W., Nairn, R., Characteristics of a Human Cell Line Transformed by DNA from Human Adenovirus Type 5. *J. Gen. Virol.*, *36*, 59–72, 1977.
19. Chavda, V.P., Bezbaruah, R., Valu, D., Patel, B., Kumar, A., Prasad, S., Kakoti, B.B., Kaushik, A., Jesawadawala, M., Adenoviral Vector-Based Vaccine Platform for COVID-19: Current Status. *Vaccines*, *11*, 432, 2023, doi: 10.3390/vaccines11020432.
20. Yei, S., Mittereder, N., Tang, K., O'Sullivan, C., Trapnell, B., Adenovirus-Mediated Gene Transfer for Cystic Fibrosis: Quantitative Evaluation of Repeated *in Vivo* Vector Administration to the Lung. *Gene Ther.*, *1*, 192–200, 1994.
21. Yang, Y., Su, Q., Wilson, J.M., Role of Viral Antigens in Destructive Cellular Immune Responses to Adenovirus Vector-Transduced Cells in Mouse Lungs. *J. Virol.*, *70*, 7209–7212, 1996.
22. Dedieu, J.-F., Vigne, E., Torrent, C., Jullien, C., Mahfouz, I., Caillaud, J.-M., Aubailly, N., Orsini, C., Guillaume, J.-M., Opolon, P., Long-Term Gene Delivery into the Livers of Immunocompetent Mice with E1/E4-Defective Adenoviruses. *J. Virol.*, *71*, 4626–4637, 1997.
23. Bischoff, J.R., Kirn, D.H., Williams, A., Heise, C., Horn, S., Muna, M., Ng, L., Nye, J.A., Sampson-Johannes, A., Fattaey, A., An Adenovirus Mutant That Replicates Selectively in P53-Deficient Human Tumor Cells. *Science*, *274*, 373–376, 1996.
24. Robbins, P.D., Tahara, H., Ghivizzani, S.C., Viral Vectors for Gene Therapy. *Trends Biotechnol.*, *16*, 35–40, 1998.
25. Miller, D.G., Adam, M.A., Miller, A.D., Gene Transfer by Retrovirus Vectors Occurs Only in Cells That Are Actively Replicating at the Time of Infection. *Mol. Cell. Biol.*, 10, 8, 4239–4242, 1990.

26. Deng, S., Liang, H., Chen, P., Li, Y., Li, Z., Fan, S., Wu, K., Li, X., Chen, W., Qin, Y., Viral Vector Vaccine Development and Application during the COVID-19 Pandemic. *Microorganisms, 10*, 1450, 2022.
27. Patterson, L.J. and Robert-Guroff, M., Replicating Adenovirus Vector Prime/Protein Boost Strategies for HIV Vaccine Development. *Expert Opin. Biol. Ther., 8*, 1347–1363, 2008.
28. Ferreira, T., Alves, P., Aunins, J., Carrondo, M., Use of Adenoviral Vectors as Veterinary Vaccines. *Gene Ther., 12*, S73–S83, 2005.
29. Weinberg, J., Matthews, T., Cullen, B., Malim, M., Productive Human Immunodeficiency Virus Type 1 (HIV-1) Infection of Nonproliferating Human Monocytes. *J. Exp. Med., 174*, 1477–1482, 1991.
30. Lewis, P., Hensel, M., Emerman, M., Human Immunodeficiency Virus Infection of Cells Arrested in the Cell Cycle. *EMBO J., 11*, 3053–3058, 1992.
31. Gallay, P., Swingler, S., Song, J., Bushman, F., Trono, D., HIV Nuclear Import Is Governed by the Phosphotyrosine-Mediated Binding of Matrix to the Core Domain of Integrase. *Cell, 83*, 569–576, 1995.
32. Kim, V.N., Mitrophanous, K., Kingsman, S.M., Kingsman, A.J., Minimal Requirement for a Lentivirus Vector Based on Human Immunodeficiency Virus Type 1. *J. Virol., 72*, 811–816, 1998.
33. Naldini, L., Blömer, U., Gallay, P., Ory, D., Mulligan, R., Gage, F.H., Verma, I.M., Trono, D., *In Vivo* Gene Delivery and Stable Transduction of Nondividing Cells by a Lentiviral Vector. *Science, 272*, 263–267, 1996.
34. Zufferey, R., Nagy, D., Mandel, R.J., Naldini, L., Trono, D., Multiply Attenuated Lentiviral Vector Achieves Efficient Gene Delivery *in Vivo. Nat. Biotechnol., 15*, 871–875, 1997.
35. Zheng, C., Wang, S., Bai, Y., Luo, T., Wang, J., Dai, C., Guo, B., Luo, S., Wang, D., Yang, Y., Lentiviral Vectors and Adeno-associated Virus Vectors: Useful Tools for Gene Transfer in Pain Research. *Anat. Rec., 301*, 825–836, 2018.
36. Kimura, E., Li, S., Gregorevic, P., Fall, B.M., Chamberlain, J.S., Dystrophin Delivery to Muscles of Mdx Mice Using Lentiviral Vectors Leads to Myogenic Progenitor Targeting and Stable Gene Expression. *Mol. Ther., 18*, 206–213, 2010.
37. Park, F., Lentiviral Vectors: Are They the Future of Animal Transgenesis? *Physiol. Genomics, 31*, 159–173, 2007.
38. Bischof, D. and Cornetta, K., Flexibility in Cell Targeting by Pseudotyping Lentiviral Vectors, in: *Lentivirus Gene Engineering Protocols: Second Edition*, pp. 53–68, 2010.
39. Ferrara, F., Del Rosario, J.M.M., Da Costa, K.A., Kinsley, R., Scott, S., Fereidouni, S., Thompson, C., Kellam, P., Gilbert, S., Carnell, G., Development of Lentiviral Vectors Pseudotyped with Influenza B Hemagglutinins: Application in Vaccine Immunogenicity, mAb Potency, and Sero-Surveillance Studies. *Front. Immunol., 12*, 661379, 2021.
40. Schambach, A. and Baum, C., Clinical Application of Lentiviral Vectors-Concepts and Practice. *Curr. Gene Ther., 8*, 474–482, 2008.

41. Oldham, R.A., Berinstein, E.M., Medin, J.A., Lentiviral Vectors in Cancer Immunotherapy. *Immunotherapy*, *7*, 271–284, 2015.
42. Yamamoto, T. and Tsunetsugu-Yokota, Y., Prospects for the Therapeutic Application of Lentivirus-Based Gene Therapy to HIV-1 Infection. *Curr. Gene Ther.*, *8*, 1–8, 2008.
43. Galimi, F. and Verma, I., Opportunities for the Use of Lentiviral Vectors in Human Gene Therapy. *Lentiviral Vectors*, 245–254, 2002.
44. Blacklow, N.R., Hoggan, M.D., Kapikian, A.Z., Austin, J.B., Rowe, W.P., Epidemiology of Adenovirus-Associated Virus Infection in a Nursery Population. *Am. J. Epidemiol.*, *88*, 368–378, 1968.
45. Fisher, K.J., Gao, G.-P., Weitzman, M.D., DeMatteo, R., Burda, J.F., Wilson, J.M., Transduction with Recombinant Adeno-Associated Virus for Gene Therapy Is Limited by Leading-Strand Synthesis. *J. Virol.*, *70*, 520–532, 1996.
46. Gao, G.-P., Qu, G., Faust, L.Z., Engdahl, R.K., Xiao, W., Hughes, J.V., Zoltick, P.W., Wilson, J.M., High-Titer Adeno-Associated Viral Vectors from a Rep/Cap Cell Line and Hybrid Shuttle Virus. *Hum. Gene Ther.*, *9*, 2353–2362, 1998.
47. Xiao, X., Li, J., Samulski, R.J., Production of High-Titer Recombinant Adeno-Associated Virus Vectors in the Absence of Helper Adenovirus. *J. Virol.*, *72*, 2224–2232, 1998.
48. Kwon, I. and Schaffer, D.V., Designer Gene Delivery Vectors: Molecular Engineering and Evolution of Adeno-Associated Viral Vectors for Enhanced Gene Transfer. *Pharm. Res.*, *25*, 489–499, 2008.
49. Smith-Arica, J.R. and Bartlett, J.S., Gene Therapy: Recombinant Adeno-Associated Virus Vectors. *Curr. Cardiol Rep.*, *3*, 43–49, 2001.
50. Büning, H., Braun-Falco, M., Hallek, M., Progress in the Use of Adeno-Associated Viral Vectors for Gene Therapy. *Cells Tissues Organs*, *177*, 139–150, 2004.
51. McClure, C., Cole, K.L., Wulff, P., Klugmann, M., Murray, A.J., Production and Titering of Recombinant Adeno-Associated Viral Vectors. *JoVE (J. Visualized Experiments)*, 27, 57, e3348, 2011.
52. Snoeck, H., Tao, W., Klotman, M., Adeno-Associated Viral Vectors: Background and Technical Aspects. *Exp. Nephrol.*, *5*, 514–520, 1997.
53. Ali, R.R., Reichel, M.B., Thrasher, A.J., Levinsky, R.J., Kinnon, C., Kanuga, N., Hunt, D.M., Bhattacharya, S.S., Gene Transfer into the Mouse Retina Mediated by an Adeno-Associated Viral Vector. *Hum. Mol. Genet.*, *5*, 591–594, 1996.
54. Schwarz, E.M., The Adeno-Associated Virus Vector for Orthopaedic Gene Therapy. *Clin. Orthop. Relat. Research®*, *379*, S31–S39, 2000.
55. Mueller, C. and Flotte, T.R., Clinical Gene Therapy Using Recombinant Adeno-Associated Virus Vectors. *Gene Ther.*, *15*, 858–863, 2008.
56. Finegold, A.A., Mannes, A.J., Iadarola, M.J.A., Paracrine Paradigm for *in Vivo* Gene Therapy in the Central Nervous System: Treatment of Chronic Pain. *Hum. Gene Ther.*, *10*, 1251–1257, 1999.

57. Volpers, C. and Kochanek, S., Adenoviral Vectors for Gene Transfer and Therapy. *J. Gene Medicine Cross-disciplinary J. Res. Sci. Gene Transfer Clin. Appl.*, *6*, S164–S171, 2004.
58. Ponnazhagan, S., Curiel, D.T., Shaw, D.R., Alvarez, R.D., Siegal, G.P., Adeno-Associated Virus for Cancer Gene Therapy. *Cancer Res.*, *61*, 6313–6321, 2001.
59. Slon-Campos, J.L., Poggianella, M., Zentilin, L., Burrone, O.R., Use of Adeno-Associated Viral Vectors to Improve Delivery of a DNA Vaccine against Dengue Virus. *J. Gen. Virol.*, *101*, 73–78, 2020.
60. Vandenberghe, L. and Auricchio, A., Novel Adeno-Associated Viral Vectors for Retinal Gene Therapy. *Gene Ther.*, *19*, 162–168, 2012.
61. Ponnazhagan, S., Adenoassociated Virus Vectors for Genetic Immunization. *Immunol. Res.*, *26*, 247–253, 2002.
62. Hu, Y.-C., Baculoviral Vectors for Gene Delivery: A Review. *Curr. Gene Ther.*, *8*, 54–65, 2008.
63. Fitzgerald, D.J., Berger, P., Schaffitzel, C., Yamada, K., Richmond, T.J., Berger, I., Protein Complex Expression by Using Multigene Baculoviral Vectors. *Nat. Methods*, *3*, 1021–1032, 2006.
64. Glorioso, J., DeLuca, N., Fink, D., Development and Application of Herpes Simplex Virus Vectors for Human Gene Therapy. *Annu. Rev. Microbiol.*, *49*, 675–710, 1995.
65. Stavropoulos, T.A. and Strathdee, C.A., An Enhanced Packaging System for Helper-Dependent Herpes Simplex Virus Vectors. *J. Virol.*, *72*, 7137–7143, 1998.
66. Burton, E.A., Wechuck, J.B., Wendell, S.K., Goins, W.F., Fink, D.J., Glorioso, J.C., Multiple Applications for Replication-Defective Herpes Simplex Virus Vectors. *Stem Cells*, *19*, 358–377, 2001.
67. Moss, B., Genetically Engineered Poxviruses for Recombinant Gene Expression, Vaccination, and Safety. *Proc. Natl. Acad. Sci.*, *93*, 11341–11348, 1996.
68. Bender, B.S., Rowe, C.A., Taylor, S.F., Wyatt, L.S., Moss, B., Small Jr., P.A., Oral Immunization with a Replication-Deficient Recombinant Vaccinia Virus Protects Mice against Influenza. *J. Virol.*, *70*, 6418–6424, 1996.
69. McAneny, D., Ryan, C.A., Beazley, R.M., Kaufman, H.L., Results of a Phase I Trial of a Recombinant Vaccinia Virus That Expresses Carcinoembryonic Antigen in Patients with Advanced Colorectal Cancer. *Ann. Surg. Oncol.*, *3*, 495–500, 1996.
70. Tomanin, R. and Scarpa, M., Why Do We Need New Gene Therapy Viral Vectors? Characteristics, Limitations and Future Perspectives of Viral Vector Transduction. *Curr. Gene Ther.*, *4*, 357–372, 2004.
71. Lesbats, P., Engelman, A.N., Cherepanov, P., Retroviral DNA Integration. *Chem. Rev.*, *116*, 12730–12757, 2016.
72. Vargas, J.E., Chicaybam, L., Stein, R.T., Tanuri, A., Delgado-Cañedo, A., Bonamino, M.H., Retroviral Vectors and Transposons for Stable Gene

Therapy: Advances, Current Challenges and Perspectives. *J. Transl. Med.*, *14*, 1–15, 2016.

73. Chen, Y.H., Keiser, M.S., Davidson, B.L., Viral Vectors for Gene Transfer. *Curr. Protoc. Mouse Biol.*, *8*, e58, 2018.
74. Chira, S., Jackson, C.S., Oprea, I., Ozturk, F., Pepper, M.S., Diaconu, I., Braicu, C., Raduly, L.-Z., Calin, G.A., Berindan-Neagoe, I., Progresses towards Safe and Efficient Gene Therapy Vectors. *Oncotarget*, *6*, 30675, 2015.
75. Hoffmann, D., Schott, J., Geis, F., Lange, L., Müller, F., Lenz, D., Zychlinski, D., Steinemann, D., Morgan, M., Moritz, T., Detailed Comparison of Retroviral Vectors and Promoter Configurations for Stable and High Transgene Expression in Human Induced Pluripotent Stem Cells. *Gene Ther.*, *24*, 298–307, 2017.
76. Dutrieux, J., Maarifi, G., Portilho, D.M., Arhel, N.J., Chelbi-Alix, M.K., Nisole, S., PML/TRIM19-Dependent Inhibition of Retroviral Reverse-Transcription by Daxx. *PLoS Pathog.*, *11*, e1005280, 2015.
77. Apolonia, L., The Old and the New: Prospects for Non-Integrating Lentiviral Vector Technology. *Viruses*, *12*, 1103, 2020.
78. Ghosh, S., Brown, A.M., Jenkins, C., Campbell, K., Viral Vector Systems for Gene Therapy: A Comprehensive Literature Review of Progress and Biosafety Challenges. *Appl. Biosaf.*, *25*, 7–18, 2020.
79. Bulcha, J.T., Wang, Y., Ma, H., Tai, P.W., Gao, G., Viral Vector Platforms within the Gene Therapy Landscape. *Signal Transduction Targeted Ther.*, *6*, 53, 2021.
80. Ferreira, M.V., Cabral, E.T., Coroadinha, A.S., Progress and Perspectives in the Development of Lentiviral Vector Producer Cells. *Biotechnol. J.*, *16*, 2000017, 2021.
81. Gutierrez-Guerrero, A., Cosset, F.-L., Verhoeyen, E., Lentiviral Vector Pseudotypes: Precious Tools to Improve Gene Modification of Hematopoietic Cells for Research and Gene Therapy. *Viruses*, *12*, 1016, 2020.
82. Cooray, S., Howe, S.J., Thrasher, A.J., Retrovirus and Lentivirus Vector Design and Methods of Cell Conditioning, in: *Methods in enzymology*, vol. 507, pp. 29–57, Elsevier, Amsterdam, Netherlands, 2012, ISBN 0076-6879.
83. Lee, C.S., Bishop, E.S., Zhang, R., Yu, X., Farina, E.M., Yan, S., Zhao, C., Zeng, Z., Shu, Y., Wu, X., Adenovirus-Mediated Gene Delivery: Potential Applications for Gene and Cell-Based Therapies in the New Era of Personalized Medicine. *Genes Dis.*, *4*, 43–63, 2017.
84. Cavazzana, M., Bushman, F.D., Miccio, A., André-Schmutz, I., Six, E., Gene Therapy Targeting Haematopoietic Stem Cells for Inherited Diseases: Progress and Challenges. *Nat. Rev. Drug Discovery*, *18*, 447–462, 2019.
85. Li, H., Yang, Y., Hong, W., Huang, M., Wu, M., Zhao, X., Applications of Genome Editing Technology in the Targeted Therapy of Human Diseases: Mechanisms, Advances and Prospects. *Signal Transduction Targeted Ther.*, *5*, 1, 2020.

86. Munis, A.M., Gene Therapy Applications of Non-Human Lentiviral Vectors. *Viruses, 12*, 1106, 2020.
87. Babaeimarzangou, S.S., Zaker, H., Soleimannezhadbari, E., Gamchi, N.S., Kazeminia, M., Tarighi, S., Seyedian, H., Tsatsakis, A., Spandidos, D.A., Margina, D., Vaccine Development for Zoonotic Viral Diseases Caused by Positivesense Singlestranded RNA Viruses Belonging to the Coronaviridae and Togaviridae Families. *Exp. Ther. Med., 25*, 1–24, 2023.
88. Joseph, R.E., Urakova, N., Werling, K.L., Metz, H.C., Montanari, K., Rasgon, J.L., Culex Tarsalis Is a Competent Host of the Insect-Specific Alphavirus Eilat Virus (EILV). *J. Virol., 97*, e01960–22, 2023.
89. Graham, B.S., Biological Challenges and Technological Opportunities for Respiratory Syncytial Virus Vaccine Development. *Immunol. Rev., 239*, 149–166, 2011.
90. Choi, Y. and Chang, J., Viral Vectors for Vaccine Applications. *Clin. Exp. Vaccine Res., 2*, 97–105, 2013.
91. Yamaki, Y., Fukushima, T., Yoshida, N., Nishimura, K., Fukuda, A., Hisatake, K., Aso, M., Sakasai, T., Kijima-Tanaka, J., Miwa, Y., Utilization of a Novel Sendai Virus Vector in *Ex Vivo* Gene Therapy for Hemophilia A. *Int. J. Hematol., 113*, 493–499, 2021.
92. Liu, G., David, B.T., Trawczynski, M., Fessler, R.G., Advances in Pluripotent Stem Cells: History, Mechanisms, Technologies, and Applications. *Stem Cell Rev. Rep., 16*, 3–32, 2020.
93. Takahashi, K. and Yokobayashi, Y., Reversible Gene Regulation in Mammalian Cells Using Riboswitch-Engineered Vesicular Stomatitis Virus Vector. *ACS Synth. Biol., 8*, 1976–1982, 2019.
94. Huang, J., Zhou, Y., Li, J., Lu, A., Liang, C., CRISPR/Cas Systems: Delivery and Application in Gene Therapy. *Front. Bioeng. Biotechnol., 10*, 942325, 2022.
95. Joseph, J.M., Gigliobianco, M.R., Firouzabadi, B.M., Censi, R., Di Martino, P., Nanotechnology as a Versatile Tool for 19F-MRI Agent's Formulation: A Glimpse into the Use of Perfluorinated and Fluorinated Compounds in Nanoparticles. *Pharmaceutics, 14*, 382, 2022.
96. Henkhaus, N., Bartlett, M., Gang, D., Grumet, R., Jordon-Thaden, I., Lorence, A., Lyons, E., Miller, S., Murray, S., Nelson, A., Plant Science Decadal Vision 2020–2030: Reimagining the Potential of Plants for a Healthy and Sustainable Future. *Plant Direct, 4*, e00252, 2020.
97. Kiesslich, S. and Kamen, A.A., Vero Cell Upstream Bioprocess Development for the Production of Viral Vectors and Vaccines. *Biotechnol. Adv., 44*, 107608, 2020.
98. Li, C. and Samulski, R.J., Engineering Adeno-Associated Virus Vectors for Gene Therapy. *Nat. Rev. Genet., 21*, 255–272, 2020.
99. Yom-Tov, N., Guy, R., Offen, D., Extracellular Vesicles over Adeno-Associated Viruses: Advantages and Limitations as Drug Delivery Platforms in Precision Medicine. *Adv. Drug Delivery Rev.*, 190, 114535, 2022.

100. Goyal, P. and Malviya, R., Advances in Nuclei Targeted Delivery of Nanoparticles for the Management of Cancer. *Biochim. Biophys. Acta (BBA)-Reviews Cancer*, 1978, 3, 188881, 2023.
101. Shim, G., Kim, D., Park, G.T., Jin, H., Suh, S.-K., Oh, Y.-K., Therapeutic Gene Editing: Delivery and Regulatory Perspectives. *Acta Pharmacol. Sin.*, *38*, 738–753, 2017.
102. Knezevic, I., Liu, M.A., Peden, K., Zhou, T., Kang, H.-N., Development of mRNA Vaccines: Scientific and Regulatory Issues. *Vaccines*, *9*, 81, 2021.
103. Mogler, M.A. and Kamrud, K.I., RNA-Based Viral Vectors. *Expert Rev. Vaccines*, *14*, 283–312, 2015.
104. Picanço-Castro, V., Pereira, C.G., Covas, D.T., Porto, G.S., Athanassiadou, A., Figueiredo, M.L., Emerging Patent Landscape for Non-Viral Vectors Used for Gene Therapy. *Nat. Biotechnol.*, *38*, 151–157, 2020.
105. Wolf, D.P., Mitalipov, P.A., Mitalipov, S.M., Principles of and Strategies for Germline Gene Therapy. *Nat. Med.*, *25*, 890–897, 2019.
106. Fajardo-Serrano, A., Rico, A.J., Roda, E., Honrubia, A., Arrieta, S., Ariznabarreta, G., Chocarro, J., Lorenzo-Ramos, E., Pejenaute, A., Vázquez, A., Adeno-Associated Viral Vectors as Versatile Tools for Parkinson's Research, Both for Disease Modeling Purposes and for Therapeutic Uses. *Int. J. Mol. Sci.*, *22*, 6389, 2021.
107. Ingusci, S., Verlengia, G., Soukupova, M., Zucchini, S., Simonato, M., Gene Therapy Tools for Brain Diseases. *Front. Pharmacol.*, *10*, 724, 2019.
108. Nicoll, J.A., Bloom, T., Clarke, A., Boche, D., Hilton, D., BRAIN UK: Accessing NHS Tissue Archives for Neuroscience Research. *Neuropathol. Appl. Neurobiol.*, *48*, e12766, 2022.
109. Zhao, Z., Anselmo, A.C., Mitragotri, S., Viral Vector-based Gene Therapies in the Clinic. *Bioeng. Transl. Med.*, *7*, e10258, 2022.
110. Yang, X., Fox, A., DeCarlo, C., Norris, C., Griffin, S., Wedekind, S., Flanagan, J.M., Shenker, N., Powell, R.L., Comparative Profiles of SARS-CoV-2 Spike-Specific Human Milk Antibodies Elicited by mRNA-and Adenovirus-Based COVID-19 Vaccines. *Breastfeeding Med.*, *17*, 638–646, 2022.
111. Albertsen, C.H., Kulkarni, J.A., Witzigmann, D., Lind, M., Petersson, K., Simonsen, J.B., The Role of Lipid Components in Lipid Nanoparticles for Vaccines and Gene Therapy. *Adv. Drug Delivery Rev.*, *189*, 114416, 2022.

8

Manufacturing and Control of Viral-Vector Vaccines: Challenges

Vivek P. Chavda[1]*, Dixa A. Vaghela[2], Dhunusmita Barman[3], Arzoo Newar[4] and Ahmed Nasima[5]

[1]Department of Pharmaceutics and Pharmaceutical Technology, L.M. College of Pharmacy, Navrangpura, Ahmedabad, Gujarat, India
[2]Pharmacy Section, L.M. College of Pharmacy, Ahmedabad, Gujarat, India
[3]NEF College of Pharmacy, Lokhra, Saukuchi, Guwahati, Assam, India
[4]Girijananda Chowdhury University, GIPS-Tezpur, Dekargaon, Sonitpur, Assam, India
[5]Department of Pharmaceutical Sciences, Dibrugarh University, Dibrugarh, Assam, India

Abstract
Viral vector–based vaccines are a promising class for producing immunization. The application of new advanced technology provides a good assessment in the development and production of vaccines, using viral vectors to mitigate the diseases. The progress from clinical development to industrial manufacturing involves programs, supply requirements, and measures to be taken care of for advanced vaccine development. In addition, to expand the potential, intensive critical steps would be required. The scalability of the production process is another major hurdle, requiring sophisticated bioreactors and purification techniques to ensure consistency, purity, and safety of the final product. Regulatory challenges further complicate the landscape as manufacturers must navigate diverse international guidelines and standards.

Keywords: Viral vector, challenges, vector design, stability of vaccines

**Corresponding author*: Vivek.chavda@lmcp.ac.in

Vivek P. Chavda and Vasso Apostolopoulos (eds.) Viral Vectors for Vaccine Delivery, (221–256) © 2025 Scrivener Publishing LLC

8.1 Introduction

Recombinant viral vector vaccines have been used to deliver genetic material into host cells to stimulate an immune response. The first viral vector expression was created from the SV40 virus in 1972. Adenoviruses, vaccinia virus (VACV), measles, pox, herpes, and lentivirus have been engineered into vaccine vectors to stimulate immune response [1]. The manufacturing process involves vector construction, cell line development, upstream processing, downstream processing, formulation, quality control, and regulatory approval process [2].

Replication-competent or replication-deficient viral vector vaccines have been developed to lower reactogenicity and improve safety [3]. Interestingly, the viral vector vaccine can mimic the natural pathogen infection process, resulting in immune recognition and classical acute inflammation through the synthesis of pathogen-associated molecular patterns (PAMPs). This allows for mucosal delivery and the development of both systemic and localized immunity [4]. Higher effectiveness would be achieved for mucosal administration of viral vector–based vaccines in complicated diseases such as COVID-19 [5]. Viral vector vaccines offer a huge advantage over traditional vaccines, including eliciting potential antibody and cell-mediated immune responses, and are crucial for eliminating pathogen-infected cells. At a single dose, it can produce a potent immune response without the use of an adjuvant [6].

Viral vectors are effective, but they come with inevitable issues that must be resolved. Viral vector–based vaccinations may be used more frequently shortly to combat serious illnesses like HIV-1 and malaria [7]. Viral integration techniques are utilized in certain vectors to achieve stable expression of the interesting gene. Cancer may arise from integration into the host genome. The existence of preexisting immunity against the vector adds another challenge to the clinical use of viral vectors. This is brought on by prior viral exposure and the development of neutralizing antibodies, which lessen the vaccine's effectiveness [8]. This chapter mainly emphasizes the fundamentals of manufacturing viral vector–based vaccines, the challenges associated with it, quality control, and technological innovations to overcome obstacles in vaccine design and development. The regulatory requirements and future challenges are addressed.

8.2 Fundamentals of Viral-Vectored Vaccine Manufacturing

8.2.1 Viral Vector Construction

Viral vectors were created using a variety of methods, which can be generally categorized into two: (i) the direct attachment of the foreign gene into the viral genomic DNA in a plasmid form by using specific restriction endonuclease [9]. (ii) Homologous recombination that can occur in the bacteria or in a permissive cell line [10] to recombine two plasmids. The two plasmid system consists of the shuttle plasmid containing the foreign gene cassette and virus sequences required for general recombination. The creation of an infectious viral vector, and a genomic plasmid that almost completely contains the virus genome along with the requisite deletions. To create viral vectors, recombination processes are often performed using one of two methods, the first one is Cre/lox recombination in mammalian cells, and the second is homologous recombination in bacteria. Using these two recombination techniques, the comprehensive protocols for producing and purifying viral vectors are outlined below [11]. The general formulation fundamentals for the manufacturing of viral vaccines are represented below in Figure 8.1.

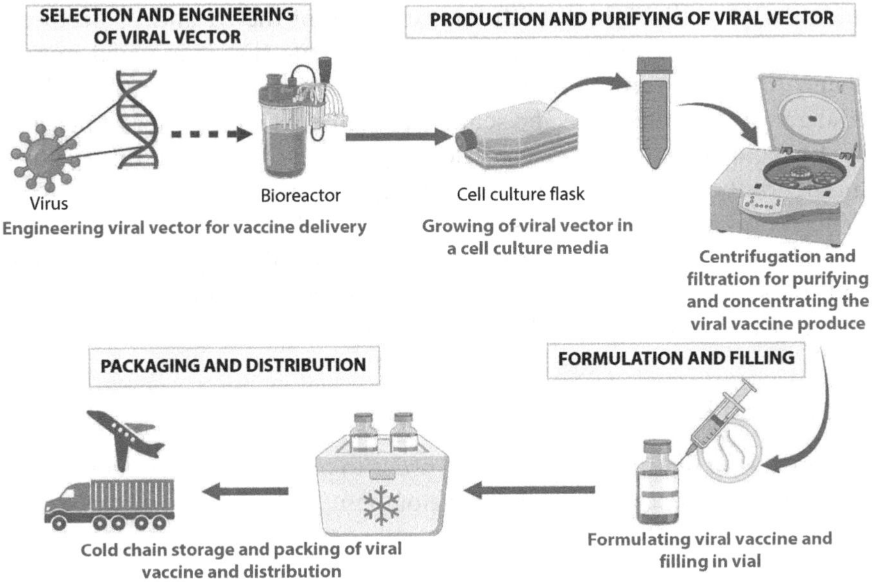

Figure 8.1 Fundamentals of viral-vectored vaccine manufacturing and distribution process.

8.2.2 Development of the Viral Vector in Bacteria Through Homologous Recombination

The full virus genome is included in the genomic plasmid pAdV-ΔE1E3, which is flanked by a special restriction enzyme (such as PacI) and has the necessary E1 and E3 deletions for the creation of first-generation viral vectors. Both ends of the viral genome are present in the shuttle plasmid, pAdV-shuttle-T [12]. After the viral sequences for the protein IX gene for homologous recombination, the deletion of E1 was restored with a eukaryotic promoter like the human cytomegalovirus (HCMV), multiple cloning sites (MCS) for the foreign gene insertion, the polyadenylation (polyA) signal such as the bovine growth hormone (BGH) polyA [13]. A special restriction enzyme site (like PacI) at either end of a virus sequence and an additional unique restriction enzyme site (like HindIII) in the middle of the left and right virus genome sequences are also present in the shuttle plasmid. pAdV-ΔE1E3 releases its genomic DNA through PacI digestion, which is then followed by gel purification [11].

8.2.2.1 Production of the Viral Vector Using Cre/loxP Recombination System

With this approach, the whole virus genome is present in the genomic plasmid pAdVΔψ, E1,E3/loxP, with the exception of the E1 and E3 sections, the packing signal (ψ) sequences, and a loxP site that is inserted immediately following recombination of the E1 deletion [14]. The two ends of viral genomes contain specific sequence, the HCMV promoter in place of the E1 region deletion, numerous cloning sites, the shuttle plasmid, pAdV-shuttle/loxP carries the numerous cloning sites and the BGH polyA. Next to BGH polyA, a loxP site is inserted. The HEK 293 cell line bearing the Cre recombinase gene (293Cre4) can be transduced with the genomic plasmid and the shuttle plasmid having a transgenic cassette in order to acquire human viral vectors via Cre/loxP recombination [11].

8.2.3 Cell Line Development

The process of manipulating genes in order to produce clonal cultures with longer lifespans is called cell line development [15].

8.2.3.1 Designer Cell Lines and Cell Line Immortalization

The development of continuous cell lines and their immortalization constituted a significant hurdle in animal cell culture. Although spontaneous immortalization in human cells is uncommon, oncogenes can stimulate it. It was discovered that certain viruses may cause immortality. Thus, viral genes or genomes are employed to immortalize cells. The majority of well-known example is the HEK 293 cell line, which was generated in the early 1970s by inducing sheared adenovirus 5 DNA into the cultures of normal human embryonic kidney cells [16].

Vectored vaccines designed based on replication-defective adenoviruses that have insufficient E1 genes (E1A and E1B) on their genome are commonly propagated using HEK 293 cells. The creation of replication-competent adenovirus (RCA) by recombining the virus genome with the adenovirus DNA utilized to prepare the immortalizing HEK 293 cells is a significant problem when employing HEK 293 cells for the manufacturing of adenoviral-vectored vaccines [17]. Then, E1-only trans-complementing "designer cell lines" emerged in response to the demand for cell lines that were safer than HEK 293. The PER.C6® cell line was developed as a result of the overall plan, which was predicated on lowering the Ad5 E1 sequences for cell immortalization. The human embryonic retinoblasts human embryonic retinoblastoma cells known as PER.C6® have undergone transformation using the Ad5 sequence 459 to 3510, which solely includes the E1A and E1B encoding sequences. Furthermore, the human PGK promoter regulates E1A and E1B, in order to compensate for the loss of the 5′ endogenous E1A promoter [15].

Any genetic modification, even if it has no direct connection to the virus that will be created, is included in cell line development. In this instance, the modified vaccinia Ankara (MVA) virus can be produced without the need for primary chicken embryo fibroblasts (CEF) because of the development of AGE1® (Probiogen) cell lines. Retinal (CR), somite (CS), and amnion membrane (CA) cells from Muscovy ducks are the source of AGE1® cell lines, which were immortalized using human Ad5 E1A and E1B genes. It was discovered that CA cells were resistant to MVA replication, although CR and CS cells showed clear distinctions in their anchorage-dependence phenotype: Whereas CS cells multiply in monolayers, CR cells can be grown without anchoring [18].

8.2.3.2 Development of Stable Cell Lines for Vaccine Constitutive Expression

In order to produce vaccines based on viral proteins or viral particles (such as VLPs) consistently, another sort of cell line creation involves the constitutive expression of viral components. The creation of Chinese hamster ovary–Hepatitis B surface antigen (CHO-HBsAG) to produce HBV vaccination is an illustration of this kind of cell line development [19]. If viral proteins are not cytotoxic, then cell line development has been employed to produce VLPs consistently. Human embryonic kidney 293 cells (HEK-G cells), which were created to produce rabies VLPs [20], and BJ-BM cells, which were created to produce VLPs from the Japanese encephalitis virus [15], are two fairly recent instances. The BEVS system's remarkable yields have created a challenging environment for stable VLP generation in animal cells [21]. However, because it may be difficult to separate the vaccine products from the baculovirus contaminants, the BEVS system might be an especially severe downstream processing challenge [22].

8.2.4 Upstream Processing

8.2.4.1 Cultivation Process and Harvest Timing of the Virus

It is important to optimize the virus cultivation temperature, which may differ from the ideal temperature for cell growth (about 37°C). When Ad5 was cultivated in 293S cells, it was found that virus output was much higher at 35°C than it was at 37°C. Additionally, it has been demonstrated that temperature influences postinfection cell death rates and cellular metabolism [23]. The viral productivity, developing cells at 33°C before virus cultivation at 36.5°C, could greatly improve PER.C6 suspension culture [24], and the ideal temperature for cultivating viruses in attached 293 cells is 35°C, while for suspension 293 cells, it is 37°C [25].

Every viral culture system should have its external pH optimized as it is a crucial process parameter. For 293S cells, no evidence of a substantial impact of pH (6.7 to 7.7) on cell proliferation was found [23]. The production of the virus would severely affect pH 6.7 and 7.7; however, only pH 7.2 exhibits significant viral productivity. While a pH of 6.8 caused a large lag phase and decreased growth of cell rate, there is no effect of pH on PER.C6 cell development between the pH range of 7.1 to 7.6 [25]. More basic circumstances resulted in greater glucose intake and lactate formation, demonstrating how sensitive cell metabolism was to pH. The timing and technique of harvesting can be adjusted to suit the needs of either the intra- or extracellular fraction or the overall population. The ideal harvest time of the virus is determined by factors such as extracellular virus stability, desired process reproducibility, and the 48 hours for the purification process [26].

8.2.5 Downstream Processing

8.2.5.1 Purification of Viral Vectors

To assess the effectiveness of the intended viral vectors, purified stocks of viral vectors are necessary for all clinical and preclinical investigations. For viral vector purification in preclinical research using animal models, the most popular and trustworthy procedure is the density-gradient centrifugation technique using cesium chloride (CsCl) [27].

8.2.5.2 Purification of a Large Stock of Viral Vector

First, divide HEK 293 cells into thirty 150-mm tissue culture plates, in the minimum essential medium (MEM) containing 10% fetal calf serum (FCS). Then, incubate the plates for the entire night at 37°C in a CO_2 incubator. After diluting the crude vector stock in phosphate buffer solution $(PBS)^{++}$, infect the cells at a multiplicity of infection (MOI) of 5 plaque-forming units (PFU) of the appropriate viral vector when they are around 90% confluent, which is normally after 24 hours of incubation. After removing the medium from each dish, add 3 ml of PBS^{++} which has the right quantity of vector to initiate the infection. After 30 minutes of CO_2 incubation at 37°C, add 25 ml of maintenance media (MEM + 2% FCS) per plate to the infected plates. The infected plates should be kept at 37°C in a CO_2 incubator until full cytopathic effect (CPE) is seen. Cell rounding and separation are the hallmarks of the CPE, which typically occurs 48 hours after infection. Using a cell lifter, remove the infected cells and culture medium, and then transfer the mixture into the sterile 500-ml centrifuge bottle. To extract the infected cells, centrifuge the contents at 2000*g* for 10 minutes at 4°C. After transferring the supernatant to a different container, autoclave it. Transmit the pellet to a 50-ml tube after resuspending it with 15 ml of 0.1 M tris solution (pH 8.0). The contents will be more viscous as a result of cell lysis and the release of cellular DNA. Add 1.5 ml of 5% sodium deoxycholate solution, followed by vortexing for 30 seconds, and then incubate the tube on ice for 30 minutes, rotating it every 10 minutes. To shear the DNA, homogenize the mixture twice at a high speed for 5 seconds and three times at a speed for 10 seconds using a tissue homogenizer.

The sample needs to be processed on ice, and this stage needs to be completed under a hood [11].

8.2.5.3 *Purification of Viral Vectors Using CsCl Density Gradient Centrifugation*

For every 1 ml of the homogenized vector suspension, add 0.58 ml of saturated CsCl solution. Mix thoroughly, and then divide the liquid between two 13-ml Beckman polyallomer tubes. After that, spin the mixture for 16 hours at 4°C and 35,000 rpm, by puncturing the tube wall nearly below the vector band with a needle connected to a 3-ml syringe, the white vector bands can be gathered. Combining the virus bands into a 5-ml Beckman polyallomer tube yields a balanced tube containing 1 ml of 0.1 M tris pH 8 and 0.58 ml of saturated CsCl (use a ratio of 1:1). Centrifuge the combined vector for 16 hours at 4°C and 35,000 rpm. After removing the white vector band from the 5-ml Beckman polyallomer tube, store it at 4°C until dialysis but not more than a day. To prepare the dialysis tube, boil 500 ml of 1 mM EDTA (pH 8.0) for 10 minutes. Once the dialysis tube has cooled, cut off one end of the tube, add the purified vector in CsCl solution, and then cut off the other end. Dialyze the vector twice for two hours at 4°C in 1 L PBS and once for two hours in 1 L PBS^{++}. Gather purified viral vector from the dialysis tube and store it in a sterile tube inside a biosafety cabinet after dialysis. To the purified viral vector preparation, now add 1/10 volume of sterile glycerol, stir, divide into aliquots (0.5 to 1 ml each), mark the vials, and store at −80°C. Using an appropriate cell line, the plaque assay can be used to titrate the viral vector. A spectrophotometer can be used to measure the organismal development (OD) at specific nm in order to count the vector particles [28].

8.2.5.4 *Stable Liquid Virus Formulation Development*

Stable formulations must be produced in order to properly utilize viruses as an avenue for vaccination applications and gene therapy. In the past, lyophilization has shown to be the most fruitful method for generating stable live viral formulations. However, they clearly fall short despite their expense, difficulty, and frequency of administration when compared to refrigerated drinks. Even though lyophilization has disadvantages, it is typically necessary for the long-term preservation of live viruses [25].

8.3 Challenges in Manufacturing Viral-Vectored Vaccines

The creation of viral vectors presents difficulties on many fronts, ranging from manufacturing methods and procedures to cost-effectiveness and safety to meeting regulatory requirements. If the manufacturing of viral vectors is to be expanded, then it is even more imperative that these obstacles be addressed. Challenges in manufacturing viral vector vaccines are the following:

Scalability: Increasing production to supply the demand for vaccinations around the world is a major problem. Establishing large-scale manufacturing facilities is necessary to produce enough in adequate quantities efficiently.
Biological Safety: Workers and the environment may be in danger when handling live viral vectors in production. Tight biosafety protocols are needed to reduce these hazards.
Quality Control: The safety and effectiveness of vaccines depend on the constant maintenance of vector quality. Strict quality control procedures must be followed to guarantee that every batch satisfies requirements.
Production Costs: It can be costly to design and maintain production procedures. Cost reduction without sacrificing quality is a never-ending concern.
Regulatory Compliance: It is critical to adhere to the strict regulations governing the manufacture of vaccines. Maintaining adherence to other standards and Good Manufacturing Practices (GMP) can be difficult [29].

8.3.1 Scale-Up and Production Yield Challenges

There are many obstacles in the area when it comes to maintaining strict GMP and fulfilling regulatory requirements established by agencies such as the FDA while scaling up viral vector manufacturing from laboratory scale to large scale. Several crucial manufacturing processes are included in these scale-up obstacles. The transition from small-scale research setups to large-scale commercial ones requires guaranteeing consistent quality and compliance with GMP requirements, thus choosing the right production platform is an important decision. The decision to scale up or down a system (increasing volume in a single system) must be carefully considered as it affects product quality, cost-effectiveness, and efficiency. For large-scale vector titers and cell densities to be achieved, the conditions for vector yield maximization and production cost minimization must be optimized. Additionally, strict adherence to safety, quality, and efficacy requirements in production is necessary to be ready for clinical trials, which are frequently dependent on a successful scale-up. To successfully move viral vector–based treatments from preclinical or research to large-scale commercial production, however, and bring the advantages of gene therapy to a wider audience, these scale-up challenges must be overcome [30].

The necessity for quick technical problem solving and speedy production leads to the complexity of manufacturing processes. Every technology has unique difficulties of its own. Conventional vaccination modalities, including live attenuated or inactivated virus vaccines, have well-established manufacturing techniques, but scaling them up takes time.

8.3.2 Ensuring Genetic Stability and Vector Integrity

AdVs are non-enveloped dsDNA viruses that are members of the Adenoviridae family [31]. AdVs can be classified into several serotypes and have a broad host origin. The size of their manipulable double-stranded linear genome is between 26 and 45 kb [32]. AdVs are becoming legitimate vaccine delivery vehicles rather than just instruments for gene replacement treatment. Because they simultaneously stimulate the innate and adaptive immune systems in their mammalian hosts, they are appealing as vaccination vectors. AdV vectors have a solid track record, are simple to use, can be produced quickly and affordably, and do not require cold chain storage. AdVs originating from humans, simians, and birds are used as vaccination vectors.

The largest enclosed DNA virus is the poxvirus. The VACV was used to successfully eradicate smallpox in the 1980s. VACV was used as a transgenic expression vector at the same time [33]. Random mutations and deletions brought about by the passage of parental VACV contributed to VACV's decreased pathogenicity [34]. By passaging 570 generations on chicken embryos, MVA is greatly reduced. MVA does not form infectious progeny but retains strong DNA replication and antigen expression capabilities in the majority of mammalian cells because of the blockage of viral assembly. Over 120,000 patients in Germany have received the superb third-generation smallpox vaccine MVA [35, 36].

Even in the presence of preexisting anti-vector immunity, recombinant MVA is safe and easily modifiable genetically and exhibits strong immunogenicity [4]. Refer to Table 8.1.

(IM- intramuscular, IN- intranasal, OR- oral, IP- intraperitoneal, SC- subcutaneous, VLPs- virus-like particles, VSV- vesicular stomatitis virus).

Table 8.1 Comparison of viral vectors.

Vector	Types of virus	Genome type	Genome size	Cargo capacity (kb)	Administration route	Predominant immune response	Weaknesses	Strengths	References
Adenovirus	Non-enveloped, DNA	Double-stranded, nonsegmented	26–45	~7.5	IM, IN, or OR	Humoral and cellular immune response	Anti-vector immunity	Well-established; high transduction efficiencies; relatively large capacities for transgenes; high titer of production	[37]
Influenza virus	Enveloped, RNA	Single-stranded, negative-sense, segmented	~13.5	<1.5	IM, IN	Humoral and cellular immune response	Limited transgene ability; genetic reassortment; safety concerns	Capable of infecting a wide range of hosts, with a genome that is easily engineered, exhibiting a low level of virulence, and supported by a well-developed manufacturing process	[38–40]
Lentivirus	Enveloped, RNA	Single-stranded positive-sense, nonsegmented	~9.2	~4	IM, IN	Humoral and cellular immune response	Safety concerns; potential batch to batch variation in manufacturing	Limited vector-specific immunity, minimal genomic integration, and sustained immune responses	[6]

(Continued)

Table 8.1 Comparison of viral vectors. (*Continued*)

Vector	Types of virus	Genome type	Genome size	Cargo capacity (kb)	Administration route	Predominant immune response	Weaknesses	Strengths	References
Measles virus	Enveloped, RNA	Single-stranded negative sense, nonsegmented	~16	~6	IM, IP, or SC	Humoral, cellular, and mucosal immune response	Limited challenge models; low viral titers	Licensed live attenuated measles vaccines have demonstrated efficacy and safety profiles. These vaccines do not integrate into the host genome and have established manufacturing processes	[41]
Newcastle disease virus	Enveloped, RNA	Single-stranded negative sense, nonsegmented	~15	~4	IM, IN	Humoral and cellular immune response	Less well immunogenic than other paramyxovirus vector–based vaccines	High viral titers, absence of genomic integration into the host, host-specific restrictions, and the lack of preexisting neutralizing antibodies against NDV in humans	[42]
Parainfluenza virus	Enveloped, RNA	Single-stranded negative-sense, nonsegmented	~15	~4	IM, IN, or OR	Humoral, cellular, and mucosal immune response	Anti-vector immunity; safety concerns	Ideal for pediatric and respiratory diseases; safe; genomic stability	[43]

(*Continued*)

Table 8.1 Comparison of viral vectors. (*Continued*)

Vector	Types of virus	Genome type	Genome size	Cargo capacity (kb)	Administration route	Predominant immune response	Weaknesses	Strengths	References
Poxvirus	Enveloped, DNA	Double-stranded, nonsegmented	130–300	~25	IM	Low/ moderate antibodies response and strong cellular immune response	Packing flexibility of the genome; without genomic integration in the host; expressing VLPs	Existence of the viral immunomodulatory genes	[44]
Rabies virus	Enveloped, RNA	Single-stranded, negative-sense, nonsegmented	~12	~6.5	IM or OR	Humoral response in dominant	A potential risk for reversion to virulence; less well immunogenicity than VSV vector	Small and easily manipulated genome; designed as inactivated bivalent vaccines	[45]
Vesicular stomatitis virus	Enveloped, RNA	Single-stranded, negative-sense, nonsegmented	~11	~6	IM, IN, or OR	Humoral and cellular immune response	Safety concerns	No concerns of virulence reversion, residual virulence, or virus recombination; small and easily manipulated genome; stable expression of foreign genes; rapid replication and high growth titer	[46]

8.3.3 Manufacturing Consideration for Different Vector Types

The cell culture and purification bioprocess technologies used for clinical product manufacture should be scalable and reliably yield high levels of product safety, purity, potency, and stability. The established processes and controls must ensure product quality by design, be founded in sound science, and comply with regulations in order to achieve optimal safety. Starting materials must adhere to strict guidelines and be recorded by lot, along with Certificates of Analysis and Origin, in order to be used for clinical vector development and purification. Animal-derived starting materials should be minimized or avoided as they may include harmful adventitious agents and be diverse, incompletely characterized, and exhibit significant variance. Animal-derived goods should only be utilized, for instance, in the early phases of clinical product development, and process development initiatives should be started to replace them if they are employed. Reputable sources with high levels of safety testing and characterization should be used to get animal-derived products. Using culture media that are approved for use in the production of biologics instead of one that has been fortified with antibiotics allows for the monitoring of the aseptic technique and guarantees sterility throughout the various stages of the cell culture process. Antibiotic use is likely to reduce contaminations caused by non-sterile methods or reagents, but it will not stop them entirely. Purity requirements can be, as a general rule, based on those created for biologic goods with licenses, like vaccines and recombinant proteins. Impurities that could limit *in vivo* transgene expression due to immune responses should be found and removed, as vectors typically seek to establish long-term gene expression. A recent clinical trial for hemophilia B revealed the loss of therapeutic transgene-expressing cells as a result of capsid-specific cytotoxic T lymphocytes [47]. The importance of making sure that vectors ready for clinical usage contain minimal amounts of potentially immunogenic contaminants. In order to support the relevant stage of clinical development, the manufacturing process should be devised and implemented at a scale that is adequate. It is important to design and execute scalable process steps or processes whose performance is constant regardless of scale. Impurities that could limit *in vivo* transgene expression due to immune responses should be found and removed, as vectors typically seek to establish long-term gene expression. A recent clinical trial for hemophilia B revealed the loss of therapeutic transgene-expressing cells as a result of capsid-specific cytotoxic T lymphocytes, highlighting the importance of making sure that vectors ready for clinical usage contain minimal amounts of potentially immunogenic contaminants. In order to support the relevant stage of clinical development, the manufacturing process should be devised and implemented at a scale that is adequate. It is important to design and execute scalable process steps or processes whose performance is constant regardless of scale [48].

8.4 Quality Control and Assurance in Vaccine Manufacturing

Vaccines and immunization represent one of the most significant advancements in public health and medicine. These biological preparations, which typically contain weakened or inactivated disease-causing microorganisms, their toxins, or specific proteins, stimulate the immune system to develop resistance against particular diseases. The widespread implementation of vaccination programs over the past half-century has led to a dramatic reduction in the global incidence of vaccine-preventable illnesses. For instance, polio incidence dropped by 99% globally; mortality in children under 5 reduced by over 50% and there has been a decrease in live births from 90 to 43 deaths per 1,000 between 1990 and 2015 [49].

The assessment, licensure, control, and surveillance of vaccine products are major challenges for regulatory authorities. To ensure continuous positive results from vaccine development and immunization, WHO has stressed the need for stringent quality assurance measures which are dependent upon control/monitoring of raw materials, adequacy of production processes, suitability of quality control methods and specifications, and control/monitoring of final finished products [50].

In the preclinical/nonclinical stage of the vaccine's development cycle, the vaccine's immunogenicity or capacity to elicit an immune response as well as its safety is examined using cell culture methods and animal testing. The nonclinical stage is followed by the submission of an IND (Investigational New Drug) application by the sponsor to the regulatory body of the particular country. Upon obtaining regulatory clearance from the Indian Drug Controller General (IND), the vaccine candidate enters the clinical development phase. A comprehensive study protocol, outlining the specific clinical trials to be conducted, is formulated. Subsequent to regulatory approval, the vaccine undergoes three distinct phases of clinical trials: phases 1, 2, and 3. Once the vaccine has been licensed, the manufacturer may elect to pursue optional phase 4 studies, which are designed to further evaluate the vaccine's safety, efficacy, and potential applications.

8.4.1 Regulatory Requirements and Quality Standards

In India, various regulatory agencies for vaccine registration are the Ministry of Health and Family Welfare (MoHFW), the National Technical Advisory Group on Immunization, the Indian Council for Medical Research (ICMR), and the Central Drugs Standard Control Organization (CDSCO). After the phase 3 clinical trial, results are to be submitted to the National Regulatory Authority (NRA) for approval. Good clinical practice (GCP) and ethical guidelines by ICMR approval are also required. Central Licencing Approval Authority (CLAA) is responsible for the central license of vaccines in India. DTAB approves the introduction of vaccines into the immunization services. All vaccine approval and clinical trials are done by CLAA which is followed by post-marketing surveillance (PMS) which is phase 4 clinical trials. Any complaint regarding the safety and efficacy of vaccine post-marketing should be directed to NRA [51].

Various regulatory bodies for vaccine registration in the US include the Centre for Biologics Evaluation and Research, Vaccines and Related Biological Products Advisory Committee, and Biologics License Application. The sponsor submits the IND to the United States Food and Drug Administration (USFDA). IND describes the vaccines, their method of manufacturing, and quality control tests. After IND approval and phase 3 trials, the producer must submit a Biologic License Application (BLA) to CBER (Centre for Biologics Evaluation and Research) of USFDA on FDA form 356h to request permission to manufacture and commercialize the vaccine for a large population. Depending on whether the application is being reviewed as a priority or under a regular review, it could take anywhere from 6 to 12 months to complete. The BLA is reviewed by a reviewer team that comprises a medical officer and a chemist. Technical advice is given by the FDA VRBPAC (vaccine and related biologics products advisory committee). Prior to marketing labeling, the examination is done to understand usage, potential benefits, and risks. Phase 4, often known as PMS, will start after the approval procedure. Within 15 days of the vaccination administration, any adverse events or effects must be notified to the authority [52].

An EU marketing authorization (MA) is required before a vaccination can be sold in the EU. The European Medicines Agency (EMA), which is in charge of the scientific assessment, oversight, and safety monitoring of pharmaceuticals in the EU, has authorized and is keeping an eye on the vaccines. The European Medicines Agency's (EMA) committee for human medicines, the Committee for Medicinal Products for Human Use (CHMP), awards the MA following a risk-benefit analysis of the vaccine product based on a dossier outlining the product's quality, safety, and efficacy. The EU approves vaccinations through nationalized, decentralized, mutual recognition, and centralized process [53]. A centralized method is usually preferred by the manufacturer when getting an MA for a vaccination product since it allows for the approval of a single MA for a vaccination product throughout the European Union. Vaccinations are easily obtainable for both patients and the healthcare system. CHMP will assess the application submitted to the European Medical Agency for the marketing of vaccination goods within the EU. Vaccines are tested for side effects after going on sale to ensure they fit the safety criteria established throughout the product development process. The strategy for risk management is also intended to detect infrequent events that would not have been apparent in the course of clinical development [54].

8.4.2 Analytical Methods for Assessing Viral Vector Purity and Potency

Since viral vectors may effectively stimulate an immune response to foreign or virus-infected cells without the addition of adjuvants, they are especially valuable for vaccine development. Vaccines including modified measles and VACVs have also been developed, although modified adenoviruses are the most widely utilized viral vectors. It is anticipated that the demand for these kinds of products will increase globally as viral-vectored vaccines against COVID-19 are successfully developed [55].

The development of analytical tools for vaccine research, whether *in vivo* or *in vitro*, follows a consistent methodology. The initial step involves defining the research question, which guides the selection of the most appropriate analytical approach. Subsequent to this, the assay design phase entails identifying assay inputs, sourcing necessary reagents, establishing a detailed protocol, and validating the assay's performance. Ultimately, the validated protocol is formalized into a standard operating procedure (SOP) that outlines specific measurements, outputs, and interpretation guidelines [56]. Refer to Figure 8.2.

Assay validation is a critical process that ensures the assay's sensitivity, specificity, and accuracy for the intended purpose. It involves rigorous evaluation using established standards and quality controls to detect any potential issues such as reagent cross-reactivity or interference. Importantly, assay assessment is an ongoing process that incorporates

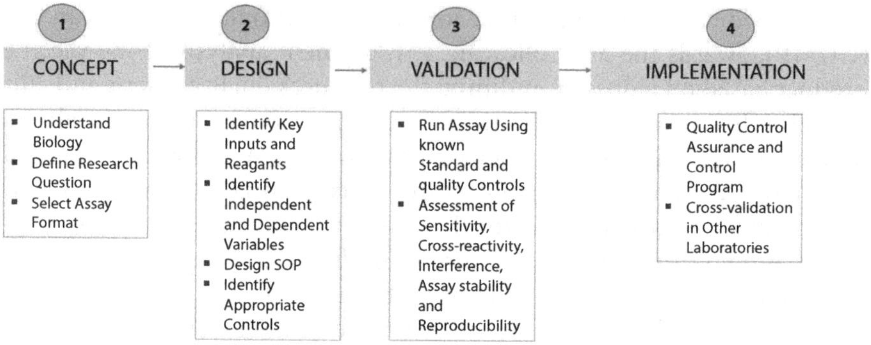

Figure 8.2 The four main phases of the analytical tool development process.

continuous validation and quality assurance [57]. In the context of a pandemic, rapid assay development is essential to keep pace with the evolving landscape of vaccine research.

A variety of vaccine platforms, including subunit protein, DNA, viral vector, mRNA, and inactivated virus, have been employed for the development of COVID-19 vaccines [58]. Given the pivotal role of coronavirus spike proteins in facilitating viral entry into host cells, the SARS-CoV-2 spike protein has emerged as a primary target for COVID-19 vaccine development [59]. Following the selection and synthesis of a vaccine antigen, it is imperative to thoroughly assess its physicochemical properties. The characteristics of the antigen formulation significantly influence the nature and efficacy of the immune response elicited. To ensure the vaccine antigen's identity, purity, structural integrity, and chemical composition, rigorous assays are necessary to identify and mitigate any potential contaminants that may compromise safety.

8.4.3 Process Validation and Quality Assurance Strategies

There are numerous definitions of "validation" in the literature. Even though the nomenclature may vary, the idea behind it is always the same: define and execute, verify that the requirements are fulfilled, and record the results. An external assessment of a system's performance and, eventually, the manufacturing process's performance is called validation. The process should result in a product that satisfies predefined standards if it runs well. Validation in vaccine production is the process of demonstrating that a given procedure, process, piece of equipment, material, activity, or system complies with GMP requirements and produces the expected outcomes [60].

8.4.3.1 Process Validation Using a Life Cycle Approach: From R&D to Clinical Trials to Commercial Scale Regulation

The validation of processes should be considered a continuous endeavor, encompassing various stages of the product life cycle. This includes the development of methodologies and processes, the validation of commercial manufacturing processes, and the ongoing maintenance of these processes throughout regular production. To ensure efficient and compliant commercial operations, process development, production capabilities, and quality systems must be integrated. According to this approach, process validation commences prior to the production of consistency batches and continues into the commercial phase. Validation activities necessitate an interdisciplinary approach, drawing upon expertise from fields such as engineering, chemistry, microbiology, statistics, manufacturing, and quality assurance. Moreover, effective planning and the unwavering support of senior management are essential.

8.4.3.2 Validation Strategy Based on Risk: Quality Risk Management System

The development of a Quality Risk Management (QRM) system in close proximity to the product life cycle is imperative in order to address the crucial inquiry of "what needs to be validated and when is the right time?" across the various validation stages. When new information becomes available, the full set of product attributes and operational parameters should be reevaluated in light of their value in relation to the particular processes and their impact on the product (in-process). This will assist in determining important operational factors. Validation efforts may therefore concentrate on the procedures that often carry the highest quality concerns. This indicates that greater levels of management are required for the characteristics that carry greater risk.

8.5 Technological Advances and Innovations in Manufacturing

8.5.1 Novel Manufacturing Platforms and Technologies

A very tiny quantity of disease-causing bacteria, viruses, or other microorganisms that are dead or weak is typically used to create vaccines. Vaccines stimulate the body's natural immune response, which lowers the risk of contracting the disease from the actual pathogen and aids in the body's effective and speedy defense against sickness [61]. The first vaccinations were somewhat basic and included either inactivated bacteria (such as pertussis) or partially purified live attenuated viruses (such as smallpox and rabies). With time, more sophisticated techniques were developed, such as the use of purified polysaccharides (such as pneumococcal vaccines), the creation of virus-like particles (such as hepatitis B and human papillomavirus), the chemical treatment of a protein toxin to form a toxoid (such as tetanus and diphtheria), and the development of a purified and inactivated virus (such as hepatitis A) [62]. Global pandemic outbreaks like COVID-19 have accelerated biotechnology's development and use, particularly in the production of vaccines. Biopharmaceutical companies have moved their focus from the conventional vaccine manufacturing techniques utilizing attenuated or inactivated viruses to the novel "biotechnology platform"-based procedures for vaccine manufacturing in order to fulfill the increased demand for vaccinations during the COVID-19 pandemic. Vaccines made using these innovative platforms have a common set of chemicals and manufacturing procedures that have been separately developed and tested by the biotechnology industry.

It might take a while to evaluate a vaccine's safety and effectiveness, get regulatory permission, manufacture the vaccine on a big scale, and distribute it widely. The creation of vaccines is a phased process. The entire procedure, which consists of two phases—the product development phase and the production phase—usually takes five to ten years.

a) ***Product Development Phase:*** In order to manufacture a vaccine, an antigen that has been determined to be the best candidate through study must first be transformed into the finished product. The components of the vaccine, the raw materials used in processing, the product's specifications, and the production procedure are all decided upon during this phase. This phase's manufacturing is conducted on a much smaller scale than that of the mass production phase. Typically, during this stage, vaccines for clinical trials are developed.

b) ***Production Phase:*** There are two steps to the production. The "drug substance" is formed in the first stage, and the "drug product" is created in the second. The prepared active component that patients are given is known as the drug product. The antigen is cultivated, extracted, and subsequently purified in the process of making the medicinal ingredient. Following their purification, the antigens are mixed with all of the other constituents and ingredients to create the finished vaccine [63]. The formulation process is at this stage. The postproduction activities that follow the vaccination's formulation process make up the majority of the second stage. A syringe or vial is filled with the vaccinations. Subsequently, it undergoes freeze-drying, after which it is packaged and labeled in compliance with regulatory standards. Next, the quality assurance department verifies that the vaccine was produced and tested in compliance with the guidelines. The product is approved for distribution and batch release following final approval. Ultimately, the vaccines are shipped all over the world in a temperature-controlled setting. This completes the traditional way of making vaccines.

Conventional vaccinations have a number of significant disadvantages, including the need for an extended culturing procedure and a significant delay between the generation of the antigen and the last-mile distribution of the vaccine. In addition, conventional vaccine production necessitates advanced containment facilities and stringent safety measures due to the infectious nature of the ingredients in order to reduce the risk to the environment and operators. Another disturbing point is that despite the efforts to modify or weaken the virus to make vaccines, live attenuated viruses can revert to their deadly variants [64]. Because none of the vaccine manufacturing procedures used in the conventional method are ideal, there is constant material loss, which lowers total productivity. Furthermore, conventional vaccine production usually entails the cooperation of several companies (contract manufacturers), each of which is in charge of a certain step or procedure in the production of vaccines. As a result, there are frequent inefficiencies in the parties' ability to coordinate effectively, particularly when it comes to following safety and quality standards and acquiring the necessary regulatory licenses. Last but not least, conventional manufacturing has never been able to quickly and effectively adjust to the shifting demand for vaccines. The rate of manufacturing must be increased, particularly during pandemics, and then reduced after the situation has stabilized. This frequently necessitates production flexibility, which is difficult to achieve in a conventional manufacturing environment.

Pandemic outbreaks, like COVID-19, are timely indicators that a better manufacturing procedure for vaccines is needed to shorten the time it takes to develop and produce vaccines. The first step in achieving this goal is the development of COVID-19 vaccines based on cutting-edge biotechnology platforms, such as mRNA and viral vector vaccines [65]. It is important to highlight that numerous biopharmaceutical firms have effectively shifted to innovative platforms during the COVID-19 pandemic, enabling the development of vaccines on a significantly faster schedule without sacrificing vaccine efficacy or safety. A recent study found that vaccines developed under the novel platform concept, like the Sputnik (viral vector vaccine), Moderna (messenger ribonucleic acid vaccines), and Pfizer/BioNTech (messenger ribonucleic acid vaccines), were very effective in protecting against COVID-19, with efficacies of 88.7%, 83.3%, and 85.7%, respectively [66]. It is important to remember that the genetic sequence of the SARS-CoV-2 virus was the only resource used in the development of these vaccines. Future vaccines to treat a wide range of infectious diseases are expected to be developed using these amazing platform methodologies, which are predicted to be easily extended, reorganized, and redesigned. Future vaccines could be produced on a wide scale quickly when it has been determined that these ones are safe and effective through testing.

The most effective way to address the various pandemic vaccine manufacturing challenges—such as speed, efficacy, and safety—is through platform-based vaccinations. A product platform can be defined as a "group" of unique elements, modules, or components that are shared by all products that are developed from it. Viral vector vaccines and mRNA vaccines are the two main types of platform-based vaccinations that are being extensively utilized to fight pandemics like COVID-19. These vaccinations have the advantage of not including the disease-causing organism in any way. This enables protection from the disease without being at risk of infection. Different Vaccine platforms are described in Figure 8.3.

CLASSICAL PLATFORMS	NEXT-GENERATION PLATFORMS
1. **Whole-inactivated Virus** Example: Polio vaccine	1. **Viral vector** Example: Ebola vaccine
2. **Live-attenuated Virus** Example: MMR vaccine	2. **DNA**
3. **Protein subunit** Example: Seasonal influenza vaccine	3. **RNA**
4. **Virus-like particle** Example: Human papillomavirus vaccine	4. **Antigen-presenting cells**

Figure 8.3 An overview of different vaccine platform.

- **Viral vector vaccines** transfer DNA (instructions) into our bodies by means of a modified harmless virus known as the vector. This DNA-carrying vector enters our cells and travels to the cell nucleus. The transcription of DNA into mRNA occurs inside the nucleus. After the mRNA leaves the nucleus, the machinery of the cell converts it into a safe fragment of the disease-causing virus, typically a protein. This foreign object triggers the immune system, which then attempts to eliminate it. This aids in the development of our body's defense mechanism against similar viral infections in the future. Vaccines derived from viral vectors typically consist of a harmless virus (vector) as the base platform carrier onto which the DNA is deposited. By tweaking the DNA information, a new vaccine can be quickly developed by combining the modified DNA onto the base platform carrier.
- **mRNA vaccines**, on the other hand, use strands of mRNA to teach our immune system how to combat illness without introducing any germs. The mRNA carries instructions on how to create a safe fragment of the pathogen, typically a protein. After the mRNA vaccination enters our cells, the cells translate the instructions and produce the protein (while remaining outside the nucleus). After identifying this protein, the immune system battles to neutralize the alien component and strengthen its defenses against further infections.
- **Antigen-presenting cells** play a crucial role in how the immune system reacts to a vaccination. The initial stages following vaccination are circumvented by loading antigen-presenting cells with peptides that would otherwise be produced by immunization. Dendritic cells are typically taken from the patient, grown, and modified to deliver the target antigen before being reinfused into the original patient. This is too time-consuming and expensive to be used as a vaccination that is widely distributed. As a result, immortalized cells have been successfully transformed into artificial antigen-presenting cells by transduction using lentiviruses.

8.5.2 Automation and Process Optimization

For the development of novel pharmaceutical products, such as virus-like particles, plasmid DNA, fragments, etc., QbD-based (quality-by-design) process development is considered the gold standard because it guarantees quality throughout the entire life cycle, permits process modifications even after approval if optimization is possible, and eliminates the need for platform processes similar to those used in the production of monoclonal antibodies [67].

But in order to apply QbD concepts to process development, a verified design space that ensures constant quality is needed, and this can be created through process understanding or experimentation. As a result, digital twins are also required for process development. The creation of a quality target product profile (QTPP) is a prerequisite for starting a QbD-based process development. To determine what is essential for the product's quality, this is required. Biologics have properties like sterility and purity, but they also have specific therapeutic effects, bioactivity, and dose. Critical quality attributes (CQAs), which are characteristics or properties that guarantee the required product quality when controlled within a certain limit, range, or distribution, must be determined based on the QTPP [68].

According to the QbD concept, CQAs are dynamic rather than static and must be updated as new information about processes and products becomes available throughout the course of a product's life cycle. CQAs are produced via risk management and experimentation, and they serve as a roadmap for future process development. Early in the process development phase, risk assessment should be carried out as part of risk management. Its goal is to create real and imagined connections between process, material, and equipment factors and CQAs. By doing this, it creates the foundation for additional process design [69].

8.6 Supply Chain and Distribution Challenges

Vaccines are challenging biological products that might become less effective and also they can mutate and change their properties if exposed to inappropriate environmental conditions. Hence, cold storage is crucial [70]. Keeping the cold chain undisturbed, vaccines will stay effective from the production phase to the administration inpatient phase. The vaccine cold chain is the practice of storing vaccines at specific temperatures throughout their storage life, supply, and delivery [71]. In order to guarantee vaccination safety and efficacy, proper cold chain management is essential as different vectored vaccine requires different cold storage conditions. Certain vaccines, like COVID-19 mRNA vaccines, require ultra-cold storage, while others may perhaps be stored in a regular refrigerator (2°C to

8°C) [72]. Viral vector vaccines are required to be stored at extremely cold temperatures with −70°C to −80°C which is known as Ultra-cold chain (UCC) vaccines system [73]. This UCC system is having multiple challenges because of the work requirement demands. The UCC system or ULT (ultra-low temperature) freezers are essential, which consume major power energy. These types of freezers must be maintained at a controlled temperature below 27°C and at low humidity which is below 50%. Other challenges of the cold chain system are the requisite of skilled technical personnel to appropriately handle vaccine storage and this involves the use of cold boxes, thermal packing, and high-quality refrigeration equipment. Passive cooling systems and transportable refrigeration units may be necessary in areas with inadequate infrastructure. For initial vaccine storage, large-scale storage facilities close to production and distribution centers are crucial [74].

In regional and local distribution, centers need to have the necessary equipment to provide constant cold chain conditions, which often require secondary and tertiary storage services [75]. Refrigerated vans and trucks are being used for local and regional distribution areas, whereas air transport is commonly utilized for long-distance and global distribution of vaccines but it might be difficult to deliver the vaccines to medical organizations or immunization sites, mainly in rural places where road or air connectivity is difficult. The community-based distribution techniques and protected transit crates are examples of solutions for the distribution of viral vaccines [74]. Nowadays, ultra-cold freezers and temperature-controlled containers, the development of mobile vaccination units and the drone technology for remote place vaccine delivery, the Internet of Things (IoT), and GPS to track consignments in real-time are extensively used, which helps in keeping an eye on supply chain temperature conditions and by using mechanisms to gather, examine, and react to data about the dissemination of vaccines, assuring that any difficulties can be timely resolved [76].

Maintaining compliance of goods/products with legal supplies and certifications, comprising Good Distribution Practices (GDP) for viral vaccine, across all sides of the distribution process, effectively handling customs clearance and following significance laws, which might vary greatly across countries [77]. For the distribution of vaccines to function well, producers, governments, logistics companies, and healthcare organizations must harmonize together and establish backup strategies in case of unpredicted circumstances like shortages of supply, road traffic jams, or interruptions in cold chain storage due to unavoidable circumstances [78]. To overcome all the challenges, certain steps need to be followed such as disseminating information to the public on vaccine availability, distribution dates, and vaccination significance and providing instructions to medical professionals on how to handle, control, administer, and store viral vector vaccines. Inadequate skills among workers, distributors, and consumers can lead to improper storage and reduced potency of the viral-vectored vaccine. By placing strong logistical structures and technology to use, it is likely to optimize the distribution of these vaccinations and ensure the rapid and secure delivery of these viral vaccines to people around the globe [70].

8.7 Regulatory Hurdles and Compliances

As stipulated in 21 Code of Federal Regulations (CFR) sections 210 and 211 and section 501(a)(2)(B) of the Federal Food, Drug, and Cosmetic Act (FD&C Act), the manufacture of investigational novel pharmaceuticals, including viral vectors used in gene therapy, must adhere to the CGMP.

8.7.1 Regulatory Approval Challenges

The following lists five instances of post-approval modifications made to vaccine manufacture, along with a description of how the WHO categorizes them. The national guidelines of one or more of the blocks selected for this study do not take into account three of these changes: "Generation of a new Master Cell Bank (MCB)," "Change in the manufacturing process of diluent," and "Qualification of a new reference standard." Modest modifications to the final product's production process are classified as "moderate" by the WHO and "major" in regional blocks. A similar disparity is shown when a diluent's production process is altered; the WHO classifies this alteration as "moderate/minor," but the EU rules do not address it, and the other two regional blocks classify it as "minor." There are variations in the criteria for approving the modification as a result of this classification variability [79].

8.7.2 Compliances with Good Manufacturing Practices (GMP)

Early in the clinical development process, it is well acknowledged that it is challenging to establish all components of GMP due to the significant investments required to set up a fully compliant GMP manufacturing unit. Certain product characterization assays may employ non-validated methodologies and broad specifications. Regulatory bodies anticipate that these assays will undergo full validation and progressively narrower specifications during clinical development. However, quality control testing for critical safety attributes, such as sterility, mycoplasma absence, and adventitious viral contamination, must be established and validated at the outset of clinical development. Likewise, it is acknowledged that during the clinical development of the majority of investigational items, process modifications, such as process optimization and scale-up, are probably going to happen.

In order to differentiate phase 1 pharmaceuticals from those produced commercially and for later phase clinical trials, the FDA released a guideline for industry in 2008 called CGMP for phase 1 investigational pharmaceuticals. This document formally acknowledged that some of the requirements found in part 211—such as the requirements for warehousing and manufacturing process validation—might not apply to the production of the majority of investigational drugs used in phase 1 clinical trials. The guidelines take into account the differences in some manufacturing controls between commercial and investigational manufacturing, as well as between different stages of the clinical trial life cycle. The manufacturing of phase 1 experimental pharmaceuticals is exempt from full cGMP compliance under the requirements, as long as sufficient controls are in place to guarantee that the drug satisfies the necessary standards for safety, identity, strength, quality, and purity. This exclusion, however, conflicts with European criteria, which require items to be completely compliant with cGMP regardless of the stage of clinical trials. When a multinational pharmaceutical corporation audits US-based academic manufacturers of phase 1 experimental medications, these disparities frequently come to light. One instance is the mandate for raw material identity testing. While ICH Q7A-7.30 mandates testing of all pharmaceutical ingredients meant for human use, independent of the clinical phase, the FDA acknowledges that at the Phase-1 stage of product development, all pertinent characteristics or acceptability criteria might not be known for certain materials [80].

8.7.3 Strategies for Navigating Regulatory Pathways

The stages of product development are accelerated by appropriate production methods. A well-designed process will minimize inefficiencies and mistakes that result in lost effort, closely coordinate to find efficiencies and avoid hazards, and speed up development by optimizing parallel processes to provide the most effective project plan. Successful engineering, testing, clinical, and regulatory strategy development result from matching the appropriate people with the correct processes. This comprises planning and carrying out bench and animal testing, as well as creating strategies around user needs, test models, simulations, and acceptance criteria. Early clinical and regulatory planning, done concurrently with product development, enables requirements and discoveries to be fed back into the process to produce a more effective approach overall [81].

8.8 Future Perspectives and Emerging Solutions

The future of viral vector–based vaccines holds significant promise due to advances in biotechnology and immunology. The progressing need for vaccine formation for infectious and other health-challenging diseases increases the understanding of complex mechanisms.

The stringent regulatory compliance includes comprehensive testing for potency, safety, sterility, and stability which must meet rigorous criteria before approval [82]. Cold chain logistics and easy distribution facilities have been required for effective chain supply management and reduced pathogen severity. The accessibility and affordability of vaccines reduce the progression of pathogens and are effective in achieving immunization within a short time limit, which can further help in the management of various symptoms. Affordability is a key factor in focusing on the lower-cost vaccines that can be produced by minimizing unnecessary steps and by achieving a crucial understanding of complex mechanisms [83].

Technological advancements can also aid in reducing human errors and maintaining effective sterilization of vaccines. Innovations in vector design, manufacturing technologies, and regulatory frameworks will be pivotal in addressing current challenges. Collaborative efforts among researchers, manufacturers, and regulatory bodies are essential to streamline processes and expedite the availability of these critical vaccines [84]. By continuously improving manufacturing practices and control measures, the field of viral-vectored vaccines will advance, contributing significantly to the prevention and treatment of infectious diseases and beyond.

8.9 Conclusion

Viral-vectored vaccine production and management offer special and challenging prospects as well as substantial problems for improving global health. From vector design and cell line generation to rigorous downstream processing and quality control, the procedure involves a number of complex phases. Quality control is a crucial step to reduce contamination and achieve the best-quality vaccine with standard optimization parameters.

Through processing using technological advancement and applying innovations at an industrial scale, the time and cost would be minimized and the error of contamination also be reduced. Addressing regulatory aspects and maintaining an effective supply chain would be useful for reducing hurdles.

Careful optimization of each step is necessary to guarantee vaccination safety, efficacy, and scalability. The concerted efforts and ongoing innovation, these vaccines will play a vital role in enhancing global health and combating emerging and existing health threats.

References

1. Ura, T., Okuda, K., Shimada, M., Developments in Viral Vector-Based Vaccines. *Vaccines*, *2*, 624–641, 2014, doi: 10.3390/vaccines2030624.
2. Tripathi, N.K. and Shrivastava, A., Recent Developments in Bioprocessing of Recombinant Proteins: Expression Hosts and Process Development. *Front. Bioeng. Biotechnol.*, *7*, 420, 2019, doi: 10.3389/fbioe.2019.00420.
3. Folegatti, P.M., Jenkin, D., Morris, S., Gilbert, S., Kim, D., Robertson, J.S., Smith, E.R., Martin, E., Gurwith, M., Chen, R.T., Vaccines Based on the Replication-Deficient Simian Adenoviral Vector ChAdOx1: Standardized Template with Key Considerations for a Risk/Benefit Assessment. *Vaccine*, *40*, 5248–5262, 2022, doi: 10.1016/j.vaccine.2022.06.008.
4. Wang, S., Liang, B., Wang, W., Li, L., Feng, N., Zhao, Y., Wang, T., Yan, F., Yang, S., Xia, X., Viral Vectored Vaccines: Design, Development, Preventive and Therapeutic Applications in Human Diseases. *Signal Transduct. Target. Ther.*, *8*, 1–38, 2023, doi: 10.1038/s41392-023-01408-5.
5. Chavda, V.P., Baviskar, K.P., Vaghela, D.A., Raut, S.S., Bedse, A.P., Nasal Sprays for Treating COVID-19: A Scientific Note. *Pharmacol. Rep.*, *75*, 249–265, 2023, doi: 10.1007/s43440-023-00463-7.
6. Travieso, T., Li, J., Mahesh, S., Mello, J.D.F.R.E., Blasi, M., The Use of Viral Vectors in Vaccine Development. *npj Vaccines*, *7*, 1–10, 2022, doi: 10.1038/s41541-022-00503-y.
7. Li, S., Locke, E., Bruder, J., Clarke, D., Doolan, D.L., Havenga, M.J.E., Hill, A.V.S., Liljestrom, P., Monath, T.P., Naim, H.Y., *et al.*, Viral Vectors for Malaria Vaccine Development. *Vaccine*, *25*, 2567–2574, 2007, doi: 10.1016/j.vaccine.2006.07.035.
8. Lundstrom, K., Viral Vectors in Gene Therapy. *Diseases*, *6*, 42, 2018, doi: 10.3390/diseases6020042.
9. Vemula, S.V. and Mittal, S.K., Production of Adenovirus Vectors and Their Use as a Delivery System for Influenza Vaccines. *Expert Opin. Biol. Ther.*, *10*, 1469–1487, 2010, doi: 10.1517/14712598.2010.519332.

10. Wu, C., Lei, X., Wang, J., Hung, T., Generation of a Replication-Deficient Recombinant Human Adenovirus Type 35 Vector Using Bacteria-Mediated Homologous Recombination. *J. Virol. Methods*, *177*, 55–63, 2011, doi: 10.1016/J.JVIROMET.2011.06.016.
11. Sayedahmed, E.E., Kumari, R., Mittal, S.K., Current Use of Adenovirus Vectors and Their Production Methods. *Methods Mol. Biol.*, *1937*, 155–175, 2019, doi: 10.1007/978-1-4939-9065-8_9.
12. Sayedahmed, E.E., *Adenovirus Vector-Based Vaccine Approach for Emerging Influenza Viruses*, Purdue University, West Lafayette, Indiana, 2018, Dissertation & Theses.
13. Mitchell, D.P., Savaryn, J.P., Moorman, N.J., Shenk, T., Terhune, S.S., Human cytomegalovirus UL28 and UL29 open reading frames encode a spliced mRNA and stimulate accumulation of immediate-early RNAs. *J. Virol.*, 83, 19, 10187–97, 2009 Oct. doi: 10.1128/JVI.00396-09. Epub 2009 Jul 22. PMID: 19625400; PMCID: PMC2748044.
14. Sena-Esteves, M. and Gao, G., Introducing Genes into Mammalian Cells: Viral Vectors. *Cold Spring Harb. Protoc.*, 2020, 8, 2020, pdb.top095513, doi:10.1101/pdb.top095513.
15. Rodrigues, A.F., Soares, H.R., Guerreiro, M.R., Alves, P.M., Coroadinha, A.S., Viral Vaccines and Their Manufacturing Cell Substrates: New Trends and Designs in Modern Vaccinology. *Biotechnol. J.*, *10*, 1329–1344, 2015, doi: 10.1002/BIOT.201400387.
16. Rodrigues, A.F., Carrondo, M.J.T., Alves, P.M., Coroadinha, A.S., Cellular Targets for Improved Manufacturing of Virus-Based Biopharmaceuticals in Animal Cells. *Trends Biotechnol.*, *32*, 602–607, 2014, doi: 10.1016/J.TIBTECH.2014.09.010.
17. Leikas, A.J., Ylä-Herttuala, S., Hartikainen, J.E.K., Adenoviral Gene Therapy Vectors in Clinical Use—Basic Aspects with a Special Reference to Replication-Competent Adenovirus Formation and Its Impact on Clinical Safety. *Int. J. Mol. Sci.*, *24*, 16519, 2023, doi: 10.3390/ijms242216519.
18. Jordan, I., Vos, A., Beilfuß, S., Neubert, A., Breul, S., Sandig, V., An Avian Cell Line Designed for Production of Highly Attenuated Viruses. *Vaccine*, *27*, 748–756, 2009, doi: 10.1016/J.VACCINE.2008.11.066.
19. Zhou, B., Xia, L., Zhang, T., You, M., Huang, Y., He, M., Su, R., Tang, J., Zhang, J., Li, S., *et al.*, Structure Guided Maturation of a Novel Humanized Anti-HBV Antibody and Its Preclinical Development. *Antiviral Res.*, *180*, 104757, 2020, doi: 10.1016/j.antiviral.2020.104757.
20. Fontana, D., Kratje, R., Etcheverrigaray, M., Prieto, C., Rabies Virus-like Particles Expressed in HEK293 Cells. *Vaccine*, *32*, 2799–2804, 2014, doi: 10.1016/J.VACCINE.2014.02.031.
21. Cox, M.M.J., Recombinant Protein Vaccines Produced in Insect Cells. *Vaccine*, *30*, 1759–1766, 2012, doi: 10.1016/J.VACCINE.2012.01.016.
22. Van Oers, M.M., Pijlman, G.P., Vlak, J.M., Thirty Years of Baculovirus-Insect Cell Protein Expression: From Dark Horse to Mainstream Technology. *J. Gen. Virol.*, *96*, 6–23, 2015, doi: 10.1099/VIR.0.067108-0.

23. Jardon, M. and Garnier, A., pH, pCO2, and Temperature Effect on R-Adenovirus Production. *Biotechnol. Prog.*, *19*, 202–208, 2003, doi: 10.1021/BP025585A.
24. Xie, L., Metallo, C., Warren, J., Pilbrough, W., Peltier, J., Zhong, T., Pikus, L., Yancy, A., Leung, J., Auniņš, J.G., *et al.*, Large-Scale Propagation of a Replication-Defective Adenovirus Vector in Stirred-Tank Bioreactor PER. C6 Cell Culture under Sparging Conditions. *Biotechnol. Bioeng.*, *83*, 45–52, 2003, doi: 10.1002/BIT.10644.
25. Altaras, N.E., Aunins, J.G., Evans, R.K., Kamen, A., Konz, J.O., Wolf, J.J., Production and Formulation of Adenovirus Vectors. *Adv. Biochem. Eng./Biotechnol.*, *99*, 193–260, 2005, doi: 10.1007/10_008.
26. Moleirinho, M.G., Silva, R.J.S., Alves, P.M., Carrondo, M.J.T., Peixoto, C., Current Challenges in Biotherapeutic Particles Manufacturing. *Expert Opin. Biol. Ther.*, *20*, 451–465, 2020, doi: 10.1080/14712598.2020.1693541.
27. Graumann, D.M.F., *Studies on Biodistribution and Pharmacokinetics of Capsid-Modified Adenoviral Vectors*, Universität Ulm, 2023.
28. Rux, J.J. and Burnett, R.M., Large-Scale Purification and Crystallization of Adenovirus Hexon. *Methods Mol. Med.*, *131*, 231–250, 2007, doi: 10.1007/978-1-59745-277-9_17.
29. Ulmer, J.B., Valley, U., Rappuoli, R., Vaccine Manufacturing: Challenges and Solutions. *Nat. Biotechnol.*, *24*, 1377–1383, 2006, doi: 10.1038/nbt1261.
30. Alam, S.T., Ahmed, S., Ali, S.M., Sarker, S., Kabir, G., Ul-Islam, A., Challenges to COVID-19 Vaccine Supply Chain: Implications for Sustainable Development Goals. *Int. J. Prod. Econ.*, *239*, 108193, 2021, doi: 10.1016/j.ijpe.2021.108193.
31. Norrby, E., Bartha, A., Boulanger, P., Dreizin, R.S., Ginsberg, H.S., Kalter, S.S., Kawamura, H., Rowe, W.P., Russell, W.C., Schlesinger, W., *et al.*, Adenoviridae. *Intervirology*, *7*, 117–125, 1976, doi: 10.1159/000149945.
32. Davison, A.J., Benkő, M., Harrach, B., Genetic Content and Evolution of Adenoviruses. *J. Gen. Virol.*, *84*, 2895–2908, 2003, doi: 10.1099/vir.0.19497-0.
33. Mackett, M., Smith, G.L., Moss, B., Vaccinia Virus: A Selectable Eukaryotic Cloning and Expression Vector. *Proc. Natl. Acad. Sci. U.S.A.*, *79*, 7415–7419, 1982, doi: 10.1073/pnas.79.23.7415.
34. Sánchez-Sampedro, L., Perdiguero, B., Mejías-Pérez, E., García-Arriaza, J., Di Pilato, M., Esteban, M., The Evolution of Poxvirus Vaccines. *Viruses*, *7*, 1726–1803, 2015, doi: 10.3390/v7041726.
35. von Krempelhuber, A., Vollmar, J., Pokorny, R., Rapp, P., Wulff, N., Petzold, B., Handley, A., Mateo, L., Siersbol, H., Kollaritsch, H., *et al.*, A Randomized, Double-Blind, Dose-Finding Phase II Study to Evaluate Immunogenicity and Safety of the Third Generation Smallpox Vaccine Candidate IMVAMUNE. *Vaccine*, *28*, 1209–1216, 2010, doi: 10.1016/j.vaccine.2009.11.030.
36. Hochstein-Mintzel, V., Huber, H.C., Stickl, H., Virulence and immunogenicity of a modified vaccinia virus (strain MVA) (author's transl). *Z. Immunitatsforsch. Exp. Klin. Immunol.*, *144*, 104–156, 1972.

37. Sakurai, F., Tachibana, M., Mizuguchi, H., Adenovirus Vector-Based Vaccine for Infectious Diseases. *Drug Metab. Pharmacokinet.*, *42*, 100432, 2022, doi: 10.1016/j.dmpk.2021.100432.
38. Gerlach, T., Elbahesh, H., Saletti, G., Rimmelzwaan, G.F., Recombinant Influenza A Viruses as Vaccine Vectors. *Expert Rev. Vaccines*, *18*, 379–392, 2019, doi: 10.1080/14760584.2019.1582338.
39. McDonald, S.M., Nelson, M.I., Turner, P.E., Patton, J.T., Reassortment in Segmented RNA Viruses: Mechanisms and Outcomes. *Nat. Rev. Microbiol.*, *14*, 448–460, 2016, doi: 10.1038/nrmicro.2016.46.
40. Su, S., Wong, G., Shi, W., Liu, J., Lai, A.C.K., Zhou, J., Liu, W., Bi, Y., Gao, G.F., Epidemiology, Genetic Recombination, and Pathogenesis of Coronaviruses. *Trends Microbiol.*, *24*, 490–502, 2016, doi: 10.1016/j.tim.2016.03.003.
41. Ganar, K., Das, M., Sinha, S., Kumar, S., Newcastle Disease Virus: Current Status and Our Understanding. *Virus Res.*, *184*, 71–81, 2014, doi: 10.1016/j.virusres.2014.02.016.
42. Chen, Z., Parainfluenza Virus 5–Vectored Vaccines against Human and Animal Infectious Diseases. *Rev. Med. Virol.*, *28*, e1965, 2018, doi: 10.1002/rmv.1965.
43. García-Arriaza, J., Cepeda, V., Hallengärd, D., Sorzano, C.O.S., Kümmerer, B.M., Liljeström, P., Esteban, M.A., Novel Poxvirus-Based Vaccine, MVA-CHIKV, Is Highly Immunogenic and Protects Mice against Chikungunya Infection. *J. Virol.*, *88*, 3527–3547, 2014, doi: 10.1128/JVI.03418-13.
44. Scher, G. and Schnell, M.J., Rhabdoviruses as Vectors for Vaccines and Therapeutics. *Curr. Opin. Virol.*, *44*, 169–182, 2020, doi: 10.1016/j.coviro.2020.09.003.
45. Gomme, E.A., Wanjalla, C.N., Wirblich, C., Schnell, M.J., Rabies Virus as a Research Tool and Viral Vaccine Vector. *Adv. Virus Res.*, *79*, 139–164, 2011, doi: 10.1016/B978-0-12-387040-7.00009-3.
46. Fathi, A., Dahlke, C., Addo, M.M., Recombinant Vesicular Stomatitis Virus Vector Vaccines for WHO Blueprint Priority Pathogens. *Hum. Vaccines Immunother.*, *15*, 2269–2285, 2019, doi: 10.1080/21645515.2019.1649532.
47. Manno, C.S., Pierce, G.F., Arruda, V.R., Glader, B., Ragni, M., Rasko, J.J., Ozelo, M.C., Hoots, K., Blatt, P., Konkle, B., *et al.*, Successful Transduction of Liver in Hemophilia by AAV-Factor IX and Limitations Imposed by the Host Immune Response. *Nat. Med.*, *12*, 342–347, 2006, doi: 10.1038/nm1358.
48. Wright, J.F., Manufacturing and Characterizing AAV-Based Vectors for Use in Clinical Studies. *Gene Ther.*, *15*, 840–848, 2008, doi: 10.1038/gt.2008.65.
49. Taj, M.B., Adeel, S.S., Malik, M.W., Najam, A., Batool, K., Assurance of Quality, Safety and Efficacy of Vaccines through Compliance of Quality Management Processes. *J. Anal. Pharm. Res.*, *8*, 188–191, 2019, doi: 10.15406/japlr.2019.08.00337.
50. Baylor, N.W. and Marshall, V.B., Regulation and Testing of Vaccines. *Vaccines*, 1427–1446, 2013, doi: 10.1016/B978-1-4557-0090-5.00073-2.

51. Gogtay, N.J., Dhingra, M.S., Yadav, A., Chandwani, H., Vaccine Policy, Regulations and Safety in India. *Int. J. Risk Saf. Med.*, *21*, 23–30, 2009, doi: 10.3233/JRS-2009-0457.
52. Pashikanti, S., A.N.V.L, S., Durga V, J.S., Regulatory Requirements for Vaccine Registration in United States. *Int. J. Drug Regul. Aff.*, *6*, 85–91, 2018, doi: 10.22270/ijdra.v6i2.253.
53. Ponnapalli, R., Divya, M.S.L., Raju, K.V., Nori, L.P., Regulatory Framework: Vaccine Development in US, India and EU. *Int. J. Appl. Pharm.*, 15, 2, 63–71, 2023, doi: 10.22159/ijap.2023v15i2.46723.
54. Clinical Research Regulation For India, ClinRegs Available online: https://clinregs.niaid.nih.gov/country/india#scope_of_assessment (accessed on 7 October 2024).
55. Chavda, V.P., Balar, P., Vaghela, D., Solanki, H.K., Vaishnav, A., Hala, V., Vora, L., Omicron Variant of SARS-CoV-2: An Indian Perspective of Vaccination and Management. *Vaccines, 11*, 160, 2023, doi: 10.3390/vaccines11010160.
56. Baldwin, J., Piplani, S., Sakala, I.G., Honda-Okubo, Y., Li, L., Petrovsky, N., Rapid Development of Analytical Methods for Evaluating Pandemic Vaccines: A COVID-19 Perspective. *Bioanalysis*. 24, 1805–1826, 2021, 10.4155/bio-2021–0096, doi:10.4155/bio-2021-0096.
57. Burd, E.M., Validation of Laboratory-Developed Molecular Assays for Infectious Diseases. *Clin. Microbiol. Rev.*, *23*, 550–576, 2010, doi: 10.1128/CMR.00074-09.
58. Thanh Le, T., Andreadakis, Z., Kumar, A., Gómez Román, R., Tollefsen, S., Saville, M., Mayhew, S., The COVID-19 Vaccine Development Landscape. *Nat. Rev. Drug Discov.*, *19*, 305–306, 2020, doi: 10.1038/d41573-020-00073-5.
59. Dai, L. and Gao, G.F., Viral Targets for Vaccines against COVID-19. *Nat. Rev. Immunol.*, *21*, 73–82, 2021, doi: 10.1038/s41577-020-00480-0.
60. Alici, E. and Blomberg, P., GMP Facilities for Manufacturing of Advanced Therapy Medicinal Products for Clinical Trials: An Overview for Clinical Researchers. *Curr. Gene Ther.*, *10*, 508–515, 2010, doi: 10.2174/156652310793797757.
61. Kumar, V., Srinivasan, V., Kumara, S., Smart Vaccine Manufacturing Using Novel Biotechnology Platforms: A Study During COVID-19. *J. Comput. Inf. Sci. Eng.*, *22*, 040903, 2022, doi: 10.1115/1.4053273.
62. Josefsberg, J.O. and Buckland, B., Vaccine Process Technology. *Biotechnol. Bioeng.*, *109*, 1443–1460, 2012, doi: 10.1002/bit.24493.
63. Chavda, V.P., Gogoi, N.R., Vaghela, D.A., Balar, P.C., Dawre, S., Dave, D.J., Parenteral Microemulsions for Drug Delivery: Advances and Update. *J. Drug Deliv. Sci. Technol.*, *89*, 104991, 2023, doi: 10.1016/j.jddst.2023.104991.
64. Charlton Hume, H.K. and Lua, L.H.L., Platform Technologies for Modern Vaccine Manufacturing. *Vaccine*, *35*, 4480–4485, 2017, doi: 10.1016/j.vaccine.2017.02.069.
65. Van Riel, D. and De Wit, E., Next-Generation Vaccine Platforms for COVID-19. *Nat. Mater.*, *19*, 810–812, 2020, doi: 10.1038/s41563-020-0746-0.

66. Vokó, Z., Kiss, Z., Surján, G., Surján, O., Barcza, Z., Pályi, B., Formanek-Balku, E., Molnár, G.A., Herczeg, R., Gyenesei, A., *et al.*, Nationwide Effectiveness of Five SARS-CoV-2 Vaccines in Hungary—the HUN-VE Study. *Clin. Microbiol. Infect.*, *28*, 398–404, 2022, doi: 10.1016/j.cmi.2021.11.011.
67. Helling, C. and Strube, J., Quality-by-Design with Rigorous Process Modeling as Platform Technology of the Future. *Chem. Ing. Tech.*, *84*, 1334–1334, 2012, doi: 10.1002/cite.201250297.
68. Yu, L.X., Amidon, G., Khan, M.A., Hoag, S.W., Polli, J., Raju, G.K., Woodcock, J., Understanding Pharmaceutical Quality by Design. *AAPS J.*, *16*, 771–783, 2014, doi: 10.1208/s12248-014-9598-3.
69. Schmidt, A., Helgers, H., Vetter, F.L., Zobel-Roos, S., Hengelbrock, A., Strube, J., Process Automation and Control Strategy by Quality-by-Design in Total Continuous mRNA Manufacturing Platforms. *Processes*, *10*, 1783, 2022, doi: 10.3390/pr10091783.
70. Pambudi, N.A., Sarifudin, A., Gandidi, I.M., Romadhon, R., Vaccine Cold Chain Management and Cold Storage Technology to Address the Challenges of Vaccination Programs. *Energy Rep.*, *8*, 955–972, 2022, doi: 10.1016/j.egyr.2021.12.039.
71. Lloyd, J. and Cheyne, J., The Origins of the Vaccine Cold Chain and a Glimpse of the Future. *Vaccine*, *35*, 2115–2120, 2017, doi: 10.1016/j.vaccine.2016.11.097.
72. Fahrni, M.L., Ismail, I.A.-N., Refi, D.M., Almeman, A., Yaakob, N.C., Saman, K.M., Mansor, N.F., Noordin, N., Babar, Z.-U.-D., Management of COVID-19 Vaccines Cold Chain Logistics: A Scoping Review. *J. Pharm. Policy Pract.*, *15*, 16, 2022, doi: 10.1186/s40545-022-00411-5.
73. Zhang, B., Sim, W.K., Shen, T.-L., Lim, S.K., Engineered EVs with Pathogen Proteins: Promising Vaccine Alternatives to LNP-mRNA Vaccines. *J. Biomed. Sci.*, *31*, 9, 2024, doi: 10.1186/s12929-024-01000-1.
74. Lugelo, A., Hampson, K., Bigambo, M., Kazwala, R., Lankester, F., Controlling Human Rabies: The Development of an Effective, Inexpensive and Locally Made Passive Cooling Device for Storing Thermotolerant Animal Rabies Vaccines. *Trop. Med. Infect. Dis.*, *5*, 130, 2020, doi: 10.3390/tropicalmed5030130.
75. Hanson, C.M., George, A.M., Sawadogo, A., Schreiber, B., Is Freezing in the Vaccine Cold Chain an Ongoing Issue? A Literature Review. *Vaccine*, *35*, 2127–2133, 2017, doi: 10.1016/j.vaccine.2016.09.070.
76. Iyer, P. and Robb, D., Cold Chain Optimisation Models: A Systematic Literature Review, 2023.
77. Rupprecht, C.E., Abela-Ridder, B., Abila, R., Amparo, A.C., Banyard, A., Blanton, J., Chanachai, K., Dallmeier, K., De Balogh, K., Del Rio Vilas, V., *et al.*, Towards Rabies Elimination in the Asia-Pacific Region: From Theory to Practice. *Biologicals*, *64*, 83–95, 2020, doi: 10.1016/j.biologicals.2020.01.008.
78. National Academies of Sciences, E., Division, H. and M., Policy, B. @ on H.S., Chain, C. @ on S. @ of A.M.P.S., Shore, C., Brown, L., Hopp, W.J.,

Causes and Consequences of Medical Product Supply Chain Failures, in: *Building Resilience into the Nation's Medical Product Supply Chains*, National Academies Press (US), 2022.

79. Dellepiane, N., Pagliusi, S., Akut, P., Comellas, S., De Clercq, N., Ghadge, S., Gastineau, T., McGoldrick, M., Nurnaeni, I., Scheppler, L., *et al.*, Alignment in Post-Approval Changes (PAC) Guidelines in Emerging Countries May Increase Timely Access to Vaccines: An Illustrative Assessment by Manufacturers. *Vaccine X*, *6*, 100075, 2020, doi: 10.1016/j.jvacx.2020.100075.
80. van der Loo, J.C.M. and Wright, J.F., Progress and Challenges in Viral Vector Manufacturing. *Hum. Mol. Genet.*, *25*, R42–52, 2016, doi: 10.1093/hmg/ddv451.
81. Lottes, A.E., Cavanaugh, K.J., Chan, Y.Y.-F., Devlin, V.J., Goergen, C.J., Jean, R., Linnes, J.C., Malone, M., Peat, R., Reuter, D.G., *et al.*, Navigating the Regulatory Pathway for Medical Devices-a Conversation with Clinicians, Researchers, and Industry Experts. *J. Cardiovasc. Transl. Res.*, *15*, 927–943, 2022, doi: 10.1007/s12265-022-10232-1.
82. Kumru, O.S., Joshi, S.B., Smith, D.E., Middaugh, C.R., Prusik, T., Volkin, D.B., Vaccine Instability in the Cold Chain: Mechanisms, Analysis and Formulation Strategies. *Biologicals*, *42*, 237–259, 2014, doi: 10.1016/j.biologicals.2014.05.007.
83. Chavda, V.P., Balar, P.C., Bezbaruah, R., Vaghela, D.A., Rynjah, D., Bhattacharjee, B., Sugandhi, V.V., Paiva-Santos, A.C., Nanoemulsions: Summary of a Decade of Research and Recent Advances. *Nanomed.*, *19*, 519–536, 2024, doi: 10.2217/nnm-2023-0199.
84. Singh, S., Pandey, A.K., Malemnganba, T., Prajapati, V.K., Technological advancements in viral vector designing and optimization for therapeutic applications, *Adv. Protein Chem. Struct. Biol.*, 139, 57–87, 2024. https://doi.org/10.1016/bs.apcsb.2023.11.013

9

Viral Vectors in Veterinary Vaccine Development

Anup Kumar[1], Pooja Pandita[2], Harsh Modi[3,4], Shahnaz Alom[5,6] and Vivek P. Chavda[7]*

[1]Department of Medical Biotechnology, University of Technology Sydney (UTS), Sydney, New South Wales, Australia
[2]Department of Pharmaceutics, Delhi Institute of Pharmaceutical Science and Research (DIPSAR), Delhi Pharmaceutical Sciences and Research University (DIPSRU), New Delhi, India
[3]Department of Chemistry and Biochemistry, University of Windsor, Windsor, Ontario, Canada
[4]Girijananda Chowdhury Institute of Pharmaceutical Sciences, Girijananda Chowdhury University-Tezpur Campus, Sonitpur, Assam, India
[5]Department of Pharmaceutical Sciences, Dibrugarh University, Dibrugarh, Assam, India
[6]Department of Chemistry and Biochemistry, Medical Biotechnology, University of Windsor, Windsor, Ontario, Canada
[7]Department of Pharmaceutics and Pharmaceutical Technology, L.M. College of Pharmacy, Ahmedabad, Gujarat, India

Abstract

Viral vectors have revolutionized veterinary vaccine development, offering advantages over traditional methods. These vectors utilize viruses to deliver genetic material, inducing targeted immune responses. Adenoviruses, retroviruses, lentiviruses, and poxviruses are examples each with unique properties. Viral vectors can elicit both humoral and cellular immunity, enabling the development of multivalent vaccines against multiple pathogens. They offer precise antigen delivery, enhancing safety and efficacy. While challenges such as preexisting immunity exist, ongoing research aims to overcome these limitations and fully harness the potential of viral vector vaccines in veterinary medicine.

**Corresponding author*: vivek.chavda@lmcp.ac.in

Vivek P. Chavda and Vasso Apostolopoulos (eds.) Viral Vectors for Vaccine Delivery, (257–316) © 2025 Scrivener Publishing LLC

Keywords: Viral vectors, veterinary vaccines, vaccine development, genetic material, immune response, adenoviruses, lentiviruses

9.1 Introduction

A critical component of maintaining animal health and guaranteeing the welfare of both domestic and wild animals is the development of veterinary vaccines [1]. As the field develops, technological breakthroughs have been crucial in improving vaccine delivery systems and efficacy. In order to provide insight into the importance and possible uses of viral vectors, this chapter will examine their pivotal role in the development of veterinary vaccines [2].

Historically, the creation of veterinary vaccinations has played a significant role in the prevention and management of infectious illnesses in animals. Vaccines are effective means of boosting the immune system and providing defense against infections. Conventional vaccination strategies use infections that have been inactivated or attenuated; nevertheless, novel methods have become more prevalent in recent years [3].

Recombinant DNA technology is used in the development of modern veterinary vaccines, allowing for the creation of vaccinations with enhanced safety profiles and tailored immune responses. This change has sped up the creation of vaccinations to protect against a broad range of infections that affect different kinds of animals. Re-emerging and developing diseases provide problems that call for flexible and reliable vaccination platforms [4].

Because of their exceptional capacity to effectively transfer genetic information into host cells, viral vectors have become revolutionary tools in the generation of veterinary vaccines. These vectors, which are frequently generated from viruses that exist in nature, can be altered to express and convey foreign antigens, stimulating the body's defenses [5]. The ability of viral vectors to imitate natural infection and elicit humoral and cellular immune responses is one of their main benefits [6].

Adenoviruses, lentiviruses, and poxviruses are a few of the often-used viral vectors in the production of veterinary vaccines. They are flexible platforms for vaccine creation because of their capability to transgene and their ability to infect a wide variety of cell types. Furthermore, a polyvalent method of vaccination may be implemented by engineering viral vectors that express antigens from numerous infections at the same time [7]. Numerous studies have shown that viral vectors in veterinary vaccinations are safe and effective. For instance, adenovirus-vectored vaccinations have demonstrated potential in protecting pigs against respiratory illnesses, while poxvirus vectors have been used to create vaccines for birds. These achievements highlight how adaptable viral vectors are in treating a range of animal health issues [8].

An extensive summary of the critical role that viral vectors have played in furthering the development of veterinary vaccines is given in this chapter. The goals include gaining an understanding of viral vector platforms through an examination of the traits and attributes of popular vectors utilized in veterinary vaccinations, with a focus on their advantages and disadvantages. The chapter looks at particular instances of effective veterinary vaccinations that use viral vectors via illuminating case studies, emphasizing their significant influence on disease prevention and control. In addition, the chapter explores the difficulties and prospects for veterinary vaccines based on viral vectors, outlining present barriers and suggesting future lines of inquiry and development. Moreover, regulatory factors are discussed, providing insight into the crucial elements involved in the creation and authorization of viral vector vaccinations for use in veterinary medicine. By achieving these goals, the chapter adds insightful information to the changing field of veterinary vaccine development. It highlights the vital role that viral vectors play in the field's advancement and provides a nuanced viewpoint that helps practitioners, researchers, and policymakers navigate the difficulties of this ground-breaking method of preserving animal health.

9.2 Basics of Viral Vectors

In genetic engineering, viral vectors are flexible instruments that are essential to the generation of veterinary vaccines. This section offers a thorough examination of the definition, traits, kinds, benefits, and drawbacks of the viral vectors utilized in veterinary vaccinations.

9.2.1 Definition and Characteristics of Viral Vectors

Genetically modified viruses called viral vectors are intended to introduce genetic material into target cells in order to promote the production of particular proteins. These vectors are perfect for delivering genes because they preserve the inherent capacity of viruses to infect cells with efficiency [9]. Viral vectors have the capacity to infect a variety of cell types, effectively express transgenes, and may be modified to improve both safety and effectiveness.

9.2.2 Types of Viral Vectors Used in Veterinary Vaccines

1. *Retroviruses:*
RNA genomes of retroviruses are reverse-transcribed into DNA after infection. The host genome incorporates this DNA, allowing transgenic expression to be steady and persistent [10]. Retroviruses are used in veterinary vaccines because they may incorporate transgenes into the host genome, which makes them appropriate for eliciting durable immune responses.

2. *Adenoviruses:*
Adenoviruses may infect a wide variety of dividing and nondividing cells. Their genome is made of double-stranded DNA. Their remarkable transduction efficiency is well known. Because adenoviral vectors may elicit potent immune responses, especially in cases of respiratory illnesses in animals, they are frequently used in veterinary vaccinations [11].

3. *AAVs or Adeno-Associated Viruses:*
AAVs have the characteristics of single-stranded DNA viruses. They can create persistent transgenic expression without assimilating into the host DNA and are not harmful. AAVs are employed in several vaccination applications because of their safety profile and capacity to provide persistent transgene expression [12].

4. *Lentiviruses:*
Upon infection, the RNA genome of lentiviruses is converted to DNA, just as that of retroviruses. Both dividing and nondividing cells can incorporate them. Lentiviral vectors are used because of their capacity to infect different cell types and promote transgene expression in both short- and long-term uses [13].

5. *Herpesviruses:*
Herpesviruses are known for their enormous double-stranded DNA genomes and ability to cause latent infections. Their ability to infect neurons is well established. The ability of herpesviral vectors to stimulate immunological responses and serve as carriers for specific veterinary vaccinations is being investigated [14].

9.2.3 Advantages and Limitations of Viral Vectors

Table 9.1 Various viral vector types and their benefits and drawbacks.

Viral vector type	Advantages	Limitations	References
Retroviruses	- Stable integration into host genome	- Limited cargo capacity	[15]
	- Long-lasting transgene expression	- Risk of insertional mutagenesis	[16]
Adenoviruses	- High transduction efficiency	- Short-lived transgene expression	[17]
	- Induces strong immune responses	- Preexisting immunity in the host	[18]
Adeno-associated viruses (AAVs)	- Nonpathogenic	- Limited cargo capacity	[12]
	- Sustained transgene expression	- Immune response against AAVs themselves	[19]
Lentiviruses	- Broad cell tropism	- Risk of insertional mutagenesis	[20]
	- Integration into both dividing and nondividing cells	- Manufacturing challenges for large-scale production	[21]
Herpesviruses	- Large cargo capacity	- Potential for latency and reactivation in the host	[22]
	- Potential for neuronal transduction	- Safety concerns related to viral spread and host interactions	[23]

To sum up, in order to fully use viral vectors in the production of veterinary vaccines, it is imperative to grasp their fundamentals. Every form of viral vector has unique benefits and drawbacks that affect which applications they are appropriate for when protecting animal health. When choosing viral vectors, researchers need to take these parameters into account carefully in order to maximize the safety and effectiveness of veterinary vaccinations (refer to Table 9.1).

9.3 Genetic Engineering of Viral Vectors

Viral vector genetic engineering is essential for customizing these vehicles for intended uses, especially when it comes to developing veterinary vaccines. The design and manufacturing of viral vectors, gene insertion methods, the function of enhancers and promoters, safety precautions, biosafety concerns, and the significance of quality control and characterization are all covered in this part [24].

9.3.1 Design and Construction of Viral Vectors

9.3.1.1 Gene Insertion Techniques

The exact insertion of foreign genes into the viral genome is a necessary step in the genetic engineering of viral vectors [25]. Conventional techniques involve the cleavage of the viral genome and insertion of the target gene by restriction enzyme-based cloning. However, advances in molecular biology have also brought more advanced technologies, such as site-specific recombination and CRISPR/Cas9-based approaches. By enabling precise and focused gene insertion, these methods lower the possibility of inadvertent genetic changes [26]. The particular needs of the vaccination will determine which insertion technique is used. For example, exact control over the position of the inserted gene is essential to prevent unforeseen effects in animal vaccinations, where safety and effectiveness are vital.

9.3.1.2 Promoters and Enhancers

The selection of promoters and enhancers has a significant impact on the effectiveness of gene expression in viral vectors. Enhancers are DNA sequences that improve a promoter's transcriptional activity, whereas promoters are DNA sequences that start transcription. Achieving the best levels of transgenic expression requires careful consideration when choosing enhancers and promoters [27]. Tissue-specific promoters that are powerful are frequently used in veterinary vaccinations, where it is essential to precisely regulate antigen expression. The temporal regulation of gene expression made possible by the use of inducible promoters improves safety and makes it possible to modify immunological responses [28].

9.3.2 Safety Measures and Biosafety Considerations

Strict safety precautions must be taken when genetically modifying viral vectors to reduce the possibility of unexpected outcomes. It is crucial to take biosafety into account, particularly when creating vaccinations for use in animals.

1. *Containment Measures:* Researchers use containment measures to stop genetically engineered vectors from unintentionally leaking into the environment. These include the use of designed vectors with decreased environmental stability and physical confinement in secure facilities [29].
2. *Risk Assessment:* To determine any possible risks connected to the genetic alterations, a comprehensive risk assessment is carried out. This entails assessing the possibility of horizontal gene transfer, vector recombination, and any unforeseen consequences on species that are not the intended targets [30].
3. *Ethical Considerations:* The correct application of genetic engineering in the creation of viral vectors is guided by ethical principles. Ethical veterinary vaccine development necessitates openness in research procedures, conformity to moral standards, and assessment of any effects on animal welfare [31].

9.3.3 Quality Control and Characterization

Strict quality control and characterization procedures are needed to guarantee the safety, effectiveness, and repeatability of viral vectors. This entails evaluating the viral vectors' potency, purity, stability, and identification, among other characteristics [32].

1. *Purity:* Verifying that the viral vector is free of impurities such as adventitious agents guarantees its security. Methods such as PCR, ELISA, and sequencing are used to confirm the virus preparations' purity.

2. *Potency:* A key component of vaccination effectiveness is the viral vector's capacity to elicit the intended immunological response. The potency of the vaccine is determined in part by measuring the inserted gene's expression, analyzing immunogenicity, and assessing antigen presentation.
3. *Stability:* Vaccine success depends on the viral vectors' capacity to remain stable throughout manufacture, distribution, and storage. Stability studies evaluate how different circumstances affect the viability and functionality of the vector.
4. *Identification:* Verifying the viral vector's identification guarantees that the appropriate genetic alterations have been produced. PCR and sequencing are two molecular methods used for identification verification (refer to Table 9.2).

Table 9.2 Considerations in viral vector design and construction.

Consideration	Description	Reference
Gene insertion techniques	- Restriction enzyme-based cloning - Site-specific recombination - CRISPR/Cas9	[33]
Promoters and enhancers	- Selection of strong and tissue-specific promoters - Use of inducible promoters	[34]
Safety measures and biosafety considerations	- Physical containment in secure laboratories - Thorough risk assessment	[35]
	- Adherence to ethical guidelines - Transparency in research practices	[29]
Quality control and characterization	- Purity assessment using PCR, ELISA, and sequencing - Evaluation of potency	[36]
	- Stability studies during production, storage, and transportation - Identity confirmation through PCR and sequencing	[37]

To sum up, the process of genetically modifying viral vectors is intricate and demands meticulous evaluation of several aspects to guarantee reliability, effectiveness, and safety. The creation of veterinary vaccines that not only fulfill high safety criteria but are also efficacious is made possible by breakthroughs in gene insertion methods, suitable promoter selection, and strong safety controls. In the realm of veterinary medicine, stringent quality control and characterization further ensure the dependability of these viral vectors.

9.4 Delivery System for Viral Vector Vaccines

9.4.1 Application of Nanotechnology in Vaccine Delivery

Notably, several vaccinations have previously been effective in preventing serious infectious diseases. Yet, despite several vaccinations, people are still unable to effectively defend themselves against certain illnesses, including AIDS, TB, and malaria [38]. According to Zhou *et al.* (2020), nanotechnology research has made it possible to create vaccine formulations that are more potent than those made with traditional methods [39]. The development, production, and manipulation of materials on a nanometric scale gave rise to nanotechnology in the 1980s. Nanotechnology made it possible to see how molecules interact with one another and to create nanostructures that would remove barriers and drawbacks from more conventional pharmacological methods [40]. Accordingly, nanotechnology research has been done to create new vaccines and support their global distribution [38]. Nanopharmacology is the application of nanotechnology in pharmacology to enhance therapeutic efficacy through the use of nanoscale particles. This enhancement results from modifications in the pharmacokinetic profile of formulations, which raise bioavailability and/or half-life, and from alterations in the pharmacodynamics that raise efficacy [41].

A vaccine's effectiveness is determined by its capacity to stimulate immunological responses that diverge from those brought on by an illness that occurs naturally. Because of their highly defined composition and length scale, nanomaterials, also known as nanoscale materials, are beneficial and can safely engage main immune pathways [38]. Antigens may be specifically delivered by nanoparticles (NPs) to immune system cells, particularly those whose surfaces have been altered by the addition of specific ligands or antibodies. By promoting absorption and a gradual release of antigens, this type of delivery enhances the effectiveness of vaccinations by stimulating cellular and humoral immune responses [42]. According to Zhu *et al.* (2014), nanocarriers have the capacity to carry immunostimulating components in addition to active pharmacological components; hence, they promote a synergistic effect on the immune system [43]. Moreover, NPs can stimulate APCs, particularly dendritic cells (DCs), which boosts the effectiveness of vaccinations [41]. Thus, the use of nanomaterials as vaccine delivery systems involves both antigen delivery and formulation adjuvant functions. In this manner, the combination of nanomaterial delivery and immunomodulatory effects promotes highly relevant immunological outcomes for vaccination [43]. Lastly, Zhou *et al.* (2020) point out that the special size of NPs is particularly helpful since it allows for more effective drainage to lymphoid organs, which are the sites of antigen uptake and processing. This improves the delivery of vaccine components [39].

Viral vectors are one type of nanocarrier that is currently being researched as a delivery platform. When combined with improvements in antigen design, these nanocarriers help to create highly effective vaccines that elicit immune responses for diseases that are still underdiagnosed [38]. The ability of NPs to load, protect, target, and deliver an immunotherapeutic payload to immune cells of interest, particularly to desirable antigen-presenting cells (APCs) is one way that they contribute to the field of vaccination [44]. By enhancing the solubility, stability, and surface characteristics of vaccination antigens to improve the immune response, nanotechnological vaccines have made it possible to transport antigens across mucosal surfaces in a targeted manner [45]. Nanomaterials have the advantages of being biocompatible, mucosally absorbable, and mainly biodegradable as carriers of vaccine formulations [41].

Additionally, they can be modified and controlled in their surface qualities, which enable chemicals to enter cells and shield formulations from deterioration [46]. The use of NPs in vaccine formulation facilitates targeted delivery of the antigen and increases its immunogenicity and durability. Currently, there are many ways to shield vaccinations from the harsh gastrointestinal environment. One such method is to carry the vaccines inside of or adsorb them onto the surfaces of nanoparticulate systems. Antigens that are adsorbed on the surface offer less protection, but they are more readily recognized by the immune system. Furthermore, an enteric surface coating on particles can provide extra protection in both situations [47]. By boosting immune responses, NPs are useful in enhancing the administration of nasal vaccinations. The nasal-associated lymphoid tissue (NALT) system also preferentially absorbs these particles [41].

9.4.2 Targeted Delivery Approaches: Viral Vectors as Nanocarriers for Targeted Mucosal and Systemic Vaccine Delivery System

Nanoscale (1000 nm) carriers are already employed in vaccine formulations that are either licensed or undergoing clinical studies [48]. Certain NPs can penetrate APCs through various routes, which allows them to modify immune responses later on. Furthermore, antigens and certain adjuvants, like TLR ligands, can be delivered simultaneously via nano-based delivery systems; carriers can occasionally operate as adjuvants on their own [49]. Three essential elements typically make up nanoscale vaccine carrier systems: an adjuvant to enhance the interaction between innate and adaptive immune systems upon encountering the antigen(s), an antigen to stimulate adaptive immune responses, and a delivery or targeting system to guarantee that the adjuvant(s) and antigen(s) are delivered in tandem to the appropriate site at the appropriate time [50].

Since vaccines or antigen-engineered nanocarriers can be manufactured for specific targets, such as tissue-specific delivery to local lymph nodes, cell-specific targeting to APCs, or targeting subcellular compartments like the nucleus for DNA vaccines and be retained at the desired site of action, they are expected to be immunologically more effective than conventional dosage forms [49]. More significantly, vaccinations and nanocarrier antigens can induce immunity at various mucosal barriers through mucosal delivery, which is the body's essential first line of defense in addition to the systemic immune response. In this regard, a significant number of productive mucosal and systemic delivery systems that make use of nano- and microscale carriers have been thoroughly studied up to the point of clinical trials in recent years [51].

Viral vaccine vectors are already nanocarriers that have PAMP adjuvants integrated into them. Viral vector vaccines contain viruses that transmit antigens at the nanoscale and stimulate both humoral and cellular immune responses [49]. Nanoscale structures are already present in certain adjuvant formulations. Modern vaccine development has made the formulation of adjuvants containing vaccine antigens necessary to boost the immunogenicity of highly purified antigens with inadequate immunostimulatory potential. Although early adjuvants (such as aluminum and oil-in-water emulsions) were used empirically, the understanding of how the immune system interacts with pathogens has improved with time. This has allowed the researchers to better understand the role of adjuvants and how to formulate modern vaccines in a way that will maximize the intended clinical benefit [52].

Vaccines using viral vectors are a flexible way to introduce the genetic code into cells of vaccinated individuals, causing the viruses to create antigens. These vaccines can improve the production, targeting, and processing of antigens by directly delivering genetic information to cells through the use of attenuated and nonreplicating viral vectors. In this manner, the synthesis and processing of the antigen within the cell will resemble that of a spontaneous infection [49]. Moreover, vaccinations with viral vectors can be given without the need for extra adjuvants and can tolerate variations depending on the vector employed. In high-stress scenarios like the COVID-19 pandemic, they are crucial because they can elicit a strong, targeted cellular and humoral immune response against the target antigen, with a better safety profile and high-yield production procedures [49, 51, 53].

9.4.3 Novel Delivery Platforms and Technologies

When it comes to the traditional method of administering vaccines, the parenteral route is the most preferred method [54]. However, due to its invasive nature and need for careful cold chain storage, noninvasive immunization routes and novel drug delivery systems are also required. Consequently, preclinical research is being done on liposomes, nanoemulsions, and patches based on the microneedle (MN), which could prove to be effective substitutes for invasive procedures [54]. According to Moderna and BioNTech/Pfizer, lipidic NPs have demonstrated remarkable efficacy in the delivery of the mRNA vaccine against COVID-19 infection [55]. Furthermore, Nuvec®, a new silica NP, has the potential to be used as a delivery vehicle or viral vector to introduce genetic material into host cells [56].

9.4.3.1 Transdermal Vaccine Delivery System

The transdermal (TD) route gained attention recently for immunization purposes, and this is worth addressing. The largest organ in humans, the skin, has a high population of immune cells and easy access to the lymphatic and circulatory systems, making it a prime candidate for targeted vaccination delivery [57]. Since the skin's outer layer, or stratum corneum, is nearly impenetrable to medications and antigens due to its unique structure, the primary obstacles in creating vaccine formulations for the TD route are those associated with resolving this penetration problem. Researchers have tackled this problem in many ways over the years, primarily involving the use of physical processes or penetration enhancers to break down this barrier and enable the transport of drugs and antigens [57].

9.4.3.2 *Microneedle Arrays Delivery System for Viral Vector Vaccine*

Developing better administration techniques to increase vaccination efficacy is still a challenge, and expanding the spectrum of antigens for new vaccines is just one aspect of the vital field of vaccine development in both research and pharmaceuticals. Numerous vaccinations utilizing viral vectors hold significant potential for triggering the humoral and cellular components of adaptive immunity specific to certain antigens. More sophisticated clinical trials are still required to address issues with the pre-existing immunity, immunogenicity, genetic stability, and genotoxicity of viral vector vaccines [58]. Modern vaccine design heavily relies on DCs, the primary immune response regulators. Since the skin contains a large number of these cells, it is thought to be a desirable target for vaccination. But there is still a lot of work to be done in terms of effectively delivering antigens to skin APCs (DCs in particular) and activating them afterward. Targeting these specialized skin APCs could be possible with MA technology [58].

In recent decades, there has been an increased interest in MN arrays (MAs), which are patches with a variable number of needle-like projections in different shapes and dimensions (usually less than 1 mm in height), including for immunization [59, 60]. MAs are made up of several micro-projections that are embedded in base support and vary in height from 25 to 2000 μm [61, 62]. Applying MAs topically increases the likelihood of piercing the stratum corneum barrier and is a desirable method of delivering vaccines intradermally (ID) [63]. The use of MA creates micropores that easily allow the passage of a variety of macromolecules and micro-molecules, including proteins and immunotherapeutic substances like vaccines [64]. Since Henry *et al.* (1998) proposed the idea of MAs, there has been continuous academic and corporate research on their development and implementation [65]. Materials used to create MAs include metals, glass, silicon, sugars, and polymers permitted by the USA Food and Drug Administration (FDA) [58].

Due to their small size, ease of administration (no sharp waste is produced), ability to deliver vaccines to specific skin depths, and effective delivery of various vaccine formulations including viral vectors, MA platforms are promising technologies for vaccine delivery [58]. By allowing antigens and adjuvants to interact with the population of dermal immune cells and making it easier for them to enter draining lymphatics, these structures offer a painless substitute for vaccine TD delivery. This interaction may trigger both local and systemic immune responses [57, 66].

The four main modes of action of MAs are as follows: poke-and-patch, coat-and-poke, poke-and-flow, and poke-and-release [67]. In the poke-and-patch approach, solid MAs are used to puncture the skin and then antigen is applied to the treated area to allow antigen to diffuse into the skin; in the coat-and-poke approach, solid MAs are coated with a target antigen that can be delivered in a single step; the poke-and-flow method depends on the diffusion of vaccine through conduits of solid MAs; on the other hand, the poke-and-release mechanism of action is a feature of dissolving MAs made from water-soluble polymers or carbohydrate material that encapsulates vaccine within the needle matrix. A review by Al-Zahrani *et al.* thoroughly details the different release methods of vaccines from MAs [67]. These soluble MAs dissolve upon implantation into the skin, releasing their payload.

Although the traditional approaches have been around for more than 150 years, they might not necessarily be the best ones. These old methods could be replaced with MAs, which should enhance the body's reaction to a range of illnesses. There are still difficulties in transferring this technological platform for the production of industrial vaccines. The goal of future work is to maximize the dose, repeatable application, and loading capacity of MA [58]. Significant vaccine loss during MAs production is yet another issue that vaccine manufacturers must deal with; one possible solution could be to look for ways to recycle vaccines as they are being manufactured. It appears that several techniques for fabricating MA, including layer-by-layer assembly and droplet air blowing, offer the additional benefit of allowing for precise control of the loaded vaccine quantity without appreciable vaccine loss [68]. Using an applicator that has been shown to increase the efficiency and reproducibility of the insertion of the vaccine-loaded MA in comparison to hand insertion may be able to overcome the variability in skin elasticity and conformability [69].

9.4.3.3 Viral Vector for DNA Vaccine Delivery

DNA vaccines are made using bacterial plasmids that have particular sequences added to them. The cytomegalovirus promoter and its neighboring intron stimulate the expression of genes. Together with components like a prokaryotic antibiotic resistance gene and a transcription termination signal, a sequence guarantees high transcription efficiency [70]. By functioning as a pathogen-associated molecular pattern (PAMP) with a strong affinity for Toll-like receptors (TLRs), DNA introduced into the plasmid boosts immunity. "Pattern recognition receptors," or TLRs, can recognize the conserved molecular patterns in DNA that are linked to infections. One such sequence, the hypomethylated CpG dinucleotide, which primarily binds to TLR-9, is prevalent in bacterial DNA but uncommon in mammalian DNA. Activation, proliferation, and differentiation of natural killer cells, T cells, and monocytes/macrophages are the results of stimulating a variety of TLR9-expressing cells, such as B cells and DCs. The industry is currently attempting to employ artificial CpG phosphorothioate oligonucleotides as adjuvants for several vaccinations. However, TLR9 is exclusively expressed on mammalian plasmacytoid DCs, not myeloid DCs, which is one reason DNA vaccines might not be effective for use in humans. It is interesting to note that DNA vaccines work effectively in $Tlr9^{-/-}$ mice, suggesting that immunological responses might be induced by routes other than TLR-9 stimulation [70, 71].

Because of their well-characterized surface features and nanoscale dimensions, which enable the insertion of immunogenic components (e.g., virosomes), viral vectors, including retrovirus, adenovirus, herpes simplex virus, and vaccinia virus, are effective in transferred DNA. However, their usage is justified by limitations such as their high cost, toxicity, immunogenicity, limited capacity to carry DNA, and ability to cause insertional alterations in host DNA [70].

9.4.3.4 Needle-Free Vaccination for Viral Vector Vaccine Delivery

Needle-free injections can be delivered by liquid jet injectors and ballistic injectors [72, 73], which are driven by a high-pressure gas or spring, and can respectively deliver liquid-based vaccines and powder vaccine particles intradermally, subcutaneously, or intramuscularly [74]. Compared to traditional needle injection, vaccines delivered by jet injection may lead to superior vaccine efficacy by enabling a wider dispersion of the vaccine in the tissue for better uptake by APCs [75]. The immunogenicity results, however, have not always been superior for jet injection, partly due to variations in injection site and depth, although several studies have shown superior efficacy with jet injection relative to intramuscular or subcutaneous route, as was the case for a hepatitis A vaccine [75, 76] and a trivalent influenza virus vaccine [77]. Additionally, preclinical and clinical research showed that jet injection could more successfully administer viral vector and DNA vaccines to improve immune responses against a variety of infections, such as HIV and malaria, among others [78, 79]. A human adenovirus-5 vaccine [80] and other investigations showed jet injection to have either equivalent or lower efficiency [80, 81]. Jet/ballistic injection has many benefits over traditional needle and syringe injections, but it can also be more painful than the traditional method. For example, trivalent influenza vaccines have higher rates of pain during injection and injection site reactions [77], hepatitis A vaccines have greater local reactions in all categories [75], and DNA vaccines have twice as many adverse events per immunization [82].

9.4.3.5 *Combination Vaccine Regimen for Viral Vector Vaccine Delivery*

One popular immunization strategy is the prime-boost regimen. As previously stated, due to the formation of anti-vector immunity, multiple vaccines with a single viral vector are deemed ineffective. A viral vector boost and DNA prime approach is frequently employed to get around this issue [83]. Numerous studies have demonstrated that this tactic triggers a CTL response that is protective. A different strategy is to employ several viral vector types in combination. Compared to other approaches, this one may produce a stronger immunological response. Given their high immunogenicity, modified vaccinia Ankara (MVA) and adenovirus (Ad) vectors are typically utilized in combination regimens. When a prime-boost regimen is used, these vectors elicit a substantially greater immune response [84, 85]. On the other hand, it was found that the co-administration of Ad and MVA vectors inhibited the production of transgenes through soluble substances released by virus-infected cells. The MVA vector was demonstrated to infect cell culture supernatant and decrease Ad vector transgene expression in an *in vitro* experiment [86]. Combining a viral vector with an already-available vaccination is an additional strategy. For example, the live, attenuated BCG vaccine for tuberculosis generates only a limited level of protection, particularly in adults and adolescents. It was investigated if an MVA85A boost regimen may improve protective immunity after receiving a BCG vaccination. Although the MVA85A Phase 2b experiment was unsuccessful, using viral vectors to improve priming immunization is still an option [87].

9.5 Routes of Administration for Viral Vector Vaccines

The delivery system and administration route have an impact on the effectiveness of the response produced by viral vector vaccines [88]. Clinical investigations for different viruses have demonstrated the multiple routes that viral vectors can be administered through the parenteral route such as intramuscular, subcutaneous, and intradermal application, and the mucosal route such as intranasal and oral administration [88]. The following section discusses the various delivery mechanisms that are being developed to ensure the highest level of safety and efficacy for the developing vaccines.

9.5.1 Parenteral Route of Administration

Historically, parenteral routes have been used to administer vaccines, specifically the intramuscular (IM), intradermal (ID), and subcutaneous (SC) routes. Most of the time, this makes it possible to create a local depot at the injection site from which the local lymph node (LN) can receive the antigen and any adjuvants that may be present. Depending on the characteristics, this process can occur passively or through immune cell capture and transport to the LN. SC and transdermal (TD) routes have been proposed as IM alternatives specifically because of the potential benefits they may offer in terms of vaccine drainage to the lymphatics and overall immunogenicity. Still, people prefer IM injections over other parenteral options since adjuvants in vaccine formulations have occasionally enhanced the amount of local side effects that are experienced after SC and TD administration [57].

9.5.1.1 Intravenous Route

Even though intravenous injection is the most widely used method of medication delivery, it is not the most effective vaccination method, particularly during a pandemic. Since intravenous injection might result in anaphylaxis, which includes an allergic reaction and toxicity, and generally elicits a comparatively weaker immune response than other injection methods, it is not typically utilized for vaccinations [74]. It is commonly known that calves who unintentionally receive an intravenous immunization may experience a deadly severe pulmonary reaction [74]. AdCLD-CoV19, created by Cellid Co., Ltd., and COH04S1, created by the City of Hope Medical Centre in the United States of America, are replicating viral vector vaccines meant to be administered parenterally via injection [89].

9.5.1.2 Intramuscular Route

The majority of COVID-19 viral vector vaccines are designed to be injected intramuscularly [66]. The intramuscular approach is the basis for the newly created replicating viral vector-based COVID-19 vaccines, such as ERUCOV-VAC from the Health Institutes of Turkey [90] and Brilife from the Israel Institute for Biological Research [66].

9.5.1.3 *Subcutaneous Route*

In response to the success of the intramuscular route, scientists have created replicating viral vector vaccines that can be injected subcutaneously. One such vaccine is AV-COVID-19, which is distributed by Aivita Biomedical, Inc. in Indonesia [66].

9.5.1.4 *Intradermal Route*

In clinical investigations, the immunological responses elicited by SC and IM immunizations are relatively equal, although intradermal (ID) immunization produces stronger responses than IM injection. This could be due to the fact that the dermis has a higher concentration of DCs, which help to capture antigens. Additionally, local inflammation triggers the maturation of DCs and their migration into draining lymph nodes, which results in vaccination dosage sparing [74, 91]. Intradermal vaccination has been employed, such as the HBV vaccine in dialysis patients, for groups that do not respond well to an IM injection [92]. Using commercially available syringes and correctly positioning the needle is a significant challenge when delivering IDs. Utilizing ID delivery devices is an additional choice for enabling more precise ID delivery [91]. Even while a vaccine administered by ID injection is more successful at eliciting immunological responses, local adverse reactions appear to be more severe when administered via ID, with the least amount of local reaction occurring with SC and IM. For instance, in human subjects, mild local pruritus (itchiness), superficial skin lesions, and injection site nodules were similarly associated with either SC delivery of a full dose or ID delivery of a DNA vaccine at a lower dose (10% of a full dose). However, no local site reactions were observed following IM injection [74].

9.5.2 Mucosal Route of Administration

Parenteral routes of immunization, although widely used, have several drawbacks. These include the costs and manpower involved in preparing, administering, and discarding injectable materials, as well as the hazards related to needle stick injuries and handling sharp waste. Due to these factors, mucosal routes of delivery for vaccinations have also been investigated, especially in light of the critical function that the mucosal-associated lymphatic tissue (MALT) plays in triggering mucosal immunity locally [93]. In this regard, the oral and nasal routes have been the most extensively studied, with an emphasis on the development of the local immune response after APCs, such as macrophages and DCs, present an antigen to tissue-resident T and B cells. The release of antigen-specific immunoglobulin A (IgA) antibodies, which can identify the antigen at the entry point and stop the disease from spreading further throughout the body, is a sign that this kind of immune response is very significant [94, 95]. The scientific community must concentrate on creating formulations for mucosal vaccine delivery because achieving this degree of protection with parenteral immunization procedures is frequently challenging.

9.5.2.1 Intranasal Route

Given its simplicity and reliability, the nasal route is better for eliciting a mucosal response than the parenteral route [88, 96]. Focusing on the intranasal (IN) route of administration as an alternative to GI barriers would have several benefits for vaccine delivery, such as high vascularization of the nasal mucosa and quick absorption of antigens into the systemic circulation [97]. Furthermore, several infections enter through this route and cause serious respiratory illnesses, which increases the region's significance and allure for the development of vaccinations against these infectious agents. For example, greater mucosal immunity in the nose and lungs may be provided by the IN administration of a coronavirus vaccine, protecting the site of entry [98]. The influenza FluMist vaccine has demonstrated the potential benefits of a nasal spray vaccine as a less intrusive delivery route in the past. However, while creating vaccine formulations, it is also important to take into account the drawbacks of the IN-administration route, such as the quick mucus clearance that shortens the antigens' residence time in the nasal mucosa and the size-restricted permeation of adjuvants and antigens across the epithelial barrier [97].

Mucosal formulations for the COVID-19 vaccine have been developed by numerous pharmaceutical companies and researchers due to the importance of the local mucosal immune response in preventing the replication of the SARS-CoV-2 virus in nasal epithelia. However, it should be noted that the nasal route is preferred for providing direct action in COVID-19 vaccinations. A vaccine that is based on an intranasal nonreplicating viral vector that has successfully completed a phase 1 clinical trial is BBV154, which was created by Bharat Biotech in India and Washington University School of Medicine in St. Louis, USA (NCT04751682). The replicating viral vector-based vaccine, DelNS1-2019-nCoV-RBD-OPT1, developed by Wishai Bio-Pharm in China, is the most advantageous of all the vaccines. It is intended to be sprayed intranasally and may be useful for convenient administration and patient compliance vaccination during outbreaks [66, 99].

9.5.2.2 Oral Route

The hostile gastrointestinal (GI) environment must be taken into account by vaccine scientists when creating a formulation for the oral route. In particular, when creating current vaccines with peptide, protein, or nucleic acid antigens, antigen protection against low gastric pH, strong enzymatic presence, and large mucus layer throughout the GI tract is crucial [100]. When administered directly to the GI tract infection site, oral vaccination has been demonstrated to be an effective method for eliciting the necessary immune responses. For instance, local immune responses in the intestinal mucosa, where the poliovirus replicates, have been linked to the effectiveness of the oral polio vaccine (OPV) in lowering infection and the transmission of polio [101]. In addition to the intranasal mucosal routes, the oral vaccine VXA-CoV2-1.1-S, produced by Vaxart, USA, is undergoing phase 2 clinical trials (NCT05067933). Moreover, iosBio Pharma, in the UK, is working with BioCell Corporation, in Auckland, New Zealand, to develop and study OraPro-COVID-19, an oral formulation based on capsules, to expedite vaccination coverage [66, 102].

9.6 Comparative Analysis of Different Administration Routes

9.6.1 Parenteral Vaccine Delivery System

There have been multiple successful reports of individual protection against serious diseases associated with parenteral vaccinations. However, due to improper reuse of these materials worldwide, parenteral administration of vaccines via needle and syringe has low acceptability by children and babies and has a high risk of infection [103]. Apart from the concerns of safety and low acceptability, a noteworthy limitation of this technique could be its inability to trigger immunity at the point of entry that is, mucosal surfaces when the pathogen enters the body [104].

While some vaccinations are authorized for subcutaneous (SC) or intradermal (ID) administration, the bulk of licensed vaccines are administered via intramuscular (IM) injection. Since intramuscular administration is simple to carry out, generally well accepted, and has a minimal chance of causing negative reactions at the injection site, it is frequently chosen. But administering vaccines to the skin, which is more immunocompetent than the muscle, has long been thought to be a tactic for boosting immune responses to vaccinations. When administered topically rather than intramuscularly, the yellow fever virus or influenza vaccinations produce better reactions in healthy persons as well as in influenza patients [105]. It has also been proven that antigen dosage reduction is possible with intradermal immunization without sacrificing effectiveness. In some studies, it was found that injecting an mRNA vaccine intradermally (ID) activated APCs at the injection site more effectively than injecting it intramuscularly (IM). This was accompanied by temporarily elevated levels of T cell responses specific to the vaccine and antibody (Ab) titers [50, 106]. When compared with IM administration, SC and ID vaccination is believed to produce superior immune cell targeting and enhanced vaccine responses. But when it comes to producing humoral immune responses to hepatitis B, hepatitis A, herpes zoster virus, influenza, diphtheria toxin, measles, mumps, rubella, varicella, and tick-borne encephalitis virus, all of these clinical trials have shown no significant variations between SC and IM vaccination. These results have supported IM vaccination as the preferred mode of delivery, along with the fact that adverse effects, including reactogenicity at the injection site, were more common in SC immunized persons in most clinical trials [107].

By administering an RBD-based peptide immunogen intradermally to BALB/c mice and comparing it side by side with the intramuscular immunization route, Yadav and his coworkers evaluated the humoral and cellular responses. They discovered that, like intramuscular (IM) immunization, intradermal (ID) vaccination is well tolerated and produces humoral antibody responses of a notable size. Furthermore, compared to the IM approach, the ID immunization produced more IFN-g and IL-2, indicating a better cellular response. Overall, their data suggest that the ID method of immunization offers a viable substitute strategy for the development of candidates for the self-administrative SARS-CoV-2 vaccine [108].

9.6.2 Mucosal Vaccine Delivery System

Consequently, mucosal vaccination delivery stands out as a useful, noninvasive, and efficient substitute to trigger systemic and local reactions [109]. Because mucosal delivery induces secretory immunoglobulin A (IgA), cell-mediated immunity in mucosal tissues, and immunization at mucosal locations where pathogens enter the body, it can elicit more effective protective immune responses than parenteral vaccinations [49]. All immune system components can be stimulated by mucosal vaccinations, preventing infections from entering the host through the mucosal surface as well as other pathways. To be more precise, systemic IgG antibodies and IgA antibodies against particular antigens at infection sites are both stimulated by mucosal vaccination. It is necessary to induce the production of secretory IgA because, in the intestinal region, for instance, these antibodies have a secretory component that gives them greater stability. They also aid in preventing the formation of pathogenic colonies in intestinal tissues by agglutinating, entrapping, and eliminating pathogens [110]. Moreover, mucosal vaccination can trigger cellular responses mediated by $CD4^+$ T helper lymphocytes and $CD8^+$ T cytotoxic lymphocytes, which are critical in the fight against intracellular pathogens, as well as the expression of particular receptors by lymphocytes, which can also trigger immune responses at more distant sites [109].

As a result, mucosal immunization is particularly important for a number of reasons: (1) higher individual adherence and greater capacity for mass immunization; (2) simpler methods of production and storage as it does not require strict sterilization protocols and has a high purity level; (3) the potential for self-administration as it does not require specialized professionals, resulting in a significant decrease in vaccination costs; (4) induction of mucosal and systemic humoral immunity through antigen-specific IgA and IgG antibody responses; (5) no interference with concerns related to culture or religion; and (6) elimination of potential disease asymptomatic carriers, thereby halting the spread of infections among people [111].

9.6.3 Challenges of the Mucosal Delivery System

However, despite all of its benefits, the method still faces difficulties related to immunological tolerance, enzymatic degradation, and ineffective immunogenicity, absorption, and presentation of antigens [112]. Overall, successful mucosal immunization strategies must have three key components: (a) efficiently targeting APCs in the mucosa to properly process antigens that activate particular T and B cells; (b) overcoming the mucosa's physiological barriers; and (c) controlling the kinetics of antigen and adjuvant delivery to support the development of a protective adaptive immune memory that lasts for a long time [113].

9.6.3.1 Advantages of the Oral Route

Compared to traditional parenteral vaccinations, oral vaccines have several benefits, including easy administration, large-scale, low-cost manufacture, and the induction of immunity in the gut mucosa, which prevents the spread of disease and boosts herd immunity [114]. Oral vaccinations are appealing for mass immunization programs because they have the possibility for self-administration, higher adherence, and a decreased incidence of adverse responses [49].

9.6.3.2 *Challenges of Oral Route*

Important requirements that must be met for the development of effective oral vaccines include high safety, long-term systemic and mucosal memory, prolonged exposure of antigens to APCs, high loads of antigens or other vehicles with encapsulation capacity, and the ability to reach intestinal cells. According to Kang *et al.* (2018), one crucial tactic to address these issues has been the research and use of oral vaccine delivery system technologies [115]. Different delivery systems have been developed for targeted delivery to immunological induction sites, which allow antigens to be absorbed by APCs and enhance immune response robustness. This is in addition to protecting antigens against the gastrointestinal environment [110].

9.6.3.3 *Advantages of Intranasal Route*

As with the oral method, intranasal administration is noninvasive, painless, requires no sterilization, and can be self-administered for both local and systemic distribution of medicinal substances. In addition to these benefits, the nasal pathway's many microvilli, porous endothelium membranes, and highly vascularized epithelium contribute to its enormous mucosal surface area [116]. One benefit of intranasal vaccination is the induction of protection against respiratory tract pathogens; long-term protection is provided by responses produced in the nose cavity's lymphoid tissue. Numerous illnesses, including measles, influenza, respiratory infections, and meningitis, are caused by bacteria entering the body through the respiratory mucosa. Given this, a vaccination that permits defense via this pathway is ideal since it guards against infection of the environment as well as the individual. Furthermore, since it is an easier form of application, decreased degradation enzyme activity, improved patient compliance, and cost savings should also be taken into account [117, 118].

9.6.3.4 *Challenges of Intranasal Route*

Inefficient absorption of soluble antigens by the local immune cells, quick mucociliary clearance, short antigen residence time, restricted molecular size penetration through epithelial barriers, lack of human-safe adjuvants, low pH, low stability of formulation against nasal enzymes, and reduced delivery volume due to the nasal cavity's low capacity (from 100 to 150 μl) are some of the challenges associated with the development of nasal vaccines. In light of these obstacles, the implementation of sophisticated delivery mechanisms may aid in prolonging the duration of vaccine administration in the nasal cavity, as well as improving formulation stability and vaccine component absorption [97, 119].

9.7 Applications of Viral Vectors in Veterinary Vaccine Development

The many ways that viral vectors are being used to generate veterinary vaccines demonstrate how important a role they play in treating a wide spectrum of infectious illnesses that affect animals. This thorough investigation explores a variety of viral vector vaccines, such as recombinant, DNA-based, inactivated, live attenuated, and subunit vaccines. A comprehensive table with an additional column detailing particular instances of viral vector-based veterinary vaccinations is also supplied to offer a practical viewpoint on the effective application of these novel strategies.

9.7.1 Live Attenuated Viral Vector Vaccines

Vaccines using weakened or altered viruses used in live attenuated viral vectors elicit an immune response without causing illness. These vaccines work on the idea of imitating natural illnesses to produce strong, lifelong protection. The capacity of live attenuated vaccines to generate humoral as well as cellular immune responses adds to their overall effectiveness and is one of their main benefits [120].

Not only is the modified poxvirus vector example previously discussed, but live attenuated vaccines have also been effectively used to protect animals against a variety of respiratory viral illnesses. For example, the induction of protective immunity in cattle has demonstrated encouraging results using a live attenuated bovine respiratory syncytial virus (BRSV) vector. There may be uses for this strategy in the prevention of respiratory illnesses in animals [121].

9.7.2 Inactivated Viral Vector Vaccines

Vaccines using inactivated viral vectors employ virus vectors that have been made non-infectious, usually by physical or chemical methods. These vaccines can nevertheless elicit an immunological response despite not being able to replicate as well as live vectors. Vaccines using inactivated viral vectors are appropriate in scenarios where safety is the main priority since they are frequently thought to be safer than live attenuated vaccines [122].

The use of an inactivated adenovirus vector expressing important antigens serves as an example of an inactivated viral vector vaccination. Compared to live vectors, inactivated vaccines have better safety profiles, even if they need booster doses to sustain protection over time [7].

Other inactivated viral vector vaccines have demonstrated potential, apart from adenoviruses. For example, it has been shown that an inactivated lentiviral vector encoding feline immunodeficiency virus (FIV) antigens is effective in triggering cat immunological responses. This strategy offers a possible way to fight retroviral infections in domestic cat populations [123].

9.7.3 DNA-Based Viral Vector Vaccines

Vaccines based on DNA-based viral vectors use the genetic makeup of the virus to induce host cells to express antigens. This method enables the activation of immunological responses, both cellular and humoral. The simplicity of design and manufacture is one benefit of DNA-based vaccinations [124].

Plasmid DNA vectors expressing viral antigens are a prime example of DNA-based viral vector vaccines. Vaccines based on DNA have the potential to be developed and customized quickly. A DNA vaccination against the equine West Nile virus has shown effective in eliciting protective immune responses in horses when it comes to vector-borne infections [125].

Other DNA-based vectors, such as bacterial artificial chromosomes (BACs) carrying the viral genome, have also been investigated in addition to plasmid DNA. For instance, a novel strategy to manage herpesvirus infections has been demonstrated using a BAC-based DNA vaccine that expresses the glycoprotein D of the bovine herpesvirus-1 (BoHV-1) and has shown promise in inducing immunological responses in cattle [126].

9.7.4 Subunit Viral Vector Vaccines

Vaccines employing subunit viral vectors concentrate on exploiting certain viral proteins or components rather than the complete viral genome. With this method, the important antigens that might trigger an immunological response are focused on. Adjuvants may be necessary for subunit vaccinations to improve their immunogenicity, as they are frequently thought to be safer than live vectors [127].

Using a lentiviral vector to produce a particular viral protein is an example of a subunit viral vector vaccine. Subunit vaccines can be specifically designed to elicit desired immune responses by focusing on certain virus proteins [128].

Subunit viral vector vaccines against a variety of infections have been investigated in addition to lentiviruses. A subunit vaccine based on a porcine circovirus type 2 (PCV2) vector expressing PRRSV antigens has demonstrated effectiveness in lowering clinical symptoms associated with the porcine reproductive and respiratory syndrome virus (PRRSV) in pigs [129].

9.7.5 Recombinant Viral Vector Vaccines

Vaccines made with recombinant viral vectors combine genetic material from several sources to produce a vaccine with improved characteristics. This tactic offers a polyvalent method that targets numerous infections at once by allowing the inclusion of beneficial traits from various viruses [4].

The use of a recombinant adenovirus vector expressing antigens from several infections is an example of a recombinant viral vector vaccine. Recombinant viral vector vaccines are useful tools for tackling challenging infectious diseases because they may be made to offer broad-spectrum protection [120].

Other recombinant viral vector vaccines have demonstrated efficacy in addition to adenoviruses. The potential of this strategy to stop avian influenza outbreaks is proven by the protective immunity that a recombinant herpesvirus vector carrying the hemagglutinin gene of the avian influenza virus has shown in chickens [130].

9.7.6 Examples of Veterinary Vaccines Using Viral Vectors

These enlarged illustrations offer a more thorough understanding of the many uses of viral vectors in the creation of veterinary vaccines. The target pathogen's characteristics, the intended immune response, and safety concerns all play a role in the choice of particular viral vector types (refer to Table 9.3).

In conclusion, the use of viral vectors in the creation of veterinary vaccines demonstrates a vibrant and cutting-edge industry. Every strategy has different benefits and things to consider, ranging from live attenuated vaccines to recombinant viral vector vaccinations. The enlarged examples highlight how effective vaccinations based on viral vectors are at preventing and managing infectious illnesses in a variety of animal species.

Table 9.3 Main features and examples of veterinary vaccines using viral vectors.

Viral vector type	Target pathogen	Vaccine type	Key features	Examples of veterinary vaccines	References
Live attenuated viral vectors	Modified poxvirus	Respiratory viral infections	Induces robust and prolonged immunity	Fowlpox-based vaccine for avian influenza (H5N1)	[131]
			Mimics natural infections	Live attenuated bovine respiratory syncytial virus (BRSV) vector for cattle	[132]
Inactivated viral vectors	Inactivated adenovirus	Gastrointestinal infections	Safer profile than live attenuated vectors	Inactivated adenovirus vector for bovine coronavirus	[133]
			May require booster doses	Inactivated lentiviral vector for feline immunodeficiency virus (FIV)	[134]
DNA-based viral vectors	Plasmid DNA	Vector-borne diseases	Induces both humoral and cellular immune responses	DNA vaccine for Equine West Nile Virus	[135]
			Requires optimization for efficient expression	BAC-based DNA vaccine for bovine herpesvirus-1 (BoHV-1)	[136]

(Continued)

Table 9.3 Main features and examples of veterinary vaccines using viral vectors. *(Continued)*

Viral vector type	Target pathogen	Vaccine type	Key features	Examples of veterinary vaccines	References
Subunit viral vectors	Lentiviral Vector	Vector-borne diseases	Focuses on specific viral proteins	Subunit vaccine for porcine reproductive and respiratory syndrome virus (PRRSV)	[122]
			May require adjuvants for increased efficacy	Subunit vaccine based on PCV2 vector for PRRSV	[137]
Recombinant viral vectors	Recombinant adenovirus	Polyvalent vaccination	Targets multiple pathogens simultaneously	Recombinant adenovirus vector for Canine distemper virus and canine parvovirus	[2]
			Incorporates features from different viruses	Recombinant herpesvirus vector for avian influenza virus	[138]

9.8 Immunology and Immune Response

Optimizing the effectiveness of viral vector vaccines requires an understanding of their immunological components. The processes of the immune system's reaction to vaccinations with viral vectors, the function of adjuvants in boosting immunity, and the idea of immunological memory and longevity are all covered in this section.

9.8.1 Mechanisms of Immune Response to Viral Vector Vaccines

Innate and adaptive immune systems interact in a well-coordinated manner during the immunological response to viral vector vaccinations. The viral vector delivers foreign antigens during immunization, setting off a series of processes.

1. *Innate Immune Response:* Immune cells that identify pathogen-associated molecular patterns (PAMPs) mount an initial defense through the innate immune response. Pattern recognition receptors (PRRs) on DCs identify vector components in the context of viral vectors, which triggers the activation of innate immune pathways [139].
2. *Adaptive Immune Response:* Presenting viral antigens to T cells is a critical function of DCs, which sets off the adaptive immune response. In order to coordinate the humoral immune response, CD4+ T cells stimulate B cells to generate antibodies. Conversely, CD8+ T lymphocytes are essential for cellular immunity because they specifically target and destroy infected cells [140].
3. *Production of Antibodies:* Vaccines utilizing viral vectors frequently elicit strong antibody reactions. Antibodies, specifically neutralizing antibodies, are essential in impeding the entrance of viruses into host cells. This is an essential defense mechanism against viral infections [141].
4. *Cellular Immunity:* The identification and eradication of virally infected cells depends on CD8+ cytotoxic T cells. Long-term immunity is aided by this cellular component of the immune response, which offers protection against intracellular infections [142].

9.8.2 Adjuvants and Immune Enhancement

Substances known as adjuvants are used in vaccinations in order to improve the immune system's reaction to the antigens. Adjuvants can work in a variety of ways, including enhancing the presentation and transport of antigens, igniting the innate immune system, regulating the production of cytokines, or encouraging the development and upkeep of memory cells. Adjuvants have the potential to enhance the immunogenicity, effectiveness, and durability of viral vector vaccines, particularly those that are susceptible to preexisting immunity or tolerance, have poor immunogenicity, or lack transgene expression [143].

Table 9.4 The main features and examples of adjuvants for viral vector vaccines.

Adjuvant category	Mechanism of action	Examples of adjuvants	Examples of veterinary vaccines using viral vectors	References
Immunostimulants	Activate the innate immune system by binding to specific receptors	LPS, CpG, MPL, poly(I:C)	Fowlpox-based vaccine for avian influenza (H5N1), live attenuated bovine respiratory syncytial virus (BRSV) vector for cattle, DNA vaccine for equine West Nile virus, subunit vaccine for porcine reproductive and respiratory syndrome virus (PRRSV)	[2, 146]
Delivery systems	Facilitate the antigen delivery and presentation by prolonging the bioavailability, targeting, or uptake of the antigens	MF59, AS01, virosomes	Inactivated adenovirus vector for bovine coronavirus, inactivated lentiviral vector for feline immunodeficiency virus (FIV), BAC-based DNA vaccine for Bovine Herpesvirus-1 (BoHV-1), subunit vaccine based on PCV2 vector for PRRSV	[147–149]

Immunostimulants and delivery methods are the two primary categories into which adjuvants fall. Immunostimulants are substances that bind to certain receptors, such as TLRs or other pattern recognition receptors (PRRs), to stimulate the innate immune system. Immunostimulants have the ability to stimulate the maturation and activation of APCs, including macrophages and DCs, as well as the production of pro-inflammatory cytokines and chemokines. Immunostimulants have the ability to influence T and B cell polarization and differentiation, which can result in the production of various immunological responses, including Th1, Th2, Th17, or Treg. Immunostimulants include LPS, CpG, MPL, or poly(I:C) [144].

Delivery systems are substances that help present and transport antigens by making them more bioavailable, directing them towards certain tissues or cells, or increasing the amount of APCs that absorb them. To improve the efficacy and specificity of delivery methods, immunostimulants or other adjuvants can be co-delivered. Different forms of delivery methods, such as emulsions, liposomes, NPs, or MNs, can be categorized. A few instances of delivery methods include Virosomes, AS01, and MF59 [145] (refer to Table 9.4).

9.8.3 Immune Memory and Longevity

The immune system's capacity to recall and react to an antigen that it has previously met is known as immune memory. Memory cells, which are long-lived, specialized lymphocytes that may quickly reactivate and multiply following reexposure to the same antigen, mediate immune memory. Memory B cells and memory T cells are the two primary subtypes of memory cells. Memory T cells can develop into effector T cells, which can aid B cells or eradicate the infected cells, whereas memory B cells can differentiate into plasma cells and release high-affinity antibodies [150].

The kind of viral vector, the target antigen, the dosage and mode of administration, the adjuvants' presence, and the host factors all affect the immunological memory and durability of viral vector vaccines. In general, by producing and sustaining memory cells in various compartments, such as the blood, lymph nodes, spleen, bone marrow, or mucosal tissues, viral vector vaccines can produce long-lasting immunological memory. However, the characteristics of the viral vector, such as its ability to replicate, tropism, immunogenicity, and transgenic expression, may affect the longevity and caliber of the immunological memory [151]. Certain viral vectors, like vaccinia virus or adenovirus, for instance, can stimulate both effector and central memory cells to produce robust and long-lasting memory responses. Adeno-associated virus and lentivirus are two examples of

Table 9.5 The main features and examples of immune memory and longevity of viral vector vaccines in veterinary vaccine development.

Viral vector type	Target antigen	Animal species	Memory cell type	Memory cell location	Memory duration	References
Adenovirus	Bovine coronavirus	Cattle	Memory B and T cells	Blood, lymph nodes, spleen, bone marrow	Up to 6 months	[7, 153]
	Feline immunodeficiency virus	Cats	Memory B and T cells	Blood, lymph nodes, spleen, bone marrow	Up to 7 years	[154]
Vaccinia virus	Avian influenza	Chickens	Memory B and T cells	Blood, lymph nodes, spleen, bone marrow	Up to 1 year	[155]
	Bovine herpesvirus-1	Cattle	Memory B and T cells	Blood, lymph nodes, spleen, bone marrow	Up to 2 years	[156]
Lentivirus	Porcine reproductive and respiratory syndrome virus	Pigs	Memory B and T cells	Blood, lymph nodes, spleen, bone marrow	Up to 1 year	[157]
	Feline immunodeficiency virus	Cats	Memory B and T cells	Blood, lymph nodes, spleen, bone marrow	Up to 7 years	[154]

(Continued)

Table 9.5 The main features and examples of immune memory and longevity of viral vector vaccines in veterinary vaccine development. (*Continued*)

Viral vector type	Target antigen	Animal species	Memory cell type	Memory cell location	Memory duration	References
Adeno-associated virus	Hemophilia A	Dogs	Memory B cells	Blood, lymph nodes, spleen, bone marrow	Up to 10 years	[158]
	Hemophilia B	Dogs	Memory B cells	Blood, lymph nodes, spleen, bone marrow	Up to 10 years	[156]
Measles virus	Canine distemper virus	Dogs	Mucosal and systemic memory B and T cells	Blood, lymph nodes, spleen, bone marrow, mucosal tissues	Up to 20 years	[156]
	Peste des Petits ruminants virus	Sheep and Goats	Mucosal and systemic memory B and T cells	Blood, lymph nodes, spleen, bone marrow, mucosal tissues	Up to 20 years	[159]

(*Continued*)

Table 9.5 The main features and examples of immune memory and longevity of viral vector vaccines in veterinary vaccine development. (*Continued*)

Viral vector type	**Target antigen**	**Animal species**	**Memory cell type**	**Memory cell location**	**Memory duration**	**References**
Vesicular stomatitis virus	Ebola	Non-human primates	Mucosal and systemic memory B and T cells	Blood, lymph nodes, spleen, bone marrow, mucosal tissues	Up to 5 years	[160]
	Lassa fever	Non-human primates	Mucosal and systemic memory B and T cells	Blood, lymph nodes, spleen, bone marrow, mucosal tissues	Up to 5 years	[161]

viral vectors that may integrate into the host genome and enable transgenic expression that is stable and long-lasting [128]. Certain viral vectors, including the vesicular stomatitis virus and the measles virus, can target certain tissues or receptors and cause systemic or mucosal memory reactions [152] (refer to Table 9.5).

9.9 Safety and Regulatory Considerations

In the development and application of veterinary viral vector vaccines, safety and regulatory compliance are critical considerations. This section explores the regulatory approval procedure, the thorough safety evaluation method, and the significance of post-market surveillance and monitoring.

9.9.1 Safety Assessment and Preclinical Studies

Preclinical research and safety evaluations of veterinary viral vector vaccines are conducted in an effort to determine the vaccines' potential negative effects on the target animal species as well as any potential concerns to the public's health and the environment [162]. The following elements are included in the preclinical research and safety assessment:

- The viral vector's identity, purity, potency, stability, and transgenic expression are among its characteristics.
- Assessment of the viral vector's biodistribution, shedding, and persistence in the intended animal species, as well as any possible human or animal-to-animal transmission.
- Evaluation of the viral vector vaccine's immunogenicity, effectiveness, and defense against the intended pathogen, as well as any potential interactions with other immunizations or innate diseases.
- Evaluation of the viral vector vaccine's toxicity, local responses, and systemic adverse effects, as well as any potential reversion to virulence, recombination, or viral vector integration.
- Evaluation of the viral vector vaccine's safety for the intended animal population, taking into account factors including developmental and reproductive toxicity, safety for immunocompromised or pregnant animals, and safety for various age groups or breeds [163] (refer to Table 9.6).

Table 9.6 Key elements and procedures of the preclinical research and safety evaluation of veterinary viral vector vaccines.

Aspect	Method	References
Characterization of the viral vector	Molecular and biological assays, such as PCR, sequencing, ELISA, Western blot, etc.	[164]
Biodistribution, shedding, and persistence of the viral vector	Animal studies, such as tissue sampling, swabbing, blood collection, etc.	[165]
Immunogenicity, efficacy, and protection of the viral vector vaccine	Animal challenge studies, such as infection, vaccination, and serology, etc.	[99]
Toxicity, local reactions, and systemic adverse events of the viral vector vaccine	Animal safety studies, such as clinical observation, pathology, histology, etc.	[162]
Safety of the viral vector vaccine for the target animal population	Animal safety studies, such as reproduction and development, immunocompromised or pregnant animals, different age groups or breeds, etc.	[134]

9.9.2 Regulatory Approval Process for Veterinary Viral Vector Vaccines

Veterinary viral vector vaccines must go through different regulatory clearance processes in different countries or regions before they may be sold. Nonetheless, a few standard procedures and prerequisites may be found, such as the following:

- Submission of the marketing authorization application, which comprises the production and control data, the product label and package insert, the environmental risk assessment, and the quality, safety, and effectiveness data of the viral vector vaccine.
- The competent authority will review the application for marketing authorization, and this review may include the viral

Table 9.7 Essential actions and specifications of the regulatory approval procedure for veterinary viral vector vaccines.

Step	Requirement	References
Submission of the marketing authorization application	Quality, safety, and efficacy data of the viral vector vaccine, manufacturing and control information, product label and package insert, and environmental risk assessment	[166]
Evaluation of the marketing authorization application	Scientific assessment, inspection, risk-benefit analysis, and public consultation of the viral vector vaccine	[167]
Authorization or rejection of the marketing authorization application	Compliance with legal and scientific standards, availability of alternative products, and public interest of the viral vector vaccine	[168]
Post-authorization obligations	Pharmacovigilance, quality control, variation, and renewal of the marketing authorization of the viral vector vaccine	[169]

vector vaccine's scientific evaluation, inspection, risk-benefit analysis, and public consultation.

- The competent authority's decision to approve or reject the marketing authorization application may be based on the viral vector vaccine's potential benefit to the public, availability of substitute goods, and adherence to legal and scientific requirements.
- Post-authorization requirements, such as pharmacovigilance, quality assurance, variation, and viral vector vaccine marketing authorization renewal (refer to Table 9.7).

9.9.3 Post-Market Surveillance and Monitoring

After being approved and sold, the goal of post-market surveillance and monitoring programs for veterinary viral vector vaccines is to guarantee the vaccines' ongoing safety, effectiveness, and quality [170]. The following elements are part of the post-market monitoring and surveillance:

- Reporting and evaluation of any unfavorable medical events that occur after vaccination, regardless of whether the events are directly caused by the vaccine (AEFI). Immunization mistakes, coincidental incidents, vaccine quality faults, and responses connected to vaccination products are the four categories into which AEFI may be divided.
- Any information that emerges from one or more sources that point to a new element of an established link, or a new possibly causative relationship, between a vaccination and a negative occurrence is considered a vaccine safety signal and has to be evaluated and managed. Various sources, including unplanned reporting, active surveillance, clinical studies, and literature reviews, can identify vaccine safety signs.
- Evaluation and enhancement of the vaccine's efficacy, or its capacity to avert illness or lessen its severity in a real-world situation. Numerous techniques, including screening

Table 9.8 The key elements and procedures of the post-market surveillance and monitoring of veterinary viral vector vaccines.

Aspect	Method	References
Reporting and analysis of the adverse events following immunization (AEFI)	Spontaneous reporting systems, such as VigiVet or VAERS, etc.	[171]
Evaluation and management of the vaccine safety signals	Signal detection and assessment, such as disproportionality analysis, causality assessment, risk management, etc.	[172]
Assessment and improvement of the vaccine effectiveness	Vaccine effectiveness studies, such as cohort studies, case-control studies, screening methods, etc.	[173]
Assessment and maintenance of the vaccine quality	Quality assurance activities, such as quality control, stability testing, batch release, good manufacturing practices, etc.	[174]

techniques, case-control studies, and cohort studies, can be used to quantify the efficacy of vaccines.

- Evaluation and upkeep of vaccination quality, or the extent to which the shot satisfies requirements and guidelines for usage as intended. Numerous procedures, including batch release, stability testing, quality control, and excellent manufacturing standards, may guarantee the quality of vaccines (refer to Table 9.8).

9.10 Notable Examples of Viral Vector Vaccines in Veterinary Medicine and Their Impact on Animal Health and Agriculture

The veterinary industry's success stories with viral vector vaccines highlight their revolutionary potential. These vaccinations have proven to be effective, safe, and versatile, protecting everything from companion animals to supporting agricultural techniques. The effects on agricultural and animal health are not only anecdotal; rather, they provide evidence of the real advantages that come from adopting cutting-edge technologies in the creation of veterinary vaccines. We provide a detailed summary of these success stories in the following table, together with information on the target infections, the viral vectors used, and the significant effects on agriculture and animal health (refer to Table 9.9).

Table 9.9 Notable examples of viral vector vaccines in veterinary medicine and their impact on animal health and agriculture.

Vaccine	Target pathogen	Viral vector used	Impact on animal health	Impact on agriculture	References
Canine DISTEMPER VIRUS (CDV) vaccine	Canine distemper virus (CDV)	Recombinant adenovirus	Robust CDV protection, mitigating economic losses in canine populations.	Advancement in dog welfare, supporting economic sustainability.	[175]

(*Continued*)

Table 9.9 Notable examples of viral vector vaccines in veterinary medicine and their impact on animal health and agriculture. (*Continued*)

Vaccine	Target pathogen	Viral vector used	Impact on animal health	Impact on agriculture	References
Porcine circovirus type 2 (PCV2) Vaccine	Porcine circovirus type 2 (PCV2)	Modified live adenovirus	Efficacious in swine, improving production efficiency and pig health.	Enhances swine farming profitability and overall industry health.	[176]
Avian influenza Vaccine	Avian influenza virus	Recombinant fowlpox virus	Revolutionizes poultry farming, ensuring sustained egg and meat production.	Bolster biosecurity, safeguarding the poultry industry.	[177]
Bovine rhinotracheitis (IBR) vaccine	Infectious bovine rhinotracheitis (IBR)	Bovine Herpesvirus Vector	Enhances cattle productivity, reducing morbidity and increasing milk production.	Improves overall cattle farming sustainability and economic returns.	[178]
Fish viral infection vaccine	Various fish viral pathogens	DNA-based viral constructs	Tailored aquaculture solutions, ensuring stability and growth of the industry.	Secures the global supply of fish products, supporting sustainable fishing.	[179]

With a focus on the target diseases, the viral vectors employed, and the implications for animal health and agriculture, this succinct presentation offers essential information for each viral vector vaccine.

9.11 Challenges and Future Directions

There are many obstacles to overcome and exciting new avenues for improvement in the field of veterinary viral vector vaccine development (refer to Tables 9.10 to 9.12).

Table 9.10 Current challenges in viral vector vaccine development.

Challenge	Description	References
Immunogenicity variability	Inconsistencies in eliciting immune responses pose hurdles; addressing variability remains a primary challenge.	[180]
Vector neutralization	Preexisting immunity to viral vectors hampers vaccine effectiveness, necessitating strategies for circumvention.	[181]
Safety concerns	Ensuring vector safety is critical; unintended adverse effects and potential risks demand rigorous safety assessments.	[182]
Manufacturing complexity	Complex manufacturing processes hinder scalability; streamlining and optimizing production are ongoing challenges.	[183]
Regulatory hurdles	Stringent regulatory requirements necessitate robust documentation; navigating regulatory frameworks remains challenging.	[184]

Table 9.11 Research directions and innovations.

Direction/ innovation	Description	References
Novel vector platforms	Exploring and developing novel viral vector platforms enhance adaptability, allowing for improved vaccine efficacy.	[185]

(Continued)

Table 9.11 Research directions and innovations. (*Continued*)

Direction/innovation	Description	References
Enhanced vector delivery systems	Advancements in delivery systems, such as nanoparticle-based carriers, aim to improve vector stability and targeting.	[186]
Personalized vaccines	Tailoring vaccines to individual species or populations enhances efficacy, focusing on specific needs and susceptibilities.	[187]
Next-generation adjuvants	Developing innovative adjuvants promotes stronger and longer-lasting immune responses, improving overall vaccine performance.	[145]
Systems Biology Approaches	Utilizing systems biology provides comprehensive insights, facilitating a deeper understanding of immune responses to vaccines.	[188]

Table 9.12 Potential for cross-species vaccines.

Cross-species potential	Description	References
Zoonotic disease prevention	Developing cross-species vaccines holds promise for preventing zoonotic diseases, addressing threats at the human-animal interface.	[189]
One Health integration	Embracing a One Health approach acknowledges the interconnectedness of human, animal, and environmental health, guiding cross-species vaccine development.	[190]
Conservation efforts	Cross-species vaccines contribute to wildlife conservation, offering tools to safeguard endangered species against infectious diseases.	[191]
Agricultural biosecurity	Implementing cross-species vaccines in agriculture enhances biosecurity, minimizing the risk of pathogen transmission between species.	[192]

The persistent difficulties in the creation of viral vector vaccines highlight the necessity for continued innovation. Key areas of emphasis include addressing the variability in immunogenicity, overcoming vector neutralization, guaranteeing safety, streamlining the manufacturing process, and negotiating regulatory challenges. Future research directions seek to investigate innovative vector platforms, enhance delivery methods, customize vaccines, create next-generation adjuvants, and apply systems biology techniques.

The possibility of cross-species vaccinations presents new opportunities for preventing zoonotic diseases, incorporating One Health concepts, promoting animal conservation, and enhancing agricultural biosecurity. Embracing these issues and future possibilities is vital for promoting veterinary vaccine research and encouraging global health across species borders.

9.12 Conclusion

Veterinarian vaccine research is being revolutionized by viral vector vaccines, which have emerged as a flexible and promising platform. Their unique features include the ability to target many diseases at once, flexibility in expressing different antigens, and the ability to elicit strong and long-lasting immune responses. Notable examples highlight the versatility of viral vectors across veterinary applications, from measles virus vector vaccines for various animals to recombinant fowlpox and turkey herpesvirus vaccines for poultry.

Viral vector vaccines have an influence on more than just the health of individual animals; they also have an impact on variables such as decreased disease incidence, better animal welfare, increased production, and increased food security. Importantly, these vaccinations support agricultural sustainability and limit the spread of zoonotic diseases, therefore adhering to the ideals of One Health.

However, problems still exist, necessitating improvements in viral vector design, production efficiency, and handling issues like immunogenicity and preexisting immunity. Viral vectors' future function depends on ongoing innovation in design, production, and control. The development of viral vectors will be fueled by the integration of multidisciplinary techniques, such as synthetic biology, genome editing, artificial intelligence, and the One Health tenets. This will confirm viral vectors' pivotal position in the advancement of veterinary vaccines.

References

1. Meeusen, E.N.T., Walker, J., Peters, A., Pastoret, P.-P., Jungersen, G., Current Status of Veterinary Vaccines. *Clin. Microbiol. Rev.*, *20*, 489–510, 2007, doi: 10.1128/CMR.00005-07.
2. Aida, V., Pliasas, V.C., Neasham, P.J., North, J.F., McWhorter, K.L., Glover, S.R., *et al.*, Novel Vaccine Technologies in Veterinary Medicine: A Herald to Human Medicine Vaccines. *Front. Vet. Sci.*, 8, 654289, 2021 Apr 15.
3. Adams, L.G., Babiuk, L., McGavin, D., Nordgren, R., Special Issues Around Veterinary Vaccines, in: *Vaccines for Biodefense and Emerging and Neglected Diseases*, pp. 225–254, Epub, 2009 Jan 30, doi: 10.1016/B978-0-12-369408-9.00016-0. PMCID: PMC7150220.
4. Nascimento, I.P. and Leite, L.C.C., Recombinant Vaccines and the Development of New Vaccine Strategies. *Braz. J. Med. Biol. Res.*, *45*, 1102–1111, 2012, doi: 10.1590/S0100-879X2012007500142.
5. Vrba, S.M., Kirk, N.M., Brisse, M.E., Liang, Y., Ly, H., Development and Applications of Viral Vectored Vaccines to Combat Zoonotic and Emerging Public Health Threats. *Vaccines (Basel)*, *8*, 680, 2020, doi: 10.3390/vaccines8040680.
6. Sheppard, M., Viral Vectors for Veterinary Vaccines. *Adv. Vet. Med.*, *41*, 145–161, 1999, doi: 10.1016/S0065-3519(99)80014-7.
7. Chavda, V.P., Bezbaruah, R., Valu, D., Patel, B., Kumar, A., Prasad, S., Kakoti, B.B., Kaushik, A., Jesawadawala, M., Adenoviral Vector-Based Vaccine Platform for COVID-19: Current Status. *Vaccines*, *11*, 432, 2023, doi: 10.3390/vaccines11020432.
8. Elkashif, A., Alhashimi, M., Sayedahmed, E.E., Sambhara, S., Mittal, S.K., Adenoviral Vector-based Platforms for Developing Effective Vaccines to Combat Respiratory Viral Infections. *Clin. Transl. Immunol.*, *10*, e1345, 2021, doi: 10.1002/cti2.1345.
9. Nayak, S. and Herzog, R.W., Progress and Prospects: Immune Responses to Viral Vectors. *Gene Ther.*, *17*, 295–304, 2010, doi: 10.1038/GT.2009.148.
10. Zhang, L., Richards, A., Barrasa, M.I., Hughes, S.H., Young, R.A., Jaenisch, R., Reverse-Transcribed SARS-CoV-2 RNA Can Integrate into the Genome of Cultured Human Cells and Can Be Expressed in Patient-Derived Tissues. *Proc. Natl. Acad. Sci. U.S.A.*, *118*, e2105968118, 2021, doi: 10.1073/pnas.2105968118.
11. Tatsis, N. and Ertl, H.C.J., Adenoviruses as Vaccine Vectors. *Mol. Ther.*, *10*, 616–629, 2004, doi: 10.1016/j.ymthe.2004.07.013.
12. Naso, M.F., Tomkowicz, B., Perry, W.L., Strohl, W.R., Adeno-Associated Virus (AAV) as a Vector for Gene Therapy. *BioDrugs*, *31*, 317–334, 2017, doi: 10.1007/s40259-017-0234-5.
13. Munis, A.M., Gene Therapy Applications of Non-Human Lentiviral Vectors. *Viruses*, *12*, 1106, 2020, doi: 10.3390/v12101106.

14. Manservigi, R., Argnani, R., Marconi, P., HSV Recombinant Vectors for Gene Therapy. *Open Virol. J.*, *4*, 123–156, 2010, doi: 10.2174/1874357901004010123.
15. Poletti, V. and Mavilio, F., Interactions between Retroviruses and the Host Cell Genome. *Mol. Ther. Methods Clin. Dev.*, *8*, 31–41, 2017, doi: 10.1016/j.omtm.2017.10.001.
16. Yi, Y., Jong Noh, M., Hee Lee, K., Current Advances in Retroviral Gene Therapy. *Curr. Gene Ther.*, *11*, 218–228, 2011, doi: 10.2174/156652311795684740.
17. Lee, C.S., Bishop, E.S., Zhang, R., Yu, X., Farina, E.M., Yan, S., Zhao, C., Zeng, Z., Shu, Y., Wu, X., *et al.*, Adenovirus-Mediated Gene Delivery: Potential Applications for Gene and Cell-Based Therapies in the New Era of Personalized Medicine. *Genes Dis.*, *4*, 43–63, 2017, doi: 10.1016/j.gendis.2017.04.001.
18. Ahi, Y.S., Bangari, D.S., Mittal, S.K., Adenoviral Vector Immunity: Its Implications and Circumvention Strategies. *Curr. Gene Ther.*, *11*, 307–320, 2011.
19. Rapti, K. and Grimm, D., Adeno-Associated Viruses (AAV) and Host Immunity – A Race Between the Hare and the Hedgehog. *Front. Immunol.*, *12*, 753467, 2021, doi: 10.3389/fimmu.2021.753467.
20. Schlimgen, R., Howard, J., Wooley, D., Thompson, M., Baden, L.R., Yang, O.O., Christiani, D.C., Mostoslavsky, G., Diamond, D.V., Duane, E.G., *et al.*, Risks Associated With Lentiviral Vector Exposures and Prevention Strategies. *J. Occup. Environ. Med.*, *58*, 1159–1166, 2016, doi: 10.1097/JOM.0000000000000879.
21. Dong, W. and Kantor, B., Lentiviral Vectors for Delivery of Gene-Editing Systems Based on CRISPR/Cas: Current State and Perspectives. *Viruses*, *13*, 1288, 2021, doi: 10.3390/v13071288.
22. Grinde, B., Herpesviruses: Latency and Reactivation – Viral Strategies and Host Response. *J. Oral Microbiol.*, *5*, 2013. doi:10.3402/jom.v5i0.22766.
23. Wilson, A.C., Impact of Cultured Neuron Models on α-Herpesvirus Latency Research. *Viruses*, *14*, 1209, 2022, doi: 10.3390/v14061209.
24. Schaffer, D.V., Koerber, J.T., Lim, K., Molecular Engineering of Viral Gene Delivery Vehicles. *Annu. Rev. Biomed. Eng.*, *10*, 169–194, 2008, doi: 10.1146/annurev.bioeng.10.061807.160514.
25. Alberts, B., Johnson, A., Lewis, J., Raff, M., Roberts, K., Walter, P., Isolating, Cloning, and Sequencing DNA, in: *Molecular Biology of the Cell, 4th edition*, Garland Science, New York, 2002.
26. Khan, S., Ullah, M.W., Siddique, R., Nabi, G., Manan, S., Yousaf, M., Hou, H., Role of Recombinant DNA Technology to Improve Life. *Int. J. Genomics*, *2016*, 2405954, 2016, doi: 10.1155/2016/2405954.
27. Nair, R.R., Blankvoort, S., Lagartos, M.J., Kentros, C., Enhancer-Driven Gene Expression (EDGE) Enables the Generation of Viral Vectors Specific to Neuronal Subtypes. *iScience*, *23*, 100888, 2020, doi: 10.1016/j.isci.2020.100888.

28. Zheng, C. and Baum, B.J., Evaluation of Promoters for Use in Tissue-Specific Gene Delivery. *Methods Mol. Biol.*, *434*, 205–219, 2008, doi: 10.1007/978-1-60327-248-3_13.
29. Kimman, T.G., Smit, E., Klein, M.R., Evidence-Based Biosafety: A Review of the Principles and Effectiveness of Microbiological Containment Measures. *Clin. Microbiol. Rev.*, *21*, 403–425, 2008, doi: 10.1128/CMR.00014-08.
30. Philips, J.G., Martin-Avila, E., Robold, A.V., Horizontal Gene Transfer from Genetically Modified Plants - Regulatory Considerations. *Front. Bioeng. Biotechnol.*, *10*, 2022.
31. Ormandy, E.H., Dale, J., Griffin, G., Genetic Engineering of Animals: Ethical Issues, Including Welfare Concerns. *Can. Vet. J.*, *52*, 544–550, 2011.
32. Dish, T., Viral Vector Characterization: A Look at Analytical Tools Available online, https://cellculturedish.com/viral-vector-characterization-analytical-tools/ (accessed on 27 January 2024).
33. Xu, Y. and Li, Z., CRISPR-Cas Systems: Overview, Innovations and Applications in Human Disease Research and Gene Therapy. *Comput. Struct. Biotechnol. J.*, *18*, 2401–2415, 2020, doi: 10.1016/j.csbj.2020.08.031.
34. Rahamkulov, I. and Bakhsh, A., Tissue-Specific and Stress-Inducible Promoters Establish Their Suitability for Containment of Foreign Gene(s) Expression in Transgenic Potatoes. *3 Biotech*, *10*, 426, 2020, doi: 10.1007/s13205-020-02350-x.
35. Bayot, M.L. and Limaiem, F., Biosafety Guidelines, in: *StatPearls*, StatPearls Publishing, Treasure Island FL, 2024.
36. Wright, J.F., Quality Control Testing, Characterization and Critical Quality Attributes of Adeno-Associated Virus Vectors Used for Human Gene Therapy. *Biotechnol. J.*, *16*, 2000022, 2021, doi: 10.1002/biot.202000022.
37. Safety, Characterization, and Release Testing Support for Viral Vectors Used for Gene Therapies Available online, https://www.eurofins.com/biopharma-services/product-testing/services-by-modality/gene-therapy-testing-services/testing-of-viral-vector-gene-therapies/ (accessed on 27 January 2024).
38. Fries, C.N., Curvino, E.J., Chen, J.-L., Permar, S.R., Fouda, G.G., Collier, J.H., Advances in Nanomaterial Vaccine Strategies to Address Infectious Diseases Impacting Global Health. *Nat. Nanotechnol.*, *16*, 1–14, 2021, doi: 10.1038/s41565-020-0739-9.
39. Zhou, J., Kroll, A.V., Holay, M., Fang, R.H., Zhang, L., Biomimetic Nanotechnology toward Personalized Vaccines. *Adv. Mater.*, *32*, 1901255, 2020, doi: 10.1002/adma.201901255.
40. Contera, S., Bernardino De La Serna, J., Tetley, T.D., Biotechnology, Nanotechnology and Medicine. *Emerging Top. Life Sci.*, *4*, 551–554, 2020, doi: 10.1042/ETLS20200350.
41. Paiva, N.F. and Vicentini, F.T.M.D.C., Oral and Nasal Vaccination: Current Prospects, Challenges, and Impact of Nanotechnology-Based

Delivery Systems. *Braz. J. Pharm. Sci.*, *59*, e21769, 2023, doi: 10.1590/s2175-97902023e21769.

42. Rai, M., Bonde, S., Yadav, A., Plekhanova, Y., Reshetilov, A., Gupta, I., Golińska, P., Pandit, R., Ingle, A.P., Nanotechnology-Based Promising Strategies for the Management of COVID-19: Current Development and Constraints. *Expert Rev. Anti-infective Ther.*, *20*, 1299–1308, 2022, doi: 10.1080/14787210.2021.1836961.
43. Zhu, M., Wang, R., Nie, G., Applications of Nanomaterials as Vaccine Adjuvants. *Hum. Vaccin. Immunother.*, *10*, 2761–2774, 2014, doi: 10.4161/hv.29589.
44. Shetab Boushehri, M., Dietrich, D., Lamprecht, A., Nanotechnology as a Platform for the Development of Injectable Parenteral Formulations: A Comprehensive Review of the Know-Hows and State of the Art. *Pharmaceutics*, *12*, 510, 2020, doi: 10.3390/pharmaceutics12060510.
45. Thakur, A., *Nanoengineered Biomaterials for Advanced Drug Delivery*, Woodhead Publishing Series in Biomaterials; Elsevier, Amsterdam, 2020, ISBN 978-0-08-102985-5.
46. Jiao, H., Yang, H., Zhao, D., Chen, J., Zhang, Q., Liang, J., Yin, Y., Kong, G., Li, G., Design and Immune Characterization of a Novel Neisseria Gonorrhoeae DNA Vaccine Using Bacterial Ghosts as Vector and Adjuvant. *Vaccine*, *36*, 4532–4539, 2018, doi: 10.1016/j.vaccine.2018.06.006.
47. Coffey, J.W., Gaiha, G.D., Traverso, G., Oral Biologic Delivery: Advances Toward Oral Subunit, DNA, and mRNA Vaccines and the Potential for Mass Vaccination During Pandemics. *Annu. Rev. Pharmacol. Toxicol.*, *61*, 517–540, 2021, doi: 10.1146/annurev-pharmtox-030320-092348.
48. Peek, L.J., Middaugh, C.R., Berkland, C., Nanotechnology in Vaccine Delivery. *Adv. Drug Deliv. Rev.*, *60*, 915–928, 2008, doi: 10.1016/j.addr.2007.05.017.
49. Kiyono, H. and Pascual, D. (Eds.), *Mucosal Vaccines: Innovation for Preventing Infectious Diseases*, 2nd, Elsevier, Cambridge, 2019, ISBN 978-0-12-811924-2.
50. Liang, F., Lindgren, G., Lin, A., Thompson, E.A., Ols, S., Röhss, J., John, S., Hassett, K., Yuzhakov, O., Bahl, K., *et al.*, Efficient Targeting and Activation of Antigen-Presenting Cells *In Vivo* after Modified mRNA Vaccine Administration in Rhesus Macaques. *Mol. Ther.*, *25*, 2635–2647, 2017, doi: 10.1016/j.ymthe.2017.08.006.
51. Shahiwala, A., Vyas, T., Amiji, M., Nanocarriers for Systemic and Mucosal Vaccine Delivery. *DDF*, *1*, 1–9, 2007, doi: 10.2174/187221107779814140.
52. Pasquale, A., Preiss, S., Silva, F., Garçon, N., Vaccine Adjuvants: From 1920 to 2015 and Beyond. *Vaccines*, *3*, 320–343, 2015, doi: 10.3390/vaccines3020320.
53. Schultze, V., D'Agosto, V., Wack, A., Novicki, D., Zorn, J., Hennig, R., Safety of MF59™ Adjuvant. *Vaccine*, *26*, 3209–3222, 2008, doi: 10.1016/j.vaccine.2008.03.093.
54. Kumar, A. and Kumar, A., Mucosal and Transdermal Vaccine Delivery Strategies against COVID-19. *Drug Deliv. Transl. Res.*, *12*, 968–972, 2022, doi: 10.1007/s13346-021-01001-9.

55. Abd Elkodous, M., Olojede, S.O., Morsi, M., El-Sayyad, G.S., Nanomaterial-Based Drug Delivery Systems as Promising Carriers for Patients with COVID-19. *RSC Adv.*, *11*, 26463–26480, 2021, doi: 10.1039/d1ra04835j.
56. Theobald, N., Emerging Vaccine Delivery Systems for COVID-19. *Drug Discov. Today*, *25*, 1556–1558, 2020, doi: 10.1016/j.drudis.2020.06.020.
57. Cordeiro, A.S., Patil-Sen, Y., Shivkumar, M., Patel, R., Khedr, A., Elsawy, M.A., Nanovaccine Delivery Approaches and Advanced Delivery Systems for the Prevention of Viral Infections: From Development to Clinical Application. *Pharmaceutics*, *13*, 2091, 2021, doi: 10.3390/pharmaceutics13122091.
58. Zaric, M., Ibarzo Yus, B., Kalcheva, P.P., Klavinskis, L.S., Microneedle-Mediated Delivery of Viral Vectored Vaccines. *Expert Opin. Drug Deliv.*, *14*, 1177–1187, 2017, doi: 10.1080/17425247.2017.1230096.
59. Coquerelle, C. and Moser, M., DC Subsets in Positive and Negative Regulation of Immunity. *Immunol. Rev.*, *234*, 317–334, 2010, doi: 10.1111/j.0105-2896.2009.00887.x.
60. Sutter, G. and Staib, C., Vaccinia Vectors as Candidate Vaccines: The Development of Modified Vaccinia Virus Ankara for Antigen Delivery. *CDTID*, *3*, 263–271, 2003, doi: 10.2174/1568005033481123.
61. Garland, M.J., Migalska, K., Mahmood, T.M.T., Singh, T.R.R., Woolfson, A.D., Donnelly, R.F., Microneedle Arrays as Medical Devices for Enhanced Transdermal Drug Delivery. *Expert Rev. Med. Devices*, *8*, 459–482, 2011, doi: 10.1586/erd.11.20.
62. Kim, Y.-C., Park, J.-H., Prausnitz, M.R., Microneedles for Drug and Vaccine Delivery. *Adv. Drug Deliv. Rev.*, *64*, 1547–1568, 2012, doi: 10.1016/j.addr.2012.04.005.
63. Donnelly, R.F., Majithiya, R., Singh, T.R.R., Morrow, D.I.J., Garland, M.J., Demir, Y.K., Migalska, K., Ryan, E., Gillen, D., Scott, C.J., *et al.*, Design, Optimization and Characterisation of Polymeric Microneedle Arrays Prepared by a Novel Laser-Based Micromoulding Technique. *Pharm. Res.*, *28*, 41–57, 2011, doi: 10.1007/s11095-010-0169-8.
64. Chen, X., Fernando, G.J.P., Crichton, M.L., Flaim, C., Yukiko, S.R., Fairmaid, E.J., Corbett, H.J., Primiero, C.A., Ansaldo, A.B., Frazer, I.H., *et al.*, Improving the Reach of Vaccines to Low-Resource Regions, with a Needle-Free Vaccine Delivery Device and Long-Term Thermostabilization. *J. Control. Release*, *152*, 349–355, 2011, doi: 10.1016/j.jconrel.2011.02.026.
65. Henry, S., McAllister, D.V., Allen, M.G., Prausnitz, M.R., Microfabricated Microneedles: A Novel Approach to Transdermal Drug Delivery. *J. Pharm. Sci.*, *87*, 922–925, 1998, doi: 10.1021/js980042+.
66. Chavda, V.P., Bezbaruah, R., Athalye, M., Parikh, P.K., Chhipa, A.S., Patel, S., Apostolopoulos, V., Replicating Viral Vector-Based Vaccines for COVID-19: Potential Avenue in Vaccination Arena. *Viruses*, *14*, 759, 2022, doi: 10.3390/v14040759.
67. Al-Zahrani, S., Zaric, M., McCrudden, C., Scott, C., Kissenpfennig, A., Donnelly, R.F., Microneedle-Mediated Vaccine Delivery: Harnessing

Cutaneous Immunobiology to Improve Efficacy. *Expert Opin. Drug Deliv.*, *9*, 541–550, 2012, doi: 10.1517/17425247.2012.676038.
68. DeMuth, P.C., Min, Y., Huang, B., Kramer, J.A., Miller, A.D., Barouch, D.H., Hammond, P.T., Irvine, D.J., Polymer Multilayer Tattooing for Enhanced DNA Vaccination. *Nat. Mater.*, *12*, 367–376, 2013, doi: 10.1038/nmat3550.
69. Van Der Maaden, K., Sekerdag, E., Jiskoot, W., Bouwstra, J., Impact-Insertion Applicator Improves Reliability of Skin Penetration by Solid Microneedle Arrays. *AAPS J.*, *16*, 681–684, 2014, doi: 10.1208/s12248-014-9606-7.
70. Lakshmi, P., Bhaskaran, S., Saroja, C., Recent Trends in Vaccine Delivery Systems: A Review. *Int. J. Pharma. Investig.*, *1*, 64, 2011, doi: 10.4103/2230-973X.82384.
71. Rice, J., Ottensmeier, C.H., Stevenson, F.K., DNA Vaccines: Precision Tools for Activating Effective Immunity against Cancer. *Nat. Rev. Cancer*, *8*, 108–120, 2008, doi: 10.1038/nrc2326.
72. Kis, E.E., Winter, G., Myschik, J., Devices for Intradermal Vaccination. *Vaccine*, *30*, 523–538, 2012, doi: 10.1016/j.vaccine.2011.11.020.
73. Giudice, E.L. and Campbell, J.D., Needle-Free Vaccine Delivery. *Adv. Drug Deliv. Rev.*, *58*, 68–89, 2006, doi: 10.1016/j.addr.2005.12.003.
74. Zhang, L., Wang, W., Wang, S., Effect of Vaccine Administration Modality on Immunogenicity and Efficacy. *Expert Rev. Vaccines*, *14*, 1509–1523, 2015, doi: 10.1586/14760584.2015.1081067.
75. Williams, J., Fox-Leyva, L., Christensen, C., Fisher, D., Schlicting, E., Snowball, M., Negus, S., Mayers, J., Koller, R., Stout, R., Hepatitis A Vaccine Administration: Comparison between Jet-Injector and Needle Injection. *Vaccine*, *18*, 1939–1943, 2000, doi: 10.1016/s0264-410x(99)00446-6.
76. Fisch, A., Cadilhac, P., Vidor, E., Prazuck, T., Dublanchet, A., Lafaix, C., Immunogenicity and Safety of a New Inactivated Hepatitis A Vaccine: A Clinical Trial with Comparison of Administration Route. *Vaccine*, *14*, 1132–1136, 1996, doi: 10.1016/0264-410x(96)00044-8.
77. Jackson, L.A., Austin, G., Chen, R.T., Stout, R., DeStefano, F., Gorse, G.J., Newman, F.K., Yu, O., Weniger, B.G., Vaccine Safety Datalink Study Group Safety and Immunogenicity of Varying Dosages of Trivalent Inactivated Influenza Vaccine Administered by Needle-Free Jet Injectors. *Vaccine*, *19*, 4703–4709, 2001, doi: 10.1016/s0264-410x(01)00225-0.
78. Aguiar, J.C., Hedstrom, R.C., Rogers, W.O., Charoenvit, Y., Sacci, J.B., Lanar, D.E., Majam, V.F., Stout, R.R., Hoffman, S.L., Enhancement of the Immune Response in Rabbits to a Malaria DNA Vaccine by Immunization with a Needle-Free Jet Device. *Vaccine*, *20*, 275–280, 2001, doi: 10.1016/s0264-410x(01)00273-0.
79. Graham, B.S., Enama, M.E., Nason, M.C., Gordon, I.J., Peel, S.A., Ledgerwood, J.E., Plummer, S.A., Mascola, J.R., Bailer, R.T., Roederer, M., *et al.*, DNA Vaccine Delivered by a Needle-Free Injection Device Improves Potency of Priming for Antibody and CD8+ T-Cell Responses after rAd5 Boost in a

Randomized Clinical Trial. *PLoS One*, *8*, e59340, 2013, doi: 10.1371/journal.pone.0059340.

80. Wesley, R.D. and Lager, K.M., Evaluation of a Recombinant Human Adenovirus-5 Vaccine Administered via Needle-Free Device and Intramuscular Injection for Vaccination of Pigs against Swine Influenza Virus. *Am. J. Vet. Res.*, *66*, 1943–1947, 2005, doi: 10.2460/ajvr.2005.66.1943.
81. McAllister, L., Anderson, J., Werth, K., Cho, I., Copeland, K., Le Cam Bouveret, N., Plant, D., Mendelman, P.M., Cobb, D.K., Needle-Free Jet Injection for Administration of Influenza Vaccine: A Randomised Non-Inferiority Trial. *Lancet*, *384*, 674–681, 2014, doi: 10.1016/S0140-6736(14)60524-9.
82. Epstein, J.E., Gorak, E.J., Charoenvit, Y., Wang, R., Freydberg, N., Osinowo, O., Richie, T.L., Stoltz, E.L., Trespalacios, F., Nerges, J., *et al.*, Safety, Tolerability, and Lack of Antibody Responses after Administration of a PfCSP DNA Malaria Vaccine via Needle or Needle-Free Jet Injection, and Comparison of Intramuscular and Combination Intramuscular/Intradermal Routes. *Hum. Gene Ther.*, *13*, 1551–1560, 2002, doi: 10.1089/10430340260201644.
83. Ura, T., Okuda, K., Shimada, M., Developments in Viral Vector-Based Vaccines. *Vaccines*, *2*, 624–641, 2014, doi: 10.3390/vaccines2030624.
84. Wang, H.-B., Kondo, A., Yoshida, A., Yoshizaki, S., Abe, S., Bao, L.-L., Mizuki, N., Ichino, M., Klinman, D., Okuda, K., *et al.*, Partial Protection against SIV Challenge by Vaccination of Adenovirus and MVA Vectors in Rhesus Monkeys. *Gene Ther.*, *17*, 4–13, 2010, doi: 10.1038/gt.2009.122.
85. Shimada, M., Wang, H.-B., Kondo, A., Xu, X.-P., Yoshida, A., Shinoda, K., Ura, T., Mizuguchi, H., Klinman, D., Luo, J.-L., *et al.*, Effect of Therapeutic Immunization Using Ad5/35 and MVA Vectors on SIV Infection of Rhesus Monkeys Undergoing Antiretroviral Therapy. *Gene Ther.*, *16*, 218–228, 2009, doi: 10.1038/gt.2008.152.
86. Yashima, S., Yoshizaki, S., Shinoda, K., Yoshida, A., Kondo, A., Mizuguchi, H., Ryo, A., Okuda, K., Shimada, M., Co-Administration of Viral Vector-Based Vaccines Suppresses Antigen-Specific Effector CD8 T Cells. *Vaccine*, *28*, 3257–3264, 2010, doi: 10.1016/j.vaccine.2010.01.065.
87. Tameris, M.D., Hatherill, M., Landry, B.S., Scriba, T.J., Snowden, M.A., Lockhart, S., Shea, J.E., McClain, J.B., Hussey, G.D., Hanekom, W.A., *et al.*, Safety and Efficacy of MVA85A, a New Tuberculosis Vaccine, in Infants Previously Vaccinated with BCG: A Randomised, Placebo-Controlled Phase 2b Trial. *Lancet*, *381*, 1021–1028, 2013, doi: 10.1016/S0140-6736(13)60177-4.
88. Rauch, S., Jasny, E., Schmidt, K.E., Petsch, B., New Vaccine Technologies to Combat Outbreak Situations. *Front. Immunol.*, *9*, 1963, 2018, doi: 10.3389/fimmu.2018.01963.
89. Eroglu, B., Nuwarda, R.F., Ramzan, I., Kayser, V.A., Narrative Review of COVID-19 Vaccines. *Vaccines*, *10*, 62, 2021, doi: 10.3390/vaccines10010062.
90. Ozdarendeli, A., Sezer, Z., Pavel, S.T.I., Inal, A., Yetiskin, H., Kaplan, B., Uygut, M.A., Bayram, A., Mazicioglu, M., Unuvar, G.K., *et al.*, Safety and Immunogenicity of an Inactivated Whole Virion SARS-CoV-2 Vaccine,

TURKOVAC, in Healthy Adults: Interim Results from Randomised, Double-Blind, Placebo-Controlled Phase 1 and 2 Trials. *Vaccine*, *41*, 380–390, 2023, doi: 10.1016/j.vaccine.2022.10.093.

91. Zehrung, D., Jarrahian, C., Wales, A., Intradermal Delivery for Vaccine Dose Sparing: Overview of Current Issues. *Vaccine*, *31*, 3392–3395, 2013, doi: 10.1016/j.vaccine.2012.11.021.
92. Barraclough, K.A., Wiggins, K.J., Hawley, C.M., Van Eps, C.L., Mudge, D.W., Johnson, D.W., Whitby, M., Carpenter, S., Playford, E.G., Intradermal Versus Intramuscular Hepatitis B Vaccination in Hemodialysis Patients: A Prospective Open-Label Randomized Controlled Trial in Nonresponders to Primary Vaccination. *Am. J. Kidney Dis.*, *54*, 95–103, 2009, doi: 10.1053/j.ajkd.2009.03.010.
93. Dacoba, T.G., Olivera, A., Torres, D., Crecente-Campo, J., Alonso, M.J., Modulating the Immune System through Nanotechnology. *Semin. Immunol.*, *34*, 78–102, 2017, doi: 10.1016/j.smim.2017.09.007.
94. Boyaka, P.N., Inducing Mucosal IgA: A Challenge for Vaccine Adjuvants and Delivery Systems. *J. Immunol.*, *199*, 9–16, 2017, doi: 10.4049/jimmunol.1601775.
95. Neutra, M.R. and Kozlowski, P.A., Mucosal Vaccines: The Promise and the Challenge. *Nat. Rev. Immunol.*, *6*, 148–158, 2006, doi: 10.1038/nri1777.
96. Chavda, V.P., Vora, L.K., Pandya, A.K., Patravale, V.B., Intranasal Vaccines for SARS-CoV-2: From Challenges to Potential in COVID-19 Management. *Drug Discov. Today*, *26*, 2619–2636, 2021, doi: 10.1016/j.drudis.2021.07.021.
97. Marasini, N., Skwarczynski, M., Toth, I., Intranasal Delivery of Nanoparticle-Based Vaccines. *Ther. Deliv.*, *8*, 151–167, 2017, doi: 10.4155/tde-2016-0068.
98. Moreno-Fierros, L., García-Silva, I., Rosales-Mendoza, S., Development of SARS-CoV-2 Vaccines: Should We Focus on Mucosal Immunity? *Expert Opin. Biol. Ther.*, *20*, 831–836, 2020, doi: 10.1080/14712598.2020.1767062.
99. Deng, S., Liang, H., Chen, P., Li, Y., Li, Z., Fan, S., Wu, K., Li, X., Chen, W., Qin, Y., *et al.*, Viral Vector Vaccine Development and Application during the COVID-19 Pandemic. *Microorganisms*, *10*, 1450, 2022, doi: 10.3390/microorganisms10071450.
100. Vela Ramirez, J.E., Sharpe, L.A., Peppas, N.A., Current State and Challenges in Developing Oral Vaccines. *Adv. Drug Deliv. Rev.*, *114*, 116–131, 2017, doi: 10.1016/j.addr.2017.04.008.
101. Okayasu, H., Sutter, R.W., Czerkinsky, C., Ogra, P.L., Mucosal Immunity and Poliovirus Vaccines: Impact on Wild Poliovirus Infection and Transmission. *Vaccine*, *29*, 8205–8214, 2011, doi: 10.1016/j.vaccine.2011.08.059.
102. Yan, Y., Pang, Y., Lyu, Z., Wang, R., Wu, X., You, C., Zhao, H., Manickam, S., Lester, E., Wu, T., *et al.*, The COVID-19 Vaccines: Recent Development, Challenges and Prospects. *Vaccines*, *9*, 349, 2021, doi: 10.3390/vaccines9040349.
103. Kalam, M.A., Khan, A.A., Alshamsan, A., Non-Invasive Administration of Biodegradable Nano-Carrier Vaccines. *Am. J. Transl. Res.*, *9*, 15–35, 2017.

104. Corthésy, B. and Bioley, G., Lipid-Based Particles: Versatile Delivery Systems for Mucosal Vaccination against Infection. *Front. Immunol.*, *9*, 431, 2018, doi: 10.3389/fimmu.2018.00431.
105. Roukens, A.H.E., Gelinck, L.B.S., Visser, L.G., Intradermal Vaccination to Protect Against Yellow Fever and Influenza, in: *Intradermal Immunization*, vol. 351, M.B.M. Teunissen, (Ed.), pp. 159–179, Current Topics in Microbiology and Immunology; Springer Berlin Heidelberg, Berlin, Heidelberg, 2011, ISBN 978-3-642-23689-1.
106. Lindgren, G., Ols, S., Liang, F., Thompson, E.A., Lin, A., Hellgren, F., Bahl, K., John, S., Yuzhakov, O., Hassett, K.J., *et al.*, Induction of Robust B Cell Responses after Influenza mRNA Vaccination Is Accompanied by Circulating Hemagglutinin-Specific ICOS+ PD-1+ CXCR3+ T Follicular Helper Cells. *Front. Immunol.*, *8*, 1539, 2017, doi: 10.3389/fimmu.2017.01539.
107. Ols, S., Yang, L., Thompson, E.A., Pushparaj, P., Tran, K., Liang, F., Lin, A., Eriksson, B., Karlsson Hedestam, G.B., Wyatt, R.T., *et al.*, Route of Vaccine Administration Alters Antigen Trafficking but Not Innate or Adaptive Immunity. *Cell Rep.*, *30*, 3964–3971.e7, 2020, doi: 10.1016/j.celrep.2020.02.111.
108. Yadav, N., Vishwakarma, P., Khatri, R., Siddqui, G., Awasthi, A., Ahmed, S., Samal, S., Comparative Immunogenicity Analysis of Intradermal versus Intramuscular Administration of SARS-CoV-2 RBD Epitope Peptide-Based Immunogen *In Vivo*. *Microbes Infect.*, *23*, 104843, 2021, doi: 10.1016/j.micinf.2021.104843.
109. Demagistris, M., Mucosal Delivery of Vaccine Antigens and Its Advantages in Pediatrics☆. *Adv. Drug Deliv. Rev.*, *58*, 52–67, 2006, doi: 10.1016/j.addr.2006.01.002.
110. Van der Weken, H., Cox, E., Devriendt, B., Advances in Oral Subunit Vaccine Design. *Vaccines (Basel)*, *9*, 1, 2020, doi: 10.3390/vaccines9010001.
111. Skwarczynski, M. and Toth, I., Non-Invasive Mucosal Vaccine Delivery: Advantages, Challenges and the Future. *Expert Opin. Drug Deliv.*, *17*, 435–437, 2020, doi: 10.1080/17425247.2020.1731468.
112. Srivastava, A., Gowda, D.V., Madhunapantula, S.V., Shinde, C.G., Iyer, M., Mucosal Vaccines: A Paradigm Shift in the Development of Mucosal Adjuvants and Delivery Vehicles. *APMIS*, *123*, 275–288, 2015, doi: 10.1111/apm.12351.
113. Woodrow, K.A., Bennett, K.M., Lo, D.D., Mucosal Vaccine Design and Delivery. *Annu. Rev. Biomed. Eng.*, *14*, 17–46, 2012, doi: 10.1146/annurev-bioeng-071811-150054.
114. Parker, E.P., Ramani, S., Lopman, B.A., Church, J.A., Iturriza-Gómara, M., Prendergast, A.J., Grassly, N.C., Causes of Impaired Oral Vaccine Efficacy in Developing Countries. *Future Microbiol.*, *13*, 97–118, 2018, doi: 10.2217/fmb-2017-0128.

115. Kang, S.H., Hong, S.J., Lee, Y.-K., Cho, S., , Oral Vaccine Delivery for Intestinal Immunity-Biological Basis, Barriers, Delivery System, and. *Polym. (Basel), 10*, 948, 2018, doi: 10.3390/polym10090948.
116. Kang, M.L., Cho, C.S., Yoo, H.S., Application of Chitosan Microspheres for Nasal Delivery of Vaccines. *Biotechnol. Adv., 27*, 857–865, 2009, doi: 10.1016/j.biotechadv.2009.06.007.
117. Pan, L., Zhang, Z., Lv, J., Zhou, P., Hu, W., Fang, Y., Chen, H., Liu, X., Shao, J., Zhao, F., *et al.*, Induction of Mucosal Immune Responses and Protection of Cattle against Direct-Contact Challenge by Intranasal Delivery with Foot-and-Mouth Disease Virus Antigen Mediated by Nanoparticles. *Int. J. Nanomed., 9*, 5603–5618, 2014, doi: 10.2147/IJN.S72318.
118. Köping-Höggård, M., Sánchez, A., Alonso, M.J., Nanoparticles as Carriers for Nasal Vaccine Delivery. *Expert Rev. Vaccines, 4*, 185–196, 2005, doi: 10.1586/14760584.4.2.185.
119. Riese, P., Sakthivel, P., Trittel, S., Guzmán, C.A., Intranasal Formulations: Promising Strategy to Deliver Vaccines. *Expert Opin. Drug Deliv., 11*, 1619–1634, 2014, doi: 10.1517/17425247.2014.931936.
120. Travieso, T., Li, J., Mahesh, S., Mello, J.D.F.R.E., Blasi, M., The Use of Viral Vectors in Vaccine Development. *npj Vaccines, 7*, 1–10, 2022, doi: 10.1038/s41541-022-00503-y.
121. Sánchez-Sampedro, L., Perdiguero, B., Mejías-Pérez, E., García-Arriaza, J., Di Pilato, M., Esteban, M., The Evolution of Poxvirus Vaccines. *Viruses, 7*, 1726–1803, 2015, doi: 10.3390/v7041726.
122. Brun, A., Vaccines and Vaccination for Veterinary Viral Diseases: A General Overview. *Vaccine Technol. Vet. Viral Dis., 1349*, 1–24, 2015, doi: 10.1007/978-1-4939-3008-1_1.
123. Hosie, M.J., Klein, D., Binley, JM., Dunsford, T.H., Jarrett, O., Neil, J.C., Knapp, E., Giannecchini, S., Matteucci, D., Bendinelli, M., *et al.*, Vaccination with an Inactivated Virulent Feline Immunodeficiency Virus Engineered To Express High Levels of Env. *J. Virol., 79*, 1954–1957, 2005, doi: 10.1128/JVI.79.3.1954-1957.2005.
124. Bolhassani, A. and Yazdi, S.R., DNA Immunization as an Efficient Strategy for Vaccination. *Avicenna J. Med. Biotechnol., 1*, 71–88, 2009.
125. Powell, K., DNA Vaccines—Back in the Saddle Again? *Nat. Biotechnol., 22*, 799–801, 2004, doi: 10.1038/nbt0704-799.
126. Meseda, C.A., Schmeisser, F., Pedersen, R., Woerner, A., Weir, J.P., DNA Immunization with a Herpes Simplex Virus 2 Bacterial Artificial Chromosome. *Virology, 318*, 420–428, 2004, doi: 10.1016/j.virol.2003.09.033.
127. Pollard, A.J. and Bijker, E.M.A., Guide to Vaccinology: From Basic Principles to New Developments. *Nat. Rev. Immunol., 21*, 83–100, 2021, doi: 10.1038/s41577-020-00479-7.
128. Nemirov, K., Bourgine, M., Anna, F., Wei, Y., Charneau, P., Majlessi, L., Lentiviral Vectors as a Vaccine Platform against Infectious Diseases. *Pharmaceutics, 15*, 846, 2023, doi: 10.3390/pharmaceutics15030846.

129. Liu, Z.-H., Deng, Z.-F., Lu, Y., Fang, W.-H., He, F.A., Modular and Self-Adjuvanted Multivalent Vaccine Platform Based on Porcine Circovirus Virus-like Nanoparticles. *J. Nanobiotechnol.*, *20*, 493, 2022, doi: 10.1186/s12951-022-01710-4.
130. Vemula, S.V. and Mittal, S.K., Production of Adenovirus Vectors and Their Use as a Delivery System for Influenza Vaccines. *Expert Opin. Biol. Ther.*, *10*, 1469–1487, 2010, doi: 10.1517/14712598.2010.519332.
131. García-Arriaza, J. and Esteban, M., Enhancing Poxvirus Vectors Vaccine Immunogenicity. *Hum. Vaccin. Immunother.*, *10*, 2235–2244, 2014, doi: 10.4161/hv.28974.
132. Schmidt, U., Beyer, J., Polster, U., Gershwin, L.J., Buchholz, U.J., Mucosal Immunization with Live Recombinant Bovine Respiratory Syncytial Virus (BRSV) and Recombinant BRSV Lacking the Envelope Glycoprotein G Protects against Challenge with Wild-Type BRSV. *J. Virol.*, *76*, 12355–12359, 2002, doi: 10.1128/JVI.76.23.12355-12359.2002.
133. Allam, A.M., Elbayoumy, M.K., Ghazy, A.A., Perspective Vaccines for Emerging Viral Diseases in Farm Animals. *Clin. Exp. Vaccine Res.*, *12*, 179–192, 2023, doi: 10.7774/cevr.2023.12.3.179.
134. Wang, S., Liang, B., Wang, W., Li, L., Feng, N., Zhao, Y., Wang, T., Yan, F., Yang, S., Xia, X., Viral Vectored Vaccines: Design, Development, Preventive and Therapeutic Applications in Human Diseases. *Sig. Transduct. Target Ther.*, *8*, 1–38, 2023, doi: 10.1038/s41392-023-01408-5.
135. Wahren, B. and Liu, M.A., DNA Vaccines: Recent Developments and the Future. *Vaccines (Basel)*, *2*, 785–796, 2014, doi: 10.3390/vaccines2040785.
136. Donofrio, G., Franceschi, V., Capocefalo, A., Taddei, S., Sartori, C., Bonomini, S., Cavirani, S., Cabassi, C.S., Flammini, C.F., Cellular Targeting of Engineered Heterologous Antigens Is a Determinant Factor for Bovine Herpesvirus 4-Based Vaccine Vector Development. *Clin. Vaccine Immunol.*, *16*, 1675–1686, 2009, doi: 10.1128/CVI.00224-09.
137. Zhang, H., Luo, Q., He, Y., Zheng, Y., Sha, H., Li, G., Kong, W., Liao, J., Zhao, M., Research Progress on the Development of Porcine Reproductive and Respiratory Syndrome Vaccines. *Vet. Sci.*, *10*, 491, 2023, doi: 10.3390/vetsci10080491.
138. Chen, J., Wang, J., Zhang, J., Ly, H., Advances in Development and Application of Influenza Vaccines. *Front. Immunol.*, *12*, 711997, 2021, doi: 10.3389/fimmu.2021.711997.
139. Mogensen, T.H., Pathogen Recognition and Inflammatory Signaling in Innate Immune Defenses. *Clin. Microbiol. Rev.*, *22*, 240–273, 2009, doi: 10.1128/CMR.00046-08.
140. Alberts, B., Johnson, A., Lewis, J., Raff, M., Roberts, K., Walter, P., The Adaptive Immune System, in: *Molecular Biology of the Cell, 4th edition*, Garland Science, New York, 2002.

141. Pantaleo, G., Correia, B., Fenwick, C., Joo, V.S., Perez, L., Antibodies to Combat Viral Infections: Development Strategies and Progress. *Nat. Rev. Drug Discov.*, *21*, 676–696, 2022, doi: 10.1038/s41573-022-00495-3.
142. Chaplin, D.D., Overview of the Immune Response. *J. Allergy Clin. Immunol.*, *125*, S3–23, 2010, doi: 10.1016/j.jaci.2009.12.980.
143. Coffman, R.L., Sher, A., Seder, R.A., Vaccine Adjuvants: Putting Innate Immunity to Work. *Immunity*, *33*, 492, 2010, doi: 10.1016/J.IMMUNI.2010.10.002.
144. Apostólico, J.S., Lunardelli, V.A.S., Coirada, F.C., Boscardin, S.B., Rosa, D.S., Adjuvants: Classification, Modus Operandi, and Licensing. *J. Immunol. Res.*, *2016*, 1459394, 2016, doi: 10.1155/2016/1459394.
145. Zhao, T., Cai, Y., Jiang, Y., He, X., Wei, Y., Yu, Y., Tian, X., Vaccine Adjuvants: Mechanisms and Platforms. *Signal Transduct. Target Ther.*, *8*, 283, 2023, doi: 10.1038/s41392-023-01557-7.
146. Choudhury, S.M., Ma, X., Dang, W., Li, Y., Zheng, H., Recent Development of Ruminant Vaccine Against Viral Diseases. *Front. Vet. Sci.*, *8*, 2021.
147. Davis, B.S., Chang, G.J., Cropp, B., Roehrig, J.T., Martin, D.A., Mitchell, C.J., Bowen, R., Bunning, M.L., West Nile Virus Recombinant DNA Vaccine Protects Mouse and Horse from Virus Challenge and Expresses *in Vitro* a Noninfectious Recombinant Antigen That Can Be Used in Enzyme-Linked Immunosorbent Assays. *J. Virol.*, *75*, 4040–4047, 2001, doi: 10.1128/JVI.75.9.4040-4047.2001.
148. Liu, Z.-H., Lei, K.-X., Han, G.-W., Xu, H.-L., He, F., Novel Lentivirus-Based Method for Rapid Selection of Inhibitory Nanobody against PRRSV. *Viruses*, *12*, 229, 2020, doi: 10.3390/v12020229.
149. Valarcher, J.F., Hägglund, S., Näslund, K., Jouneau, L., Malmström, E., Boulesteix, O., Pinard, A., Leguéré, D., Deslis, A., Gauthier, D., *et al.*, Single-Shot Vaccines against Bovine Respiratory Syncytial Virus (BRSV): Comparative Evaluation of Long-Term Protection after Immunization in the Presence of BRSV-Specific Maternal Antibodies. *Vaccines (Basel)*, *9*, 236, 2021, doi: 10.3390/vaccines9030236.
150. Janeway, C.A., Jr., Travers, P., Walport, M., Shlomchik, M., Immunobiology, in: *The Immune System in Health and Disease, 5th edition*, pp. 15–19, Garland Publishing, New York, 2001.
151. Auladell, M., Jia, X., Hensen, L., Chua, B., Fox, A., Nguyen, T.H.O., Doherty, P.C., Kedzierska, K., Recalling the Future: Immunological Memory Toward Unpredictable Influenza Viruses. *Front. Immunol.*, *10*, 2019.
152. Sasso, E., D'Alise, A.M., Zambrano, N., Scarselli, E., Folgori, A., Nicosia, A., New Viral Vectors for Infectious Diseases and Cancer. *Semin. Immunol.*, *50*, 101430, 2020, doi: 10.1016/j.smim.2020.101430.
153. Kumar, S., Saxena, S.K., Maurya, V.K., Tripathi, A.K., Progress and Challenges Toward Generation and Maintenance of Long-Lived Memory T Lymphocyte Responses During COVID-19. *Front. Immunol.*, *12*, 804808, 2022, doi: 10.3389/fimmu.2021.804808.

154. Moderna COVID-19 Vaccine Generates Long-Lasting Immune Memory, Available online: https://www.nih.gov/news-events/nih-research-matters/moderna-covid-19-vaccine-generates-long-lasting-immune-memory (accessed on 27 January 2024).
155. Ahluwalia, P., Vaibhav, K., Ahluwalia, M., Mondal, A.K., Sahajpal, N., Rojiani, A.M., Kolhe, R., Infection and Immune Memory: Variables in Robust Protection by Vaccines Against SARS-CoV-2. *Front. Immunol.*, 12, 660019, 2021 May 11, doi: 10.3389/fimmu.2021.660019. PMID: 34046033, PMCID: PMC8144450.
156. Vanniasinkam, T., Tikoo, S.K., Samal, S.K. (Eds.), *Viral Vectors in Veterinary Vaccine Development: A Textbook*, Springer International Publishing, Cham, 2021, ISBN 978-3-030-51926-1.
157. Viral-Vectored Vaccines | Frontiers Research Topic, Available online: https://www.frontiersin.org/research-topics/49576/viral-vectored-vaccines (accessed on 27 January 2024).
158. Viral Vector Vaccines for Animal Diseases Are Common | Eureka Blog, Available online: https://www.criver.com/eureka/viral-vector-vaccines-animal-diseases-are-common (accessed on 27 January 2024).
159. Antia, A., Ahmed, H., Handel, A., Carlson, N.E., Amanna, I.J., Antia, R., Slifka, M., Heterogeneity and Longevity of Antibody Memory to Viruses and Vaccines. *PLoS Biol.*, *16*, e2006601, 2018, doi: 10.1371/journal.pbio.2006601.
160. Chiappelli, F., Bakhordarian, A., Thames, A.D., Du, A.M., Jan, A.L., Nahcivan, M., Nguyen, M.T., Sama, N., Manfrini, E., Piva, F., *et al.*, Ebola: Translational Science Considerations. *J. Transl. Med.*, *13*, 11, 2015, doi: 10.1186/s12967-014-0362-3.
161. Russier, M., Pannetier, D., Baize, S., Immune Responses and Lassa Virus Infection. *Viruses*, *4*, 2766–2785, 2012, doi: 10.3390/v4112766.
162. Green, M.D., Al-Humadi, N.H., Preclinical Toxicology of Vaccines, in: *A comprehensive guide to Toxicology in Nonclinical Drug Development, 2nd ed.*, pp. 709–735, Epub, 2017, doi: 10.1016/B978-0-12-803620-4.00027-X. 2016 Nov 11. PMCID: PMC7161388.
163. Park, S.-J., Jang, M.S., Lim, K.-H., Seo, J.-W., Im, W.-J., Han, K.-H., Kim, S.-E., Jang, E., Park, D., Kim, Y.-B., Preclinical Evaluation of General Toxicity and Safety Pharmacology of a Receptor-Binding Domain-Based COVID-19 Subunit Vaccine in Various Animal Models. *Arch. Toxicol.*, *97*, 2429–2440, 2023, doi: 10.1007/s00204-023-03549-6.
164. Mello-Román, J., medicine, J.M.-R.-… methods in; 2019, undefined Predictive Models for the Medical Diagnosis of Dengue: A Case Study in Paraguay, hindawi.com.
165. Silva Lima, B. and Videira, M.A., Toxicology and Biodistribution: The Clinical Value of Animal Biodistribution Studies. *Mol. Ther. Methods Clin. Dev.*, *8*, 183–197, 2018, doi: 10.1016/j.omtm.2018.01.003.

166. Pre-Authorisation Guidance | European Medicines Agency, Available online: https://www.ema.europa.eu/en/human-regulatory-overview/marketing-authorisation/pre-authorisation-guidance (accessed on 27 January 2024).
167. Beretta, G. and Marelli, L., Fast-Tracking Development and Regulatory Approval of COVID-19 Vaccines in the EU: A Review of Ethical Implications. *Bioethics*, *37*, 498–507, 2023, doi: 10.1111/bioe.13151.
168. Goldberg, R., Vaccine Liability in the Light of Covid-19: A Defence of Risk–Benefit. *Med. Law Rev.*, *30*, 243–267, 2022, doi: 10.1093/medlaw/fwab053.
169. COVID-19 Guidance: Post-Authorisation | European Medicines Agency, Available online: https://www.ema.europa.eu/en/human-regulatory-overview/public-health-threats/coronavirus-disease-covid-19/covid-19-public-health-emergency-international-concern-2020-23/guidance-medicine-developers-and-other-stakeholders-covid-19/covid-19-guidance-post-authorisation (accessed on 27 January 2024).
170. Di Pasquale, A., Bonanni, P., Garçon, N., Stanberry, L.R., El-Hodhod, M., Tavares Da Silva, F., Vaccine Safety Evaluation: Practical Aspects in Assessing Benefits and Risks. *Vaccine*, *34*, 6672–6680, 2016, doi: 10.1016/j.vaccine.2016.10.039.
171. Parrella, A., Gold, M., Braunack-Mayer, A., Baghurst, P., Marshall, H., Consumer Reporting of Adverse Events Following Immunization (AEFI). *Hum. Vaccin. Immunother.*, *10*, 747–754, 2014, doi: 10.4161/hv.27459.
172. Investigation of Safety Signals, Available online: https://www.who.int/initiatives/the-global-vaccine-safety-initiative/investigation-of-safety-signals (accessed on 27 January 2024).
173. Verani, J.R., Baqui, A.H., Broome, C.V., Cherian, T., Cohen, C., Farrar, J.L., Feikin, D.R., Groome, M.J., Hajjeh, R.A., Johnson, H.L., *et al.*, Case-Control Vaccine Effectiveness Studies: Preparation, Design, and Enrollment of Cases and Controls. *Vaccine*, *35*, 3295–3302, 2017, doi: 10.1016/j.vaccine.2017.04.037.
174. Manufacturing, Safety and Quality Control of Vaccines, Available online: https://www.who.int/news-room/feature-stories/detail/manufacturing-safety-and-quality-control (accessed on 27 January 2024).
175. Martella, V., Elia, G., Buonavoglia, C., Canine Distemper Virus. *Vet. Clin. North Am. Small Anim. Pract.*, *38*, 787–797, vii–viii, 2008, doi: 10.1016/j.cvsm.2008.02.007.
176. Fort, M., Sibila, M., Allepuz, A., Mateu, E., Roerink, F., Segalés, J., Porcine Circovirus Type 2 (PCV2) Vaccination of Conventional Pigs Prevents Viremia against PCV2 Isolates of Different Genotypes and Geographic Origins. *Vaccine*, *26*, 1063–1071, 2008, doi: 10.1016/j.vaccine.2007.12.019.
177. Boyle, D.B., Selleck, P., Heine, H.G., Vaccinating Chickens against Avian Influenza with Fowlpox Recombinants Expressing the H7 Haemagglutinin. *Aust. Vet. J.*, *78*, 44–48, 2000, doi: 10.1111/j.1751-0813.2000.tb10359.x.
178. More, S., Bøtner, A., Butterworth, A., Calistri, P., Depner, K., Edwards, S., Garin-Bastuji, B., Good, M., Gortázar Schmidt, C., Michel, V., *et al.*,

Assessment of Listing and Categorisation of Animal Diseases within the Framework of the Animal Health Law (Regulation (EU) No 2016/429): Infectious Bovine Rhinotracheitis (IBR). *EFSA J.*, *15*, e04947, 2017, doi: 10.2903/j.efsa.2017.4947.

179. Kembou-Ringert, J.E., Steinhagen, D., Readman, J., Daly, J.M., Adamek, M., Tilapia Lake Virus Vaccine Development: A Review on the Recent Advances. *Vaccines (Basel)*, *11*, 251, 2023, doi: 10.3390/vaccines11020251.
180. Sauna, Z.E., Jawa, V., Balu-Iyer, S., Chirmule, N., Understanding Preclinical and Clinical Immunogenicity Risks in Novel Biotherapeutics Development. *Front. Immunol.*, *14*, 1151888, 2023, doi: 10.3389/fimmu.2023.1151888.
181. Wang, W.-C., Sayedahmed, E.E., Mittal, S.K., Significance of Preexisting Vector Immunity and Activation of Innate Responses for Adenoviral Vector-Based Therapy. *Viruses*, *14*, 2727, 2022, doi: 10.3390/v14122727.
182. Giraldo, P.A., Shinozuka, H., Spangenberg, G.C., Cogan, N.O.I., Smith, K.F., Safety Assessment of Genetically Modified Feed: Is There Any Difference From Food? *Front. Plant Sci.*, *10*, 1592, 2019, doi: 10.3389/fpls.2019.01592.
183. Plotkin, S., Robinson, J.M., Cunningham, G., Iqbal, R., Larsen, S., The Complexity and Cost of Vaccine Manufacturing – An Overview. *Vaccine*, *35*, 4064–4071, 2017, doi: 10.1016/j.vaccine.2017.06.003.
184. Mitchell, V.S., Philipose, N.M., Sanford, J.P., (Eds.), Institute of Medicine (US) Committee on the Children's Vaccine Initiative: Planning Alternative Strategies. The Children's Vaccine Initiative: Achieving the Vision, National Academies Press (US), Washington (DC), 1993. PMID: 25144104.
185. Gebre, M.S., Brito, L.A., Tostanoski, L.H., Edwards, D.K., Carfi, A., Barouch, D.H., Novel Approaches for Vaccine Development. *Cell*, *184*, 1589–1603, 2021, doi: 10.1016/j.cell.2021.02.030.
186. Mitchell, M.J., Billingsley, M.M., Haley, R.M., Wechsler, M.E., Peppas, N.A., Langer, R., Engineering Precision Nanoparticles for Drug Delivery. *Nat. Rev. Drug Discov.*, *20*, 101–124, 2021, doi: 10.1038/s41573-020-0090-8.
187. Poland, G.A., Ovsyannikova, I.G., Jacobson, R.M., Personalized Vaccines: The Emerging Field of Vaccinomics. *Expert Opin. Biol. Ther.*, *8*, 1659–1667, 2008, doi: 10.1517/14712598.8.11.1659.
188. Pezeshki, A., Ovsyannikova, I., McKinney, B., Poland, G., Kennedy, R., The Role of Systems Biology Approaches in Determining Molecular Signatures for the Development of More Effective Vaccines. *Expert Rev. Vaccines*, *18*, 253–267, 2019, doi: 10.1080/14760584.2019.1575208.
189. Carpenter, A., Waltenburg, M.A., Hall, A., Kile, J., Killerby, M., Knust, B., Negron, M., Nichols, M., Wallace, R.M., Behravesh, C.B., *et al.*, Vaccine Preventable Zoonotic Diseases: Challenges and Opportunities for Public Health Progress. *Vaccines (Basel)*, *10*, 993, 2022, doi: 10.3390/vaccines10070993.
190. Mackenzie, J.S. and Jeggo, M., The One Health Approach—Why Is It So Important? *Trop. Med. Infect. Dis.*, *4*, 88, 2019, doi: 10.3390/tropicalmed4020088.

191. Barnett, K.M. and Civitello, D.J., Ecological and Evolutionary Challenges for Wildlife Vaccination. *Trends Parasitol.*, *36*, 970–978, 2020, doi: 10.1016/j.pt.2020.08.006.
192. Vora, N.M., Hannah, L., Walzer, C., Vale, M.M., Lieberman, S., Emerson, A., Jennings, J., Alders, R., Bonds, M.H., Evans, J., *et al.*, Interventions to Reduce Risk for Pathogen Spillover and Early Disease Spread to Prevent Outbreaks, Epidemics, and Pandemics. *Emerg. Infect. Dis.*, *29*, e221079, 2023, doi: 10.3201/eid2903.221079.

10

Advantages and Challenges of Viral Vector Vaccines

Shilpa Dawre[1]*, Mahendra Prajapati[1] and Ganesh Shevalkar[2]

[1]*School of Pharmacy & Technology Management, SVKMs, NMIMS, Babulde Banks of Tapi River, Shirpur, Maharashtra, India*
[2]*Department of Pharmaceutics, Sandip Institute of Pharmaceutical Sciences, Nashik, Maharashtra, India*

Abstract
Infectious diseases and malignancies cause challenges to public health and impact socioeconomic growth as well. Among all vaccine modalities, viral vector vaccine offers several advantages over conventional vaccines. Viral vector vaccines can modulate both cellular and humoral immunity against human infections. In addition, they can be easily targeted to particular cell receptors to enhance the immunization response. However, viral vector vaccines pose many challenges such as high cost, scale-up challenges, immunomodulation, safety profile, and lack of regulatory guidelines. This book chapter discusses the viruses utilized for the development of vaccine vectors and their mechanism of action. Furthermore, this chapter overviewed the advantages and challenges of viral vector vaccines in detail.

***Keywords*:** Viral vectors, vaccine, advantages, challenges, mechanism of action of viral vectors

10.1 Introduction

The viral vectors emerged as an important tool for the delivery of genes and vaccine development. Their potential relies on the capability of viruses to invade the host cells and cause infection. As compared to other vectors,

**Corresponding author*: shilpadawre@gmail.com

Vivek P. Chavda and Vasso Apostolopoulos (eds.) Viral Vectors for Vaccine Delivery, (317–340) © 2025 Scrivener Publishing LLC

viral vectors are more specific, extremely effective in gene transduction, and trigger immunity due to stimulation of cell-based immunity [1].

The viral vector vaccines work differently than subunit vaccines, as the second-mentioned vaccines support the prevention of infections by triggering a humoral response [2]. Viral vectors based on recombinant technology have been successfully utilized for remedial applications. They can allow antigen appearance inside the cell and cause a strong cytotoxic T lymphocyte (CTL) reaction, resulting eradication of cells infected by the virus [3]. The viral vector–based vaccines have been developed for tackling several dreadful diseases such as COVID-19, malaria, and HIV-1. In spite of their effectiveness, viral vectors demonstrate many inevitable complications that require attention [1].

The major hurdle in the successful implementation of viral vector vaccines is gene integration which can cause cancer. For stable gene expression on vectors, a viral integration process is required. An additional barrier to the clinical application of vaccines based on viral vectors is the existence of prior immunity against the vector. Prior exposure to the virus can reduce the efficacy of the vaccine due to the formation of neutralizing antibodies. The formulation of viral vectors needs a specific level of biological safety for obtaining public approval [4]. Thus, low or nonpathogenic viruses need to be carefully picked. Genetically engineered viruses can reduce the chances of pathogenicity. In addition, most viral vectors show replication defective. For instance, adeno-associated virus (AAV) vectors have E1A

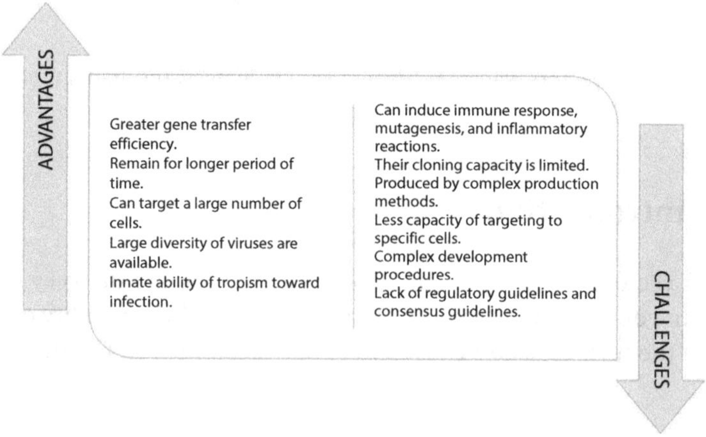

Figure 10.1 Advantages and challenges of viral vector vaccines.

and E1B encrypted areas, required for replication progression inside cells that have been infected, and are replaced and removed by the targeted gene [5]. Thus, while utilizing a viral vector, it is very crucial to analyze the risk-benefit ratio and prospective implications by studying virus characteristics and epidemiology.

In the present book chapter, we discuss several viral vectors with the highlights of their mechanism of action. Furthermore, we overviewed viral vector vaccine advantages and challenges (Figure 10.1). In addition to that in current chapter compiled a few clinical studies of vaccines based on viral vectors.

10.2 Types of Viral Vectors for Vaccine Development

In this section, we have overviewed various viral vectors that have been explored for the development of vaccines (Table 10.1).

10.2.1 Poxviruses Vectors

Vaccinia virus belongs to the family of poxvirus. It is an enveloped virus with a complex structure and large size. Commonly, these vectors have been utilized for smallpox vaccine and found safe and efficacious. Vaccinia virus has a double-stranded linear DNA 190 kb in dimension [6]. Due to its large size, foreign genes can be easily inserted in the sequence, i.e., ~25 kb. There are many reports that suggest that viral vector–based vaccines can trigger a strong immune response against antigens. It is due to the high transgene expression. Moreover, vectors can induce innate immunity response transmitted by inflammasomes and Toll-like receptors providing an adjuvant effect. Presently, many clinical trials are under progress for vaccine development using vaccinia virus–based vectors for diseases like malaria, influenza, hepatitis, HIV-1, cancer, and tuberculosis [7]. For vaccine development, highly attenuated and replication-deprived strains were designed such as NYVAC, ALVAC, TROVAC, and MVA [6].

In addition, the advantage is the feasibility of large-scale manufacturing which is already proven by the smallpox vaccine. For example, the Bavarian Nordic A/S company manufactured IMVAMUNE® (smallpox vaccine) in quantity of ~20 million doses and supplied it to the United States government for emergency use. However, the vaccinia virus has a drawback of lower immunogenicity, as observed in individuals vaccinated for smallpox.

Table 10.1 List of clinical trials using viral vectors for vaccine development.

Description of the vaccine platform	Vaccines	Number of doses	Interval between doses	Route of administration	Developers	Clinical trial phase
Nonreplicating viral vector	ChAdOx1-S – (AZD1222) (Covishield)	1–2	Day 0 + 28	Intramuscular	AstraZeneca; University of Oxford	Phase 4 (NCT04760132 NCT04775069)
Nonreplicating viral vector	Ad COV2.S	1–2	Day 0 or day 0 + 56	Intramuscular	Janssen Pharmaceutical	Phase 4 (EUCTR2021-002327-38-NL)
Nonreplicating viral vector	Hepatitis B	2	Day 0 + 21	Intramuscular	Gamaleya National Research Center for Epidemiology and Microbiology; Ministry of Health of the Russian Federation	Phase 3
Nonreplicating viral vector	Hepatitis B	1	Day 0	Intramuscular	CanSino Biological Inc./Beijing Institute of Biotechnology	Phase 4

(*Continued*)

Table 10.1 List of clinical trials using viral vectors for vaccine development. (*Continued*)

Description of the vaccine platform	Vaccines	Number of doses	Interval between doses	Route of administration	Developers	Clinical trial phase
Nonreplicating viral vector	Hepatitis B	1	Day 0	Intramuscular	ReiThera; Leukocare; Univercells	Phase 2/3
Nonreplicating viral vector	Hepatitis B	2	Day 0 + 28	Intranasal	University of Hong Kong; Xiamen University; Beijing Wantai Biological Pharmacy	Phase 2

This was due to the prior immunity against the virus. Finally, vaccinia virus vectors offer great potential to develop well-tolerated vaccines [8].

10.2.2 Adenovirus Vectors

There are around 50 human adenovirus (Ad) strains that have been recognized. Among them, an extensively studied vector for human use is Ad serotype 5 (Ad5) for the delivery of genes. Among them, an extensively studied vector for human use is Ad serotype 5 (Ad5) for the delivery of genes, due to its capability to generate high titers. Adenovirus serotype 5 is a non-enveloped virus and has a double-stranded DNA genome and linear structure of 36 kb. Adenovirus serotype 5 is a non-enveloped virus and has a double-stranded DNA genome and linear structure of 36 kb covered with a penton or hexon capsid shell. It can cause gastroenteritis, respiratory diseases, and pharyngoconjunctival fever. Recombinant adenovirus vectors are broadly used due to their excessive potential for the appearance of transgene, wide viral tropism capacity, and large transduction efficiency [9]. The majority of adenovirus vectors are deprived of duplication due to omission of genes (E1A and E1B). Furthermore, the adenovirus protein increases the effectiveness of the transduction of genes since the protein regulates the tropism of the virus. Many recombinant adenovirus vector–based vaccines are in clinical trials to combat solid tumors, influenza, and HIV-1 [10].

The disadvantage of Ad vectors is preexisting immunity because, commonly, people have been exposed to this virus and neutralizing antibodies are generated. The replication of defective Ad demonstrates decreased virulence; therefore, advancement is required in the clinical safety of adenovirus [11].

10.2.3 Retrovirus Vectors

Retrovirus (RV) contains single-stranded RNA and is an enveloped virus. RV vectors originate from avian or avian, and they have replication defective. The commonly studied virus among them is Moloney murine leukemia virus (MoMLV) [12]. Like AAV, RV also offers the expression of genes for an extended period of time. The genome size is ~7 to 11 kb and this vector can be inserted with ~7 to 8 kb of foreign DNA genome. The advantage is that it has less immunogenicity and patients do not have prior immunity to retroviral vectors. Nevertheless, these vectors are linked with many infections like leukemia and lymphoma [13].

A retroviral vector–based vaccine is already in clinical trials, for the treatment of malignant glioma or X-linked severe combined immunodeficiency (SCID-X1). However, a lot of research and investigation are required to implement RV vectors for vaccine development.

10.2.4 Lentivirus Vectors

Lentiviruses (LVs) belong to a subclass of RVs. LV offers benefits that are analogous to retroviral vectors. However, LV-based vectors can still pose a risk of tumor formation, although smaller than that of retroviral vectors. This is because LVs tend to integrate their genetic material away from cellular promoters, reducing the likelihood of oncogenic activation. LV is responsible for HIV infection [14]. HIV-based vectors are developed by removing the envelope of the HIV virus and some of the directing genes. To produce tissue and cell specificity, an envelope can be modified, or a chimeric envelope can be formed. Many viruses' envelopes such as MoMLV, measles, and filovirus have been utilized as vectors. In a clinical trial, the HIV-1–based vector, namely, VRX496, was used for HIV-1 gene therapy. However, the virulence of HIV-1 is concerning [15].

10.2.5 Cytomegalovirus Vectors

Human cytomegalovirus (HCMV) or human herpesvirus type 5 belongs to the herpesvirus family and is extensively studied as a vector. HCMV has a capsid and comprises genome double-stranded linear DNA (235 kb) [16]. The capsid has gH and gB glycoproteins that bind to receptors of the cell. In a study, the vaccine was developed using a rhesus CMV (RhCMV) vector for protection against SIV infection. The results indicate that the RhCMV-based vaccine triggers MHC-II–restricted CTLs capable of recognizing a broad range of antigen epitopes. The vaccine created using the HMCV vector has been observed effective vaccine to combat HIV-I infection [17].

10.2.6 Sendai Virus Vectors

It belongs to the family of *Paramyxoviridae*. It contains genome single-stranded RNA genome and an enveloped virus. Sendai virus (SeV) is similar to human parainfluenza type 1 (hPIV-1) virus. Thus, immunity generated against hPIV-1 further works for SeV. The SeV genome has two envelope glycoproteins F and HN that support cellular entry and encode six proteins. Thus, the F-protein–devoid virus forms a replication-deficient virus and enhances the safety profile of the vector [18].

The SeV comprises RNA-dependent RNA polymerase and its gene code within the cell plasma, facilitating rapid gene expression postinfection. The SeV vector can transduce both nondividing and dividing cells efficiently, enabling effective gene transfer. In addition, it can be delivered through an intranasal route to avoid preexisting immunity. Compared to other viral vectors, transgene volume is lesser (3.4 kb); therefore, limited use of this vector occurs [18]. A clinical trial of SeV vector–based vaccine for HIV-1 is currently going on (NCT01705990). The trial suggests that replicating SeV vector produces robust immune response than the nonreplicating vector.

10.2.7 Adeno-Associated Virus Vectors

AAVs contain DNA which is single-stranded and genome size of 4.7 kb. It is a non-enveloped virus. They belong to the *Parvoviridae* family and rely on replication-assisted viral functions [17]. Despite not being linked to any human disease, AAV has been identified in 70% to 80% of the human population through 11 serotypes, mainly defined by AAV-specific antibodies, with AAV-2 being the most prevalent [18].

Recombinant AAV vectors (rAAVs) have the capacity to trigger transgene expression across multiple tissues. In contrast to wild-type AAV, rAAVs are unable to integrate into the host cell chromosomes' safe vector site, a feature stemming from a repeat deletion within their genome [17]. Nonetheless, rAAVs have the potential to inadvertently integrate their DNA into the host cell genome, leading to the silencing of tumor suppressor genes. The rAAV genome primarily consists of an expression cassette and has a restricted insertion capacity of 5 kb.

For the development of vaccine candidates approved for human clinical use, rAAV particles are purified through chromatography. In preclinical studies, intramuscular injection of rAAV-expressing SIV antigens has been shown to elicit a protective and long-lasting antibody and T cell response against heterologous SIV antigens. rAAV candidates for the acquired immune deficiency syndrome vaccine were developed through collaboration between the International AIDS Vaccine Initiative and Targeted Genetics [19]. These candidates have completed phase 1 clinical trials in India and European countries and recently in phase 2 assessment in Africa.

Several preclinical studies have proven the efficacy of AAV vectors against papillomavirus [19], HIV-1 [20], and influenza. Nevertheless, clinical trials are fewer due to weak cellular and humoral immune triggers by the AAV virus compared with other viral vectors. Furthermore, infectious vaccines usually aim for healthy people, a large population, and an extensive age range, including adults and children. Therefore, AAV vectors for vaccines need a high safety profile and cost-effectiveness.

10.3 Mechanism of Action of Viral Vectors

Viral vector vaccines, whether replicating or nonreplicating, utilize modified viruses such as adenoviruses or poxviruses as vectors to introduce genetic material encoding a viral antigen of interest into the host cell [21]. Vaccines based on self-replicating viral vectors harness the cellular machinery of the virus vector to generate fresh viral particles within infected cells. This process enables the infection of new cells and the subsequent production of additional vaccine antigens. Contrarily, vaccines based on non-replicating viral vectors are unable to produce new viral particles; rather, they rely on the machinery of the host cell to yield antigens for the vaccine before the viral vector is eliminated [22]. Neither the administered virus nor the viral vector vaccine induces infection, as the genetic material delivered does not integrate into the host genome. This vaccine type typically benefits from stimulating the expression of viral antigens within infected host cells, thereby enabling efficient MHC class I and class II presentations [22].

Furthermore, virus-based vectors exhibit great specificity of gene transduction and an immune response with enhanced cellular responsiveness. Additionally, despite viral vector–based vaccines being commonly observed as less effective than conventional vaccines, their ability to persist as genetic material in the host offers unique advantages. They directly invade antigen-presenting cells (APCs) and exhibit strong intrinsic adjuvant activity, thereby eliciting vigorous adaptive and innate immune responses. They can generate high titers of neutralizing antibodies, which may be sufficient for adequate immunization with just one vaccine dose. Replicating and nonreplicating vectors have been employed to transport genes encoding either the SARS-CoV-2 S-glycoprotein or the receptor-binding domain for the manufacturing of COVID-19 vector–based vaccines [23, 24]. There are various mechanisms of action of viral vectors for vaccine development that have been discussed in this section.

10.3.1 Self-Adjuvanting Nature of Viral Vector Vaccines

The immune system of mammals has developed to quickly detect viral invaders and develop strong adaptive and innate immunity. As a result, researchers have identified multiple innate sensors and pathways that govern the immune response to viruses. Various pattern recognition receptors are engaged in this procedure, and the outcome varies based on the virus's characteristics and its genome replication mechanism [25]. The mitogen-activated protein (MAP) kinase and NF-κB (nuclear factor "kappa-light-chain-enhancer" of activated B cells) track are activated when viral genomes bind to these receptors, which causes the generation of cytokines and chemokines [26]. In addition, type I interferon (IFN-I) induction is mediated by the interferon regulatory factors IRF3 and IRF7 signals. These pathways have evolved primarily for the aim of antimicrobial defense, with the induction of IFN-I–medicated "antiviral state" as a model [27]. These transcriptional processes triggered by the virus also stimulate infected APCs, directing the adaptive immune system to produce potent antibody responses and helper T cell type 1 (T_H1)–biased cellular responses, which include CD8⁺ T cells. Therefore, vaccines based on virus vectors are typically "self-adjuvanted," and virus-induced inflammation is perfectly adapted to generate robust vaccine responses [28]. In some cases, reduction can even enhance the immunostimulatory capabilities observed with the wild-type version of the virus. A well-known illustration is the vaccinia virus, which encodes an IFN-I receptor and inhibitor of the production of IFN-I inside cells. On the contrary, these virulence elements are absent in modified vaccinia virus Ankara (MVA), a replication-defective variation of vaccinia virus characterized by significant genome reduction. Consequently, MVA is unable to suppress the human IFN-I response. These studies proved the self-adjuvanting properties of live viral vaccines cannot be predictably determined by the duplication capability and reduction level [28].

10.3.2 Enhanced Cytotoxic $CD8^+$ T Lymphocyte Production

Cytotoxic $CD8^+$ T lymphocytes (CTLs) are a crucial predictor of defense against a variety of intracellular infections and tumors. As a result, strong CTL immunity is an essential component that must be present for effective defense against a variety of diseases, and CTL immunity is effectively incited by viruses [29]. Viruses use the host cell's translational apparatus as "nature's own gene delivery system" to express their genes. Infected cells generate gene products, and peptide fragments and can be directly accessed by the host major histocompatibility complex (MHC) class I peptide by traversing using a transporter associated with antigen processing (TAP) complex and proteasome [30]. The term "direct presentation" is used to describe this procedure. In contrast, cross-presentation, which is the sole method used by non-live vaccines to deliver peptide fragments to MHC class I complexes of expert APCs, is a process in which phagocytic uptake delivers peptide fragments. Therefore, vectored antigens are expressed by professional APCs such as dendritic cells, which contribute, at least in part, to the robust activation, differentiation, and proliferation of CTL responses by live viral vaccines. The viral infection also activates the APCs that present the antigenic peptide. The capacity of APCs to prime powerful CTL responses will be enhanced by simultaneous functional activation [31].

It is interesting to note that a wide variety of viruses like hepatitis B, which typically demonstrate a pretty limited cell type and tissue tropism, can presumably infect or at least transduce dendritic cells. Of course, viral vectors are also capable of utilizing this mechanism. To increase CTL induction by virally vectored vaccines, each of these pathways cooperates with the inflammatory milieu that has already been self-adjuvanted.

10.3.3 Conformational Antigen Expression on Host Cell Membranes Infected by a Vector

Accurate three-dimensional twisting and mammalian glycosylation patterns are important for presenting conformational determinants necessary for inducing defensive antibodies. APCs and virions both include membrane-bound antigens, which serve as a reliable source for B lymphocytes to recognize and take up antigens [32]. A preferred method to meet these needs is by employing live viral vaccines, which enable structural antigen expression on the cell envelope of infected APCs. However, it does not seem that the presence of vaccine antigens in virions is a need for antibody formation. Unenclosed vaccination vectors can trigger immune responses against membrane-anchored conformational antigens. Therefore, the idea of "genetic vaccines" also includes the generation of antibodies.

10.3.4 Sustained Supply of Significant Amounts of Antigen

A key component of the best immune stimulation is the ability of viral vector–based vaccines to show antigens of the vaccine in large amounts and for large amounts of time. Although this primarily applies to live vaccines, the amount of antigen loaded in the vaccine can control how strong an immune response is to replication-deficient vector systems [33]. The idea behind genetic vaccination supports the idea that the antigen's persistence is not just a straightforward function of its *in vivo* half-life.

10.4 Advantages of Viral Vector Vaccines

The primary objective of vaccinations is to prime the immune system to identify the viral protein molecules or target viruses, thereby safeguarding the body from infectious diseases. To achieve this, it is essential to consider key factors such as safety, stability, and immunogenicity [24].

10.4.1 Safety

Viral vectors are altered by eradicating the gene that causes infection while retaining the ability to invade cells in order to transport target genes deprived of spreading illness. This progression resembles the spread of viral infections. Adenoviruses, influenza viruses, measles viruses, and cowpox viruses are just a few of the viruses that have been used as vectors. These viral vectors lack the genetic components that cause illness, and some of them even lack the components required for reproduction [34]. Thus, the virus vector demonstrated safety.

10.4.2 Stability

Few mRNA vaccinations are stored at extremely low temperatures in order to stop deprivation. Vaccines based on viral vectors are stable and need fewer careful handling and storing settings than other vaccination platforms. The AAV-based vaccine from Johnson & Johnson can be transported and stored at temperatures ranging from 15°C to 25°C until the date of expiration. Alternatively, it can be stored at 2°C to 8°C for up to 6 months. This significantly increases the need for ultralow temperature storage of mRNA vaccines to prevent deterioration. For up to 6 months, Pfizer-BNT162b2 BioNTech must be stored between −80°C and −60°C. Moderna's mRNA-1273 vaccination should be kept between 2°C and 8°C for up to 30 days but should be kept at or below −20°C for up to 6 months. As a result, vaccine accessibility is improved globally and vaccine availability and cost are both significantly increased [35, 36].

10.4.3 Immunogenicity

The delivery and appearance of antigens are pivotal for immunity development and defense. Both cellular and humoral immune triggers are essential for clearing SARS-CoV-2, as indicated by research findings and data collected during the COVID-19 pandemic. The antigen presentation mechanism of viral vector vaccines allows for long-lasting immunity without the requirement for frequent booster doses. Last but not least, adverse reactions to vaccination must be regularly evaluated, and our knowledge of viral vector immunology must be expanded in order to guarantee consistency in high immunogenicity and safety [33].

10.4.3.1 Humoral Immunity

Humoral immunity is an explicit immunity wherein B cells generate antibodies to offer protection upon encountering a specific antigen. It is possible to develop a humoral immunity to viruses by vaccination or acquired infection [2]. Neutralizing antibodies are among the critical indicators of the immune system against infections caused by viruses and play a pivotal role in humoral immunity. Due to variations in replication capacities, protein expression profiles, and entry kinetics among different viral vectors, they may evoke diverse immune responses and provide varying levels of protection. Due to adenoviruses' ability to infect a variety of host tissue cells, they are the viral vector most frequently employed for COVID-19 vaccine production. In addition to the measles virus, oncolytic herpes simplex virus-1 (HSV-1), vesicular stomatitis virus (VSV), and MVA, several other viral vector–based COVID-19 vaccines have undergone extensive preclinical testing [37]. Despite the fact that numerous vaccines based on viral vectors stimulate robust humoral immunity in phase 1 trials, human and animal models evaluating a potential COVID-19 vaccine candidate, Merck's rVSV-vectored, was terminated due to inadequate immunogenicity.

The humoral immunogenicity of viral vector vaccines is also influenced by immunogen designs. Animals immunized with spike proteins of SARS-CoV-2 depleted of glycan barriers exhibited more potent protective responses, according to Huang *et al.* The vaccination route, dosage, heterologous/homologous prime immunization boosting strategies, as well as individual variations among vaccine recipients, can also have an impact on the vaccine's efficacy [4].

10.4.3.2 Cell-Mediated Immunity

Viral vector vaccines can elicit potent and enduring cellular responses, such as CTLs, which are essential for eliminating virus-infected cells. When triggered by antigens, antigen-specific cytotoxic T cells ($CD8^+$) distinguish, multiply, and mature into T cells. This cellular immunity also activates NK cells and macrophages to target and destroy intracellular parasites [38].

During a clinical trial (phase 1/2) of the AZD1222 vaccine, it was observed that between days 7 and 28 after vaccination, $CD4^+$ and $CD8^+$ T cells exhibited enhanced CD69 and Ki-67 expressions, accompanied by heightened production of TNF tumor necrosis factor and interferon (IFN) by $CD4^+$ T cells. The vaccine showed immunogenicity against Ad5-nCoV, with the majority of subjects experiencing swift T cell responses. These responses reach their highest point 14 days after vaccination, indicating an early onset of detectable immune responses. Notably, antigen-specific $CD4^+$ and $CD8^+$ T cells were stimulated in vaccine recipients [39].

10.4.3.3 Mucosal Immunity

Mucosal immunity has an important role in the initial defense against viral invasion by locally producing antibodies. This mechanism serves as the first line of defense, helping to maintain immunological tolerance to non-pathogenic antigens while triggering a robust immune response against exogenous pathogenic antigens [40]. Nasal spray and nebulized inhalation vaccinations confer mucosal immunity, thereby preventing infection and interrupting the spread at the initial point of invasion of the virus. This is unlike most intramuscular vaccines, which primarily elicit cellular and humoral protection.

COVID-19 enters the human body via the nasopharynx route. It is challenging to fend off the virus invasion at this site due to the extremely limited dispersion of IgG brought on by intramuscular vaccination [41]. Additionally, observed that Omicron primarily affects the upper respiratory tract and causes infection; as a result, switching the vaccination route and relying on mucosal immunity to protect against infection may be more efficient. Clinical studies have shown that infections with the SARS-CoV-2 Omicron variant exhibit heightened activity in the upper respiratory tract. Consequently, ensuring elevated neutralizing antibody levels in the respiratory mucosa may be essential for enhancing anti-infective efficacy [42].

In the context of mucosal responses, the nasal pathway is prioritized over the parenteral route due to its dependability and simplicity. Furthermore, a localized mucosal immune reaction is imperative for impeding the replication of the SARS-CoV-2 virus in the nasal epithelium. Consequently, various pharmaceutical companies and researchers have innovated novel techniques for delivering the COVID-19 vaccine to enhance the organism's mucosal immune response, primarily through nasal spray administration and nebulized inhalation.

This study presents the first clinical outcomes for an aerosol COVID-19 vaccine. CanSino Biologics, a Chinese company, initially developed the adenovirus vector vaccine for intramuscular injection, later introducing a nebulized inhalation delivery method for clinical trials. The results demonstrate that two doses of aerosolized Ad5-nCoV are well-tolerated and do not lead to any significant adverse reactions associated with vaccination. A robust cellular response can be induced by a single dose of aerosolized Ad5-nCoV, equivalent to a fifth of an intramuscular dose. Similarly, two doses of aerosolized Ad5-nCoV can elicit a similar response.

Furthermore, the development of multi-disease or multi-pathogen vector vaccines, which utilize critical protective antigens from multiple pathogens in a single vector to immunize against various diseases, has become feasible through immunity to viral vectors [4].

10.5 Challenges of Viral Vector Vaccine

Several viral vectors, such as HSVs, AAVs, adenoviruses (Ad), RVs, and LVs have undergone testing for clinical applications [2]. Although several virus-based vaccines are safe and effective for the delivery of genes, few pose a risk of oncogenesis. Moreover, certain viral vectors, such as adenovirus and herpes viral vectors, may pose toxicity and immunogenicity concerns [5]. Despite the promise of using viral vector systems for vaccine development, there are several challenges as well. Therefore, ongoing research is being conducted to evaluate the safety and efficacy of these vectors during clinical trials.

Significantly, Institutional Biosafety Committees (IBCs) and healthcare providers face challenges due to the limited resources available for conducting risk assessments and establishing protocols to minimize exposure and risks in both research and clinical environments. The absence of consensus guidelines for these vectors in such settings underscores the importance of individualized risk assessment. This section overviewed various challenges in the development of vaccines based on viral vectors.

10.5.1 Development of Immunity Against Viral Vectors

A potential drawback of viral vector vaccines is that they may cause the recipient to develop immunity (neutralizing antibodies) to the viral vector itself. Many viral vectors are considered "self-adjuvants" because they can activate the innate immune signaling cascade within host cells through the recognition of pathogen-associated molecular patterns (PAMPs) by pattern-recognition receptors (PRRs). This stands in contrast to conventional vaccines, which typically require adjuvants to activate innate immunity [21].

10.5.2 Adverse Events

Antibody-dependent enhancement (ADE) refers to a phenomenon where antibodies aid the entry of a virus into host cells, leading to increased viral replication and higher infectivity, subsequently resulting in severe outcomes. This aspect, often underestimated in vaccine development, can potentially cause adverse events, making individuals who have been vaccinated exhibit increased susceptibility to severe symptoms following infection [43].

An instance of severe adverse effects following vaccination was observed with a formalin-inactivated RSV vaccine, which resulted in increased hospitalizations and fatalities in infants. Subsequent research suggested that the T_H2 response can trigger vaccine ADE. Furthermore, investigations established that the formalin-inactivated virus triggers ADE in monkeys, attributing the T_H2 response in mice to carbonyl groups present in the formaldehyde-inactivated RSV [44].

Moreover, formalin inactivation of viruses has been associated with antigen alteration, resulting in a generation of non-neutralizing antibodies (non-NAbs) with immature avidity and complement activation, as seen in a measles vaccine. To induce potent neutralizing antibodies, triggering TLR activation, which aids affinity maturation, has been suggested alongside the use of a T_H1-polarizing adjuvant in vaccine design.

Reports on the formation of MERS/SARS vaccines also highlighted the potential for ADE. The inclusion of antigen S-glycoprotein in vaccines was found to potentially increase susceptibility to viral infection, especially when inducing low-titer antibodies. Additionally, it has been suggested that neutralizing antibodies (NAbs) that strongly bind to the receptor-binding domain (RBD) region of the S-protein may induce alterations that increase virus entry through canonical viral receptor–dependent pathways, resembling viral receptor binding. In nonhuman primate models of SARS, it has been observed that antibodies directed at specific regions of the S-protein can potentially exacerbate viral infection. This has raised concerns regarding the development of COVID-19 vaccines based on the S-protein, given the significant sequence homology and structural resemblance shared among the SARS-CoV, MERS-CoV, and SARS-CoV-2 S-glycoproteins [45].

10.5.3 Scale-Up Hurdles in Viral Vector Production

10.5.3.1 Complexity and Variability of the Process

Viral vector vaccine production indeed involves many individualized processes, making it a complex task. Here are some key steps involved: i) Design and construction. The virus-based vector is created and modified to transport the vaccine antigen and gene. ii) Transfection: Introducing the viral vector into the production cell line is achieved through a process called transfection. iii) Isolation and purification: The viral vector is separated from the production cell line and purified to eliminate impurities.

iv) Upstream processing: This phase involves selecting suitable producer cell culture lines and defining the optimal growth conditions. v) Downstream processing: This includes the isolation and purification steps [46].

As mentioned above viral vector generation is a multistage process that involves genetic engineering, cell cultivation, virus production, harvesting, purification, and quality control. Each step requires careful optimization and regulation of various factors, such as host cell selection, transfection efficiency, bioreactor conditions, purification methods, and vector quality. The process is also affected by the choice of viral vector, such as adenovirus, AAV, herpes simplex, or LV, which have different characteristics and requirements. The complexity and variability of the process pose challenges for scalability, reproducibility, and standardization [4].

Since downstream operations can represent up to 70% of production costs, it is crucial that all phases of process development are designed in concert. However, these processes pose certain risks such as genomic integration, host-induced neutralizing antibodies against vector viruses, and the requirement of different strategies for booster vaccinations. Additionally, the manufacture of viral vectors is typically challenging due to the complexity of the production processes involved. For instance, viral vector production requires the utilization of a host cell line in addition to the intended vector, which is inherently complex [47].

10.5.3.2 Low Yield and High Cost

Viral vector production often suffers from low yield, meaning that the amount of functional vector particles obtained is much lower than the amount of input materials and resources. This is due to factors such as low transfection efficiency, low virus replication, low vector stability, and high vector loss during purification. Low yield results in high cost, as more raw materials, reagents, equipment, and labor are needed to produce the desired number of viral vectors. High cost limits the availability and accessibility of viral vector–based therapies, especially for large-scale and chronic applications [48].

10.5.3.3 Regulatory and Quality Control Challenges

Quality control and regulatory demands in viral vector vaccine production are essential aspects of ensuring the safety and efficacy of these biopharmaceutical products. Viral vector production must comply with stringent regulatory and quality standards set by authorities such as the FDA. These standards include Good Manufacturing Practices (GMP), which ensure the potency, safety, purity, and consistency of the viral vectors. This is a fundamental requirement for viral vector vaccine production, emphasizing the need for consistency, traceability, and documentation throughout the process. GMP standards also ensure compliance with regulatory requirements set by organizations like the WHO and the FDA [49].

However, meeting these standards can be challenging, as viral vector production involves biological materials and processes that are difficult to control and measure. For example, it is challenging to determine the exact number, identity, and functionality of the vector particles, as well as the presence and removal of impurities, such as host cell proteins, nucleic acids, and empty capsids. Moreover, the regulatory and quality requirements may vary depending on the type of viral vector, the target disease, and the target population [46].

Quality control involves a comprehensive evaluation of every stage of the manufacturing process, from initial cell line development to final vector product release. Quality control protocols encompass critical assessments of vector titer, purity, potency, functionality, and biosafety.

10.5.3.4 Restrictions of Frequent Culture Systems

The frequent culture systems, particularly those involving mammalian cells grown in adherent suspension, are widely used in the manufacturing of viral vectors. However, these systems face significant challenges when it comes to scaling up. The variety of containers that need to be managed during the production process leads to a bottleneck in downstream processing. Therefore, new culture systems that are more suitable for larger-scale viral vector production are being considered. Moreover, the specific type of viral vector to be produced plays a critical role in the selection of producer cell lines. For instance, in the manufacturing of gene therapies, customized processes in viral vector manufacturing are ubiquitous. This is because patient genetics are diverse, making it essential to tailor processes for each case. This requirement for high variability forces manufacturers to adapt complex procedures regularly and efficiently. Finally, the effective long-period storage of virus-based vectors is essential for their utility in gene therapy, vaccine development, and biopharmaceutical research. However, one of the primary challenges in long-term storage lies in formulation [50].

10.5.3.5 Formulation and Storage of Viral Vector Products

Developing the right formulations is intricate work, as they must preserve the integrity and functionality of viral vectors during storage.

The formulation must ensure safety and potency during storage and distribution, ensuring their suitability for clinical and research purposes. Factors such as freezing methods, excipients, stabilizers, and optimal storage conditions become paramount in this context [48].

Selecting appropriate freezing methods is equally crucial in the preservation of biopharmaceutical products based on viral vectors. Factors like the low stability of rAAVs and the different serotypes of AAVs make it necessary to store them in a frozen state. Considerations of the ideal freezing rates are equally important as logistic planning since viral vectors should not be subjected to multiple freeze/thaw cycles [49].

10.5.3.6 Requirement of High-Cost Technologies

Development of viral vectors requires sophisticated instrumentation and automated techniques which is costly. Single-use technologies, when combined with a high level of automation, can result in process optimization not only in AAV production but also in cell and gene therapy development and manufacturing in general. The automated fluid management system RoSS.FILL is part of a fully scalable platform for aseptic aliquotation, completed by RoSS.PADL for homogenization through automated kneading and cooling. The freeze/thaw process can be performed with the innovative plate freezing platform RoSS.pFTU, able to freeze single-use bags down to −80°C in a fast and controlled manner [48].

10.5.3.7 Handling and Shipment

Viral vectors are shipped frozen on dry ice and should be stored at −80°C upon arrival and for extended storage. Short-term storage at −20°C or +4°C is permissible. Whenever possible, it is recommended to aliquot vectors into single-use portions to avoid repeated freeze/thaw cycles. Vectors are ready to use upon shipment [28].

The hurdles mentioned in the manufacturing of virus-based vectors highlight the complexities and challenges associated with scaling up the process for various applications such as gene therapy, vaccine development, and biopharmaceutical research. In summary, the restrictions of frequent culture systems include challenges in scaling up the need for customization based on the type of viral vector and patient genetics, adherence to stringent quality control measures and regulatory standards, and efficient long-term storage of viral vectors [46].

10.6 Conclusion

In the case of infectious diseases and public health events, viral vector vaccine modalities provided a prompt response. It is noteworthy that the COVID-19 vaccine based on viral vectors has been undertaken for clinical trials and permitted in a short span of time for tackling the COVID-19 pandemic situation. However, the efficacy, superiorities, and unique properties of these viral vector vaccines have not been fully studied, particularly for mucosal immunization. Moreover, viral vector vaccines require a thorough understanding of viral biology and the host immunomodulatory effect of these vectors. In the future, with advancements in the field of viral vector vaccines, precision medicine is also possible. To make the viral vector vaccines successful, collaborative work between industry and research groups is required. Moreover, for approval of viral vector vaccines, clear-cut regulatory guidelines and evaluation procedures are required.

References

1. Sasso, E., D'Alise, A.M., Zambrano, N., Scarselli, E., Folgori, A., Nicosia, A., New Viral Vectors for Infectious Diseases and Cancer. *Semin. Immunol., 50*, 101430, 2020, doi: 10.1016/j.smim.2020.101430.
2. McCann, N., O'Connor, D., Lambe, T., Pollard, A.J., Viral Vector Vaccines. *Curr. Opin. Immunol., 77*, 102210, 2022, doi: 10.1016/j.coi.2022.102210.
3. Naim, H.Y., Applications and Challenges of Multivalent Recombinant Vaccines. *Hum. Vaccin. Immunother., 9*, 457–461, 2013, doi: 10.4161/hv.23220.
4. Wang, S., Liang, B., Wang, W., Li, L., Feng, N., Zhao, Y., Wang, T., Yan, F., Yang, S., Xia, X., Viral Vectored Vaccines: Design, Development, Preventive and Therapeutic Applications in Human Diseases. *Signal Transduction Targeted Ther., 8*, 149, 2023, doi: 10.1038/s41392-023-01408-5.
5. Ertl, H.C.J., Immunogenicity and Toxicity of AAV Gene Therapy. *Front. Immunol., 13*, 975803, 2022, doi: 10.3389/fimmu.2022.975803.
6. Pastoret, P.-P. and Vanderplasschen, A., Poxviruses as Vaccine Vectors. *Comp. Immunol. Microbiol. Infect. Dis., 26*, 343–355, 2003, doi: 10.1016/S0147-9571(03)00019-5.
7. Balar, P.C., Apostolopoulos, V., Chavda, V.P.A., New Era of Immune Therapeutics for Pancreatic Cancer: Monoclonal Antibodies Paving the Way. *Eur. J. Pharmacol., 969*, 176451, 2024, doi: 10.1016/j.ejphar.2024.176451.
8. Vanderplasschen, A. and Pastoret, P., The Uses of Poxviruses as Vectors. *Curr. Gene Ther., 3*, 583–595, 2003, doi: 10.2174/1566523034578168.

9. Syyam, A., Nawaz, A., Ijaz, A., Sajjad, U., Fazil, A., Irfan, S., Muzaffar, A., Shahid, M., Idrees, M., Malik, K., *et al.*, Adenovirus Vector System: Construction, History and Therapeutic Applications. *BioTechniques*, *73*, 297–305, 2022, doi: 10.2144/btn-2022-0051.
10. Sakurai, F., Tachibana, M., Mizuguchi, H., Adenovirus Vector-Based Vaccine for Infectious Diseases. *Drug Metab. Pharmacokinet.*, *42*, 100432, 2022, doi: 10.1016/j.dmpk.2021.100432.
11. Chavda, V.P., Bezbaruah, R., Valu, D., Patel, B., Kumar, A., Prasad, S., Kakoti, B.B., Kaushik, A., Jesawadawala, M., Adenoviral Vector-Based Vaccine Platform for COVID-19: Current Status. *Vaccines*, *11*, 432, 2023, doi: 10.3390/vaccines11020432.
12. Epstein, A. and Manservigi, R., Herpesvirus/Retrovirus Chimeric Vectors. *Curr. Gene Ther.*, *4*, 409–416, 2004, doi: 10.2174/1566523043345922.
13. Li, X., Le, Y., Zhang, Z., Nian, X., Liu, B., Yang, X., Viral Vector-Based Gene Therapy. *Int. J. Mol. Sci.*, *24*, 7736, 2023, doi: 10.3390/ijms24097736.
14. Ku, M.-W., Charneau, P., Majlessi, L., Use of Lentiviral Vectors in Vaccination. *Expert Rev. Vaccines*, *20*, 1571–1586, 2021, doi: 10.1080/14760584.2021.1988854.
15. Oldham, R.A., Berinstein, E.M., Medin, J.A., Lentiviral Vectors in Cancer Immunotherapy. *Immunotherapy*, *7*, 271–284, 2015, doi: 10.2217/imt.14.108.
16. Méndez, A.C., Rodríguez-Rojas, C., Del Val, M., Vaccine Vectors: The Bright Side of Cytomegalovirus. *Med. Microbiol. Immunol.*, *208*, 349–363, 2019, doi: 10.1007/s00430-019-00597-7.
17. Chang, W.L.W., Deere, J.D., Kieu, H.T., Castillo, L.D., Machmach, K., Shen, X., Tomaras, G.D., Shacklett, B.L., Barry, P.A., Hartigan-O'Connor, D.J., *et al.*, RhCMV Serostatus and Vaccine Adjuvant Impact Immunogenicity of RhCMV/SIV Vaccines. *Sci. Rep.*, *10*, 14056, 2020, doi: 10.1038/s41598-020-71075-x.
18. Bitzer, M., Armeanu, S., Lauer, U.M., Neubert, W.J., Sendai Virus Vectors as an Emerging Negative-strand RNA Viral Vector System. *J. Gene Med.*, *5*, 543–553, 2003, doi: 10.1002/jgm.426.
19. Nieto, K., Stahl-Hennig, C., Leuchs, B., Müller, M., Gissmann, L., Kleinschmidt, J.A., Intranasal Vaccination with AAV5 and 9 Vectors Against Human Papillomavirus Type 16 in Rhesus Macaques. *Hum. Gene Ther.*, *23*, 733–741, 2012, doi: 10.1089/hum.2011.202.
20. Fuchs, S.P. and Desrosiers, R.C., Promise and Problems Associated with the Use of Recombinant AAV for the Delivery of Anti-HIV Antibodies. *Mol. Ther. Methods Clin. Dev.*, *3*, 16068, 2016, doi: 10.1038/mtm.2016.68.
21. Travieso, T., Li, J., Mahesh, S., Mello, J.D.F.R.E., Blasi, M., The Use of Viral Vectors in Vaccine Development. *npj Vaccines*, *7*, 75, 2022, doi: 10.1038/s41541-022-00503-y.
22. Ura, T., Okuda, K., Shimada, M., Developments in Viral Vector-Based Vaccines. *Vaccines*, *2*, 624–641, 2014, doi: 10.3390/vaccines2030624.

23. Pulendran, B., Arunachalam, S., O'Hagan, P., D.T. Emerging Concepts in the Science of Vaccine Adjuvants. *Nat. Rev. Drug Discov.*, *20*, 454–475, 2021, doi: 10.1038/s41573-021-00163-y.
24. Deng, S., Liang, H., Chen, P., Li, Y., Li, Z., Fan, S., Wu, K., Li, X., Chen, W., Qin, Y., *et al.*, Viral Vector Vaccine Development and Application during the COVID-19 Pandemic. *Microorganisms*, *10*, 1450, 2022, doi: 10.3390/microorganisms10071450.
25. Takeuchi, O. and Akira, S., Pattern Recognition Receptors and Inflammation. *Cell*, *140*, 805–820, 2010, doi: 10.1016/j.cell.2010.01.022.
26. Hoesel, B. and Schmid, J.A., The Complexity of NF-κB Signaling in Inflammation and Cancer. *Mol. Cancer*, *12*, 86, 2013, doi: 10.1186/1476-4598-12-86.
27. Stegelmeier, A.A., Darzianiazizi, M., Hanada, K., Sharif, S., Wootton, S.K., Bridle, B.W., Karimi, K., Type I Interferon-Mediated Regulation of Antiviral Capabilities of Neutrophils. *Int. J. Mol. Sci.*, *22*, 4726, 2021, doi: 10.3390/ijms22094726.
28. Ghosh, S., Brown, A.M., Jenkins, C., Campbell, K., Viral Vector Systems for Gene Therapy: A Comprehensive Literature Review of Progress and Biosafety Challenges. *Appl. Biosaf.*, *25*, 7–18, 2020, doi: 10.1177/1535676019899502.
29. Chan, Y.K., Wang, S.K., Chu, C.J., Copland, D.A., Letizia, A.J., Costa Verdera, H., Chiang, J.J., Sethi, M., Wang, M.K., Neidermyer, W.J., *et al.*, Engineering Adeno-Associated Viral Vectors to Evade Innate Immune and Inflammatory Responses. *Sci. Transl. Med.*, *13*, 580, 2021, doi: 10.1126/scitranslmed.abd3438.
30. Thomas, C.E., Ehrhardt, A., Kay, M.A., Progress and Problems with the Use of Viral Vectors for Gene Therapy. *Nat. Rev. Genet.*, *4*, 346–358, 2003, doi: 10.1038/nrg1066.
31. Goyvaerts, C. and Breckpot, K., Pros and Cons of Antigen-Presenting Cell Targeted Tumor Vaccines. *J. Immunol. Res.*, *2015*, 1–18, 2015, doi: 10.1155/2015/785634.
32. Cruz-Reséndiz, A., Zepeda-Cervantes, J., Sampieri, A., Bastián-Eugenio, C., Acero, G., Sánchez-Betancourt, J.I., Gevorkian, G., Vaca, L.A., Self-Aggregating Peptide: Implications for the Development of Thermostable Vaccine Candidates. *BMC Biotech.*, *20*, 1, 2020, doi: 10.1186/s12896-019-0592-9.
33. Brisse, M., Vrba, S.M., Kirk, N., Liang, Y., Ly, H., Emerging Concepts and Technologies in Vaccine Development. *Front. Immunol.*, *11*, 583077, 2020, doi: 10.3389/fimmu.2020.583077.
34. Weiner, D.B. and Nabel, G.J., Development of Gene-Based Vectors for Immunization, in: *Plotkin's Vaccines*, pp. 1305–1319.e8, Elsevier, 2018. doi: 10.1016/B978-0-323-35761-6.00067-5.
35. Kudlay, D. and Svistunov, A., COVID-19 Vaccines: An Overview of Different Platforms. *Bioengineering*, *9*, 72, 2022, doi: 10.3390/bioengineering9020072.

36. Bulcha, J.T., Wang, Y., Ma, H., Tai, P.W.L., Gao, G., Viral Vector Platforms within the Gene Therapy Landscape. *Signal Transduct. Target. Ther.*, *6*, 53, 2021, doi: 10.1038/s41392-021-00487-6.
37. Turley, J.L. and Lavelle, E.C., Resolving Adjuvant Mode of Action to Enhance Vaccine Efficacy. *Curr. Opin. Immunol.*, *77*, 102229, 2022, doi: 10.1016/j.coi.2022.102229.
38. Wang, S., Liang, B., Wang, W., Li, L., Feng, N., Zhao, Y., Wang, T., Yan, F., Yang, S., Xia, X., Viral Vectored Vaccines: Design, Development, Preventive and Therapeutic Applications in Human Diseases. *Signal Transduc. Targeted Ther.*, *8*, 149, 2023, doi: 10.1038/s41392-023-01408-5.
39. Sadarangani, M., Marchant, A., Kollmann, T.R., Immunological Mechanisms of Vaccine-Induced Protection against COVID-19 in Humans. *Nat. Rev. Immunol.*, *21*, 475–484, 2021, doi: 10.1038/s41577-021-00578-z.
40. Fraser, R., Orta-Resendiz, A., Mazein, A., Dockrell, D.H., Upper Respiratory Tract Mucosal Immunity for SARS-CoV-2 Vaccines. *Trends Mol. Med.*, *29*, 255–267, 2023, doi: 10.1016/j.molmed.2023.01.003.
41. Chatterjee, S., Sullivan, H.A., MacLennan, B.J., Xu, R., Hou, Y., Lavin, T.K., Lea, N.E., Michalski, J.E., Babcock, K.R., Dietrich, S., *et al.*, Nontoxic, Double-Deletion-Mutant Rabies Viral Vectors for Retrograde Targeting of Projection Neurons. *Nat. Neurosci.*, *21*, 638–646, 2018, doi: 10.1038/s41593-018-0091-7.
42. Sullivan, D.J., Gebo, K.A., Shoham, S., Bloch, E.M., Lau, B., Shenoy, A.G., Mosnaim, G.S., Gniadek, T.J., Fukuta, Y., Patel, B., *et al.*, Early Outpatient Treatment for Covid-19 with Convalescent Plasma. *N. Engl. J. Med.*, *386*, 1700–1711, 2022, doi: 10.1056/NEJMoa2119657.
43. Lee, W.S., Wheatley, A.K., Kent, S.J., DeKosky, B.J., Antibody-Dependent Enhancement and SARS-CoV-2 Vaccines and Therapies. *Nat. Microbiol.*, *5*, 1185–1191, 2020, doi: 10.1038/s41564-020-00789-5.
44. Xu, L., Ma, Z., Li, Y., Pang, Z., Xiao, S., Antibody Dependent Enhancement: Unavoidable Problems in Vaccine Development, pp. 99–133, 2021.
45. Karthik, K., Senthilkumar, T.M.A., Udhayavel, S., Raj, G.D., Role of Antibody-Dependent Enhancement (ADE) in the Virulence of SARS-CoV-2 and Its Mitigation Strategies for the Development of Vaccines and Immunotherapies to Counter COVID-19. *Hum. Vaccin. Immunother.*, *16*, 3055–3060, 2020, doi: 10.1080/21645515.2020.1796425.
46. van der Loo, J.C.M. and Wright, J.F., Progress and Challenges in Viral Vector Manufacturing. *Hum. Mol. Genet.*, *25*, R42–R52, 2016, doi: 10.1093/hmg/ddv451.
47. Whitley, J., Zwolinski, C., Denis, C., Maughan, M., Hayles, L., Clarke, D., Snare, M., Liao, H., Chiou, S., Marmura, T., *et al.*, Development of mRNA Manufacturing for Vaccines and Therapeutics: mRNA Platform Requirements and Development of a Scalable Production Process to Support Early Phase Clinical Trials. *Transl. Res.*, *242*, 38–55, 2022, doi: 10.1016/j.trsl.2021.11.009.

48. Srivastava, A., Mallela, K.M.G., Deorkar, N., Brophy, G., Manufacturing Challenges and Rational Formulation Development for AAV Viral Vectors. *J. Pharm. Sci.*, *110*, 2609–2624, 2021, doi: 10.1016/j.xphs.2021.03.024.
49. Beattie, S., Facing Potential Chemistry, Manufacturing, & Control (CMC) Development Challenges with Recombinant Adeno-Associated Viral Vectors: Available Regulatory Guidance & Recommendations. *Cell Gene Ther. Insights*, *09*, 811–831, 2023, doi: 10.18609/cgti.2023.101.
50. Cameau, E. and Capone, J., Evolution of Culture Systems for Viral Vector Production: Advantages, Challenges and Cost Considerations. *Cell Gene Ther. Insights*, 6, 225–228, 2020, doi: 10.18609/cgti.2020.030.

11

Commercially Available Viral Vectors and Vaccines

Vasso Apostolopoulos[1]*, Pankti C. Balar[2], Arun Kumar Singh[3] and Vivek P. Chavda[4]

[1]School of Health and Biomedical Sciences, RMIT University, Bundoora, Melbourne, Australia
[2]Pharmacy Section, L.M. College of Pharmacy, Ahmedabad, Gujarat, India
[3]Amity Institute of Pharmacy, Amity University Greater Noida, Greater Noida, Uttar Pradesh, India
[4]Department of Pharmaceutics and Pharmaceutical Technology, L.M. College of Pharmacy, Ahmedabad, Gujarat, India

Abstract

The SARS-CoV-2 pandemic has spotlighted the urgent need for effective vaccine technologies against emerging pathogens. Viral vector vaccines, using recombinant viruses to deliver antigens, have emerged as a potent solution. Historically, viral vectors have evolved from pioneering studies in the 1980s, culminating in pivotal breakthroughs such as the development of the Ad5-based hepatitis B vaccine. However, it was the current pandemic that exemplified the rapid development of viral vector vaccines on a global scale. Adenovirus vectors like Ad5 and Ad26 have demonstrated remarkable efficacy against COVID-19, highlighting their scalability and impact. These vectors induce strong immune responses, laying a foundation for future vaccine strategies. Beyond COVID-19, other viral vectors such as vesicular stomatitis virus, flavivirus, measles virus, and poxvirus offer promising avenues for combating infectious diseases including dengue and Ebola which have also progressed to be approved for human use. All these highlight the important role of viral vector vaccines in addressing global health challenges.

***Keywords*:** Viral vectors, adenoviral vectors, vaccines, vaccine delivery, poxvirus vector, flavivirus vector, vesicular stomatitis vector, AdV

**Corresponding author*: vasso.apostolopoulos@rmit.edu.au

Vivek P. Chavda and Vasso Apostolopoulos (eds.) Viral Vectors for Vaccine Delivery, (341–356) © 2025 Scrivener Publishing LLC

11.1 Introduction

In 1983, an article was published describing the use of a "new" vaccine delivery system incorporating the hepatitis B surface antigen into a modified vaccinia virus [1]. This led to a publication in 1984 showing that live recombinant vaccinia virus protected chimpanzees against hepatitis B [2]. These two instrumental publications paved the way for a new era in vaccine design. Although initially prevalent in veterinary medicine, only five had progressed to human clinical trials and were licensed by 2020. These included (i) the ChimeriVax-JE in 2010 against Japanese encephalitis, (ii) CYD-TDV-Dengvaxis in 2015 against dengue virus, and three vaccines against Ebola being GamEvac-Combi in 2015, Ad5-EBOV in 2017, and VSV-EBOV in 2017 [3]. However, the landscape quickly shifted with the onset of the SARS-CoV-2 pandemic, leading to a surge in adenoviral vector vaccine development and administration, reaching billions of individuals worldwide, as discussed herein [4–7]. The widespread development of adenoviral vaccines globally provides valuable insights into their safety, immunogenicity, and efficacy, influencing the development of other viral vector vaccines approved for human use.

11.2 Viral Vector–Based Vaccines, Licensed for Humans

Adenoviruses, notably serotypes Ad5 and Ad26, serve as robust vaccine vectors due to their ability to effectively infect host cells, provoke a potent immune response, and facilitate large-scale production. Several prominent vaccines utilize these vectors, including Ad5-nCoV, Ad5-EBOV, Ad26.CoV2.S, Sputnik V, Sputnik Light, cAd3-EBO Z, and ChAdOx1-nCoV-19. Leveraging the inherent qualities of adenoviruses, these vaccines have demonstrated efficacy against various pathogens such as SARS-CoV-2 and Ebola virus. Their versatility and proven track record make them invaluable tools in the ongoing global efforts to combat infectious diseases (Figure 11.1) [4, 7, 8].

11.2.1 Adenovirus Vector Vaccines

Adenoviruses, particularly serotypes Ad5 and Ad26, are commonly used as vaccine vectors due to their efficient transduction of host cells, strong immunogenicity, and scalability.

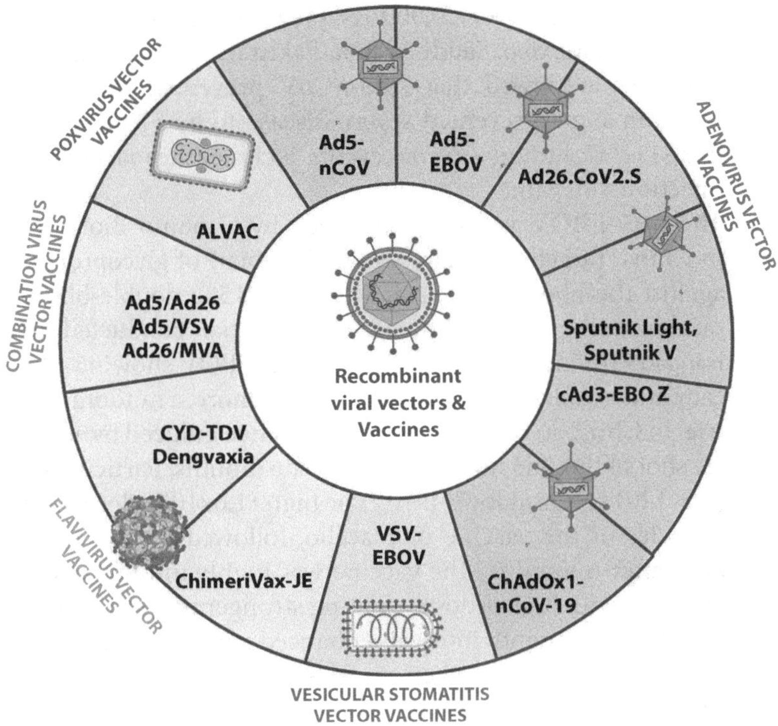

Figure 11.1 Schematic diagram of recombinant viral vectors and vaccines used in humans.

a. **The Ad5-nCoV vaccine,** also known as Convidecia, developed by CanSino Biologics in China [9, 10], targets the spike glycoprotein of SARS-CoV-2. A single dose is given intramuscularly and it is being used as an inhaled booster. In a phase 2 clinical trial, 108 participants were divided into three groups, receiving varying doses of the vaccine: low (5×10^{10}), middle (1×10^{11}), or high (1.5×10^{11}) viral particles. The vaccine showed good tolerability and elicited immune responses, with antibody responses observed by day 28 and T cell responses by day 14 [10]. In a randomized controlled clinical trial in Wuhan, China, the vaccine demonstrated significant immune responses, including specific antibodies and neutralizing antibodies, with minimal adverse reactions. Particularly, the 5×10^{10} viral particle dose exhibited both safety and efficacy, suggesting its potential as a viable single-dose COVID-19 immunization option [9]. Several phase 3 clinical trials in over 40,000 recipients were conducted in Argentina, Mexico, Saudi Arabia, Pakistan, and Russia. The global data showed that Ad5-nCoV prevented moderate symptoms and prevented severe disease to be 57.5% effective [11]. Common adverse events included headache and injection-site pain.

b. **The Ad5-EBOV vaccine**, developed by CanSino Biologics in China, targets the Zaire strain (Makona) of glycoprotein against the Ebola virus [12]. In 2014/2015, a double-blind, randomized phase 1 human clinical trial conducted in Jiangsu Province, China, evaluated Ad5-EBOV showing efficacy and no adverse effects [13]. Furthermore, a randomized trial in China assessed immune persistence induced by a single shot of the Ad5 Ebola vaccine over 6 months. Participants (n = 120) received low ($4x10^{10}$) or high ($1.6x10^{11}$) dose viral particles of the vaccine or placebo, followed by a booster dose after 6 months. The vaccine was highly immunogenic and safe, with higher doses eliciting stronger responses [12]. Boosting at 6-month intervals enhanced antibody responses, supporting durable protection strategies against Ebola. Ad5-EBOV received conditional approval from the European Commission in November 2019 and was granted prequalification status by the WHO in November 2019, signifying its efficacy and safety for use in preventing Ebola virus disease outbreaks.

c. **The Ad26.CoV2.S vaccine**, a recombinant Ad26 vector encoding SARS-CoV-2 spike protein, developed by Jansen Pharmaceutical Companies, was evaluated in a multi-center phase 1/2a clinical trial [14]. Administered in single or two doses to healthy adults, common mild adverse events were noted such as fatigue and headache, with fewer systemic reactions in older and low-dose recipients. High titers of neutralizing antibodies and T cell responses were shown, supporting the safety and immunogenicity of Ad26.CoV2.S for further development against COVID-19. Human phase 3 clinical trials with 43,000 participants showed 66% efficacy after one dose in preventing symptomatic COVID-19, with 85% efficacy against severe cases, and 100% efficacy against hospitalization or death [15]. Furthermore, in a double-blind phase 3 study with 31,300 participants, a booster dose showed an acceptable safety profile and effectiveness against severe-critical COVID-19 outcomes [16]. The FDA, EMA, and UK MHRA granted emergency or conditional authorization for the Janssen COVID-19 vaccine, but the FDA revoked its emergency use authorization in June 2023 at the manufacturer's request.

d. **The Sputnik Light vaccine** by Gamaleya Research Institute of Epidemiology and Microbiology in Russia, against SARS-CoV-2 Spike protein comprises the recombinant Ad26 vector carrying the SARS-CoV-2 spike glycoprotein gene, given as a single dose [17]. In a non-randomized phase 1/2 trial in Russia, the safety and immunogenicity were evaluated. Most adverse reactions were mild (66.4%), with no serious events reported. Sputnik Light stimulated strong humoral and cellular immune responses in both seronegative and seropositive individuals, with those who are seropositive showing even stronger responses [17]. These findings suggested Sputnik Light to be a promising candidate against the SARS-CoV-2 virus and are well-suited for areas with severe outbreaks, enabling rapid vaccination of more individuals. Additionally, it serves as a booster shot for those who received Sputnik V at least 6 months prior. By comparison, Sputnik V is a two-dose vaccine developed by the Gamaleya Research Institute of Epidemiology and Microbiology in Russia. It consists of two different adenovirus vectors (Ad5 and Ad26) administered in separate doses, given 21 days apart. Sputnik V has shown high efficacy in preventing COVID-19 infection. Sputnik Light efficacy is lower than the two-dose Sputnik V regimen [18]. Sputnik V was registered on 11 August 2020 by the Russian Ministry of Health, approved for distribution in Russian, and as of April 2021, it was approved for distribution in 59 countries.

e. The National Institute of Allergy and Infectious Diseases and Okairos, a biotechnology company for the development of vaccines acquired by GlaxoSmithKline in 2013, developed an Ebola vaccine using a chimpanzee adenovirus (cAd3) vector. The vaccine delivered Ebola Zaire genetic material (**cAd3-EBO Z**) and was proven to be safe and stimulated immune responses in phase 1 and phase 2 human clinical trials. The Sabin Vaccine Institute licensed the cAd3 platform to develop vaccines against the Sudan Ebola virus and Marburg viruses, with ongoing clinical trials for both.

f. **The ChAdOx1-nCoV-19 vaccine**, also known as Covishield or Vaxzevria, developed by the University of Oxford and AstraZeneca, targets the SARS-CoV-2 Spike protein with a tissue plasminogen leader sequence. Administered in a single-blind, randomized, controlled phase 2/3 trial, the vaccine includes a novel chimpanzee adenovirus vector, ChAdOx1, and is administered in a prime-boost regimen [19]. It was noted that ChAdOx1-nCoV-19 induced comparable immune responses, including anti-spike and anti-RBD antibodies, across all age groups, including older adults. This finding is significant given the heightened risk of severe disease in older individuals and addresses concerns regarding reduced immunogenicity with other adenoviral vaccines in this demographic. The vaccine received emergency use authorization in many countries worldwide, including the UK, the European Union, India, Brazil, and several others. The vaccine faced temporary suspensions in several countries due to concerns over rare blood clotting events, particularly cerebral venous sinus thrombosis, which prompted regulatory agencies to investigate its safety. These suspensions occurred at various times in early 2021, with countries such as Germany, France, Italy, Spain, and others pausing their use of the vaccine in March 2021 and in Australia in April 2021. However, after thorough reviews by regulatory agencies, many countries resumed administering the vaccine, often with updated guidance regarding its use, in particular to individuals over the age of 50 years. On 20 March 2023, Australia discontinued the use of Vaxzevria given its link to side effects. In the first week of May 2024, the European Union withdrew the marketing authorization of Vaxzevria given its high risk of rare cases of thrombosis with thrombocytopenia syndrome, accounting for 445 confirmed cases with 81 deaths.

11.2.2 Vesicular Stomatitis Virus Vector Vaccines

Vesicular Stomatitis Virus (VSV) vectors are known for their broad cell tropism and ability to induce strong immune responses. Derived from a naturally occurring virus that affects livestock and occasionally humans, VSV vectors have been evaluated and used for antigen delivery in vaccines [20].

The VSV-EBOV vaccine, also known as rVSV-ZEBOV or Ervebo, was initially developed by the Public Health Agency of Canada and later by Merck Inc. It targets the Ebola virus by encoding the glycoprotein of the Zaire strain [21]. A single intramuscular dose of rVSV-ZEBOV was administered to contacts and contacts of contacts in Guinea and Sierra Leone. Randomized clusters showed 100% vaccine efficacy, with no Ebola cases among immediately vaccinated individuals 10 days post-vaccination compared to 16 cases in delayed clusters. Non-randomized clusters also showed 100% efficacy. Most adverse events were mild, supporting rVSV-ZEBOV's efficacy in preventing Ebola virus disease [21]. The WHO prequalified the vaccine in less than 48 hours, marking its fastest process. It was approved for medical use in the EU in November 2019, and in the US in December 2019, Ervebo had its indication expanded by the FDA in July 2023 to include individuals >12 years.

11.2.3 Flavivirus Vector Vaccines

ChimeriVax-JE, also known as IMOJEV, is a vaccine developed by Sanofi Pasteur. It uses a chimeric technology to include the yellow fever virus as a vaccine vector (YF17D) and incorporates the viral envelope (prM and E) genes of the Japanese encephalitis virus strain SA14-14-2 [22]. In a randomized, double-blind study (n = 202), healthy adults received ChimeriVax-JE and placebo 28 days apart, with a subgroup receiving a ChimeriVax-JE booster after 6 months. Safety and antibodies persisted for up to 60 months [23]. Adverse events were comparable between ChimeriVax-JE and placebo groups, with few serious events. ChimeriVax-JE stimulates strong immune responses against Japanese encephalitis, providing protection against the disease [23]. It was approved by the United States Food and Drug Administration in 2009 and the European Medicines Agency in 2013.

YF17D vector has also been used in the CYD-TDV or Dengvaxia vaccine against dengue virus incorporating prM and E genes of DENV1-4, developed by Sanofi Pasteur [24, 25]. In a phase 3 human clinical trial, CYD-TDV vaccine efficacy was evaluated in children aged 2 to 14 in Asia-Pacific. Randomized to receive CYD-TDV or placebo at months 0, 6, and 12, 10,275 children were immunized. Vaccine efficacy against symptomatic, virologically confirmed dengue surpassed 25%, achieving 56.5% efficacy. Serious adverse events were comparable between vaccine and control groups, suggesting the vaccine's safety [24]. In another study, 20,869 healthy children receiving either vaccine or placebo showed that the efficacy against virologically confirmed dengue was 60.8%, and in the intention-to-treat group, it was 64.7%. Serotype-specific efficacy varied, ranging from 42.3

to 77.7%. Interestingly, severe virologically confirmed dengue cases were mostly observed in the control group, resulting in an efficacy of 95.5%. Additionally, the vaccine demonstrated efficacy in preventing hospitalization due to dengue at 80.3%. Importantly, the safety profile resembled that of the placebo, suggesting a favorable safety profile [25]. Dengvaxia vaccine is recommended for those with prior dengue infection or in regions where most individuals have been infected due to antibody-dependent enhancement. However, its use in non-immune populations may elevate the risk of severe dengue. Despite this, in 2017, over 733,000 children and 50,000 adults were vaccinated with Dengvaxia, irrespective of serostatus, sparking controversy. In December 2018, Dengvaxia was approved in the European Union and in the US in May 2019. QDENGA vaccine also known as TAK-003 or DENVax, against dengue virus, includes a modified vaccinia Ankara vector and is primarily used for non-immune individuals with strong and sustained immune responses generated [26]. It was approved in the European Union in 2022 for ages 4 and up and is also sanctioned in the UK, Thailand, Indonesia, Brazil, and Argentina. However, the US application in July 2023 was withdrawn due to the FDA's data request beyond the review cycle's scope.

11.2.4 Combination Virus Vectors: Ad5/Ad26

A combination of Ad5/Ad26 viral vectors is used in the Gam-COVID-Vac (Sputnik V) vaccines against SARS-CoV-2 spike protein, developed by Gamaleya Research Institute of Epidemiology and Microbiology, Russia [27]. A phase 3 clinical trial showed 91.6% efficacy against COVID-19. Conducted across 25 sites in Moscow, Russia, the double-blind, placebo-controlled trial enrolled 21,977 adults randomly allocated to either the vaccine or placebo. Two doses were given on day 1 and on day 21, and following the first dose, 16 of 14,964 (0.1%) vaccine recipients contracted COVID-19, compared to 62 of 4,902 (1.3%) in the placebo group. Adverse events were primarily mild, with few serious cases reported [27].

11.2.5 Combination Virus Vectors: Ad5/VSV

A combination of Ad5/VSV viral vectors is used in the GamEvac-Combi vaccine against Ebola virus glycoprotein, developed by Gamaleya Research Institute of Epidemiology and Microbiology, Russia [28]. In a dose-escalation clinical trial, 84 healthy adults aged 18 to 55 injected with GamEvac-Combi, in two doses, showed safety and immunogenicity. Common adverse events included injection site pain, with no serious adverse events. The seroconversion rate was 100%, with high antigen-specific IgG and neutralizing antibodies as well as strong T cell responses, suggesting long-term protection against Ebola.

11.2.6 Measles Virus Vector Vaccines

Measles virus vectors (MVAs) induce robust immune responses and can accommodate large genetic inserts. They have been evaluated as potential vaccines against HIV and cancer. However, Johnson & Johnson at its Janssen Pharmaceutical company developed a vaccine against the Ebola virus using a combination of Ad26/MVA viral vectors as delivery for antigens. The vaccines named Ad26.ZEBOV (Zabdeno) and MVA-BN-Filo (Mvabea) were evaluated in a phase 2 human clinical trial (EBOVAC2) in a randomized, observer-blind, participant-blind, and placebo-controlled design [29]. The regimen consists of two components with Ad26.ZEBOV as prime followed by a second vaccine boost of MVA-BN-Filo vaccine 8 weeks later. In this study, 423 participants aged 18 to 65 across four cohorts were enrolled. Vaccines were administered at varying intervals, and strong antibodies were induced which persisted for up to 1 year. The regimen demonstrated safety, tolerability, and immunogenicity, supporting its prophylactic use against Ebola virus. In May 2020, the European Union recommended marketing authorization for the combination Ad26.ZEBOV (Zabdeno) and MVA-BN-Filo (Mvabea) vaccines, noting that it is unsuitable for immediate outbreak response and recommended as an additional Ad26.ZEBOV booster for those at risk who had the regimen over four months prior, though human efficacy is still extrapolated from animal studies. It was approved for medical use in the European Union in July 2020.

11.2.7 Poxvirus Vector Vaccines

Modified vaccinia Ankara and canarypox virus (ALVAC) have gained interest as vaccine vectors due to their ability to accommodate large genetic inserts and elicit strong immune responses. Notably, Janssen's smallpox/monkeypox vaccine, using modified vaccinia Ankara, has been authorized for human use, demonstrating the efficacy and safety of poxvirus-based vaccines. Similarly, the HIV vaccine candidate RV144, which uses ALVAC, has advanced to human clinical trials, highlighting the potential of poxvirus vectors against infectious diseases.

11.3 Conclusion

Viral vector vaccines have emerged as potent stimulants of the immune system in combatting infectious diseases by using genetically engineered viruses. Adenovirus vectors (Ad5 and Ad26) are notable for their efficient host cell transduction and immunogenic outcomes. Vaccines such as Ad5-nCoV and Ad26.CoV2.S have demonstrated promising immune responses against COVID-19 in clinical trials. The Ad5-EBOV vaccine has shown efficacy against the Ebola virus, suggesting its potential for outbreak prevention. VSV vectors, as noted by the VSV-ZEBOV vaccine, have displayed high effectiveness in preventing Ebola virus disease. Similarly, yellow fever virus vectors, seen in vaccines like ChimeriVax-JE and CYD-TDV, have shown efficacy against Japanese encephalitis and dengue fever, respectively. Furthermore, some vaccines use a combination of viral vectors, as seen in Gam-COVID-Vac and GamEvac-Combi, with high efficacy rates against COVID-19 and Ebola virus. MVAs have also shown promise in vaccines against the Ebola virus when combined with the Ad26 viral vector. These vaccines hold promise in preventing a broad range of infectious diseases, offering effectiveness for global health security [30–33]. Continued research and development are pivotal in fully understanding the potential of viral vector vaccines in overcoming infectious diseases on a global scale. However, risk assessment is essential as viral vector–based vaccines may trigger antibody-dependent enhancement responses, increasing the risk of severe infection. Furthermore, they can result in uncommon yet significant adverse effects, such as blood clotting disorders, requiring thorough monitoring.

References

1. Smith, G.L., Mackett, M., Moss, B., Infectious vaccinia virus recombinants that express hepatitis B virus surface antigen. *Nature*, 302, 5908, 490–5, 1983.
2. Moss, B., Smith, G.L., Gerin, J.L., Purcell, R.H., Live recombinant vaccinia virus protects chimpanzees against hepatitis B. *Nature*, 311, 5981, 67–9, 1984.
3. McCann, N., O'Connor, D., Lambe, T., Pollard, A.J., Viral vector vaccines. *Curr. Opin. Immunol.*, 77, 102210, 2022.
4. Chavda, V.P., Bezbaruah, R., Athalye, M., Parikh, P.K., Chhipa, A.S., Patel, S., Apostolopoulos, V., Replicating Viral Vector-Based Vaccines for COVID-19: Potential Avenue in Vaccination Arena. *Viruses*, 14, 4, 759–780, 2022.

5. Chavda, V.P., Ghali, E., Balar, P.C., Chauhan, S.C., Tiwari, N., Shukla, S., Athalye, M., Patravale, V., Apostolopoulos, V., Yallapu, M.M., Protein subunit vaccines: Promising frontiers against COVID-19. *J. Control. Release*, 366, 761–782, 2024.
6. Chavda, V.P., Hossain, K.H., Beladiya, J., Apostolopoulos, V., Nucleic acid vaccines for COVID-19: a paradigm shift in the vaccine development arena. *Biologics*, 1, 3, 337–356, 2021.
7. Chavda, V.P., Kapadia, C., Soni, S., Prajapati, R., Chauhan, S.C., Yallapu, M.M., Apostolopoulos, V., A global picture: therapeutic perspectives for COVID-19. *Immunotherapy*, 14, 5, 351–371, 2022.
8. Chavda, V.P., Yao, Q., Vora, L.K., Apostolopoulos, V., Patel, C.A., Bezbaruah, R., Patel, A.B., Chen, Z.S., Fast-track development of vaccines for SARS-CoV-2: The shots that saved the world. *Front Immunol.*, 13, 961198, 2022.
9. Zhu, F.C., Guan, X.H., Li, Y.H., Huang, J.Y., Jiang, T., Hou, L.H., Li, J.X., Yang, B.F., Wang, L., Wang, W.J., Wu, S.P., Wang, Z., Wu, X.H., Xu, J.J., Zhang, Z., Jia, S.Y., Wang, B.S., Hu, Y., Liu, J.J., Zhang, J., Qian, X.A., Li, Q., Pan, H.X., Jiang, H.D., Deng, P., Gou, J.B., Wang, X.W., Wang, X.H., Chen, W., Immunogenicity and safety of a recombinant adenovirus type-5-vectored COVID-19 vaccine in healthy adults aged 18 years or older: a randomised, double-blind, placebo-controlled, phase 2 trial. *Lancet*, 396, 10249, 479–488, 2020.
10. Zhu, F.C., Li, Y.H., Guan, X.H., Hou, L.H., Wang, W.J., Li, J.X., Wu, S.P., Wang, B.S., Wang, Z., Wang, L., Jia, S.Y., Jiang, H.D., Wang, L., Jiang, T., Hu, Y., Gou, J.B., Xu, S.B., Xu, J.J., Wang, X.W., Wang, W., Chen, W., Safety, tolerability, and immunogenicity of a recombinant adenovirus type-5 vectored COVID-19 vaccine: a dose-escalation, open-label, non-randomised, first-in-human trial. *Lancet*, 395, 10240, 1845–1854, 2020.
11. Halperin, S.A., Ye, L., MacKinnon-Cameron, D., Smith, B., Cahn, P.E., Ruiz-Palacios, G.M., Ikram, A., Lanas, F., Lourdes Guerrero, M., Munoz Navarro, S.R., Sued, O., Lioznov, D.A., Dzutseva, V., Parveen, G., Zhu, F., Leppan, L., Langley, J.M., Barreto, L., Gou, J., Zhu, T., CanSino, C.-G.E.S.G., Final efficacy analysis, interim safety analysis, and immunogenicity of a single dose of recombinant novel coronavirus vaccine (adenovirus type 5 vector) in adults 18 years and older: an international, multicentre, randomised, double-blinded, placebo-controlled phase 3 trial. *Lancet*, 399, 10321, 237–248, 2022.
12. Li, J.X., Hou, L.H., Meng, F.Y., Wu, S.P., Hu, Y.M., Liang, Q., Chu, K., Zhang, Z., Xu, J.J., Tang, R., Wang, W.J., Liu, P., Hu, J.L., Luo, L., Jiang, R., Zhu, F.C., Chen, W., Immunity duration of a recombinant adenovirus type-5 vector-based Ebola vaccine and a homologous prime-boost immunisation in healthy adults in China: final report of a randomised, double-blind, placebo-controlled, phase 1 trial. *Lancet Glob Health*, 5, 3, e324–e334, 2017.
13. Zhu, F.C., Hou, L.H., Li, J.X., Wu, S.P., Liu, P., Zhang, G.R., Hu, Y.M., Meng, F.Y., Xu, J.J., Tang, R., Zhang, J.L., Wang, W.J., Duan, L., Chu, K., Liang, Q.,

Hu, J.L., Luo, L., Zhu, T., Wang, J.Z., Chen, W., Safety and immunogenicity of a novel recombinant adenovirus type-5 vector-based Ebola vaccine in healthy adults in China: preliminary report of a randomised, double-blind, placebo-controlled, phase 1 trial. *Lancet*, 385, 9984, 2272–9, 2015.

14. Sadoff, J., Le Gars, M., Shukarev, G., Heerwegh, D., Truyers, C., de Groot, A.M., Stoop, J., Tete, S., Van Damme, W., Leroux-Roels, I., Berghmans, P.J., Kimmel, M., Van Damme, P., de Hoon, J., Smith, W., Stephenson, K.E., De Rosa, S.C., Cohen, K.W., McElrath, M.J., Cormier, E., Scheper, G., Barouch, D.H., Hendriks, J., Struyf, F., Douoguih, M., Van Hoof, J., Schuitemaker, H., Interim Results of a Phase 1-2a Trial of Ad26.COV2.S Covid-19 Vaccine. *N. Engl. J. Med.*, 384, 19, 1824–1835, 2021.
15. Sadoff, J., Gray, G., Vandebosch, A., Cardenas, V., Shukarev, G., Grinsztejn, B., Goepfert, P.A., Truyers, C., Fennema, H., Spiessens, B., Offergeld, K., Scheper, G., Taylor, K.L., Robb, M.L., Treanor, J., Barouch, D.H., Stoddard, J., Ryser, M.F., Marovich, M.A., Neuzil, K.M., Corey, L., Cauwenberghs, N., Tanner, T., Hardt, K., Ruiz-Guinazu, J., Le Gars, M., Schuitemaker, H., Van Hoof, J., Struyf, F., Douoguih, M., Group, E.S., Safety and Efficacy of Single-Dose Ad26.COV2.S Vaccine against Covid-19. *N. Engl. J. Med.*, 384, 23, 2187–2201, 2021.
16. Hardt, K., Vandebosch, A., Sadoff, J., Le Gars, M., Truyers, C., Lowson, D., Van Dromme, I., Vingerhoets, J., Kamphuis, T., Scheper, G., Ruiz-Guinazu, J., Faust, S.N., Spinner, C.D., Schuitemaker, H., Van Hoof, J., Douoguih, M., Struyf, F., E.s. group, Efficacy, safety, and immunogenicity of a booster regimen of Ad26.COV2.S vaccine against COVID-19 (ENSEMBLE2): results of a randomised, double-blind, placebo-controlled, phase 3 trial. *Lancet Infect Dis.*, 22, 12, 1703–1715, 2022.
17. Tukhvatulin, A.I., Dolzhikova, I.V., Shcheblyakov, D.V., Zubkova, O.V., Dzharullaeva, A.S., Kovyrshina, A.V., Lubenets, N.L., Grousova, D.M., Erokhova, A.S., Botikov, A.G., Izhaeva, F.M., Popova, O., Ozharovskaia, T.A., Esmagambetov, I.B., Favorskaya, I.A., Zrelkin, D.I., Voronina, D.V., Shcherbinin, D.N., Semikhin, A.S., Simakova, Y.V., Tokarskaya, E.A., Shmarov, M.M., Nikitenko, N.A., Gushchin, V.A., Smolyarchuk, E.A., Zubkova, T.G., Zakharov, K.A., Vasilyuk, V.B., Borisevich, S.V., Naroditsky, B.S., Logunov, D.Y., Gintsburg, A.L., An open, non-randomised, phase 1/2 trial on the safety, tolerability, and immunogenicity of single-dose vaccine "Sputnik Light" for prevention of coronavirus infection in healthy adults. *Lancet Reg. Health Eur.*, 11, 100241, 2021.
18. Akrami, M., Hosamirudsari, H., Faraji, N., Behnush, B., Goudarzi, F., Hesari, E., Akbarpour, S., Najafi, A., Nateghi, S., Sputnik V vaccine-related complications and its impression on inflammatory biomarkers in healthcare providers. *Indian J. Med. Microbiol.*, 43, 79–84, 2023.
19. Ramasamy, M.N., Minassian, A.M., Ewer, K.J., Flaxman, A.L., Folegatti, P.M., Owens, D.R., Voysey, M., Aley, P.K., Angus, B., Babbage, G., Belij-Rammerstorfer, S., Berry, L., Bibi, S., Bittaye, M., Cathie, K., Chappell, H.,

Charlton, S., Cicconi, P., Clutterbuck, E.A., Colin-Jones, R., Dold, C., Emary, K.R.W., Fedosyuk, S., Fuskova, M., Gbesemete, D., Green, C., Hallis, B., Hou, M.M., Jenkin, D., Joe, C.C.D., Kelly, E.J., Kerridge, S., Lawrie, A.M., Lelliott, A., Lwin, M.N., Makinson, R., Marchevsky, N.G., Mujadidi, Y., Munro, A.P.S., Pacurar, M., Plested, E., Rand, J., Rawlinson, T., Rhead, S., Robinson, H., Ritchie, A.J., Ross-Russell, A.L., Saich, S., Singh, N., Smith, C.C., Snape, M.D., Song, R., Tarrant, R., Themistocleous, Y., Thomas, K.M., Villafana, T.L., Warren, S.C., Watson, M.E.E., Douglas, A.D., Hill, A.V.S., Lambe, T., Gilbert, S.C., Faust, S.N., Pollard, A.J., Oxford, C.V.T.G., Safety and immunogenicity of ChAdOx1 nCoV-19 vaccine administered in a prime-boost regimen in young and old adults (COV002): a single-blind, randomised, controlled, phase 2/3 trial. *Lancet*, 396, 10267, 1979–1993, 2021.

20. Suder, E., Furuyama, W., Feldmann, H., Marzi, A., de Wit, E., The vesicular stomatitis virus-based Ebola virus vaccine: From concept to clinical trials. *Hum. Vaccin. Immunother.*, 14, 9, 2107–2113, 2018.
21. Henao-Restrepo, A.M., Camacho, A., Longini, I.M., Watson, C.H., Edmunds, W.J., Egger, M., Carroll, M.W., Dean, N.E., Diatta, I., Doumbia, M., Draguez, B., Duraffour, S., Enwere, G., Grais, R., Gunther, S., Gsell, P.S., Hossmann, S., Watle, S.V., Konde, M.K., Keita, S., Kone, S., Kuisma, E., Levine, M.M., Mandal, S., Mauget, T., Norheim, G., Riveros, X., Soumah, A., Trelle, S., Vicari, A.S., Rottingen, J.A., Kieny, M.P., Efficacy and effectiveness of an rVSV-vectored vaccine in preventing Ebola virus disease: final results from the Guinea ring vaccination, open-label, cluster-randomised trial (Ebola Ca Suffit!). *Lancet*, 389, 10068, 505–518, 2017.
22. Monath, T.P., Seligman, S.J., Robertson, J.S., Guy, B., Hayes, E.B., Condit, R.C., Excler, J.L., Mac, L.M., Carbery, B., Chen, R.T., Brighton Collaboration Viral Vector Vaccines Safety Working, G., Live virus vaccines based on a yellow fever vaccine backbone: standardized template with key considerations for a risk/benefit assessment. *Vaccine*, 33, 1, 62–72, 2015.
23. Nasveld, P.E., Ebringer, A., Elmes, N., Bennett, S., Yoksan, S., Aaskov, J., McCarthy, K., Kanesa-thasan, N., Meric, C., Reid, M., Long term immunity to live attenuated Japanese encephalitis chimeric virus vaccine: randomized, double-blind, 5-year phase II study in healthy adults. *Hum. Vaccin.*, 6, 12, 1038–46, 2010.
24. Capeding, M.R., Tran, N.H., Hadinegoro, S.R., Ismail, H.I., Chotpitayasunondh, T., Chua, M.N., Luong, C.Q., Rusmil, K., Wirawan, D.N., Nallusamy, R., Pitisuttithum, P., Thisyakorn, U., Yoon, I.K., van der Vliet, D., Langevin, E., Laot, T., Hutagalung, Y., Frago, C., Boaz, M., Wartel, T.A., Tornieporth, N.G., Saville, M., Bouckenooghe, A., C.Y.D.S. Group, Clinical efficacy and safety of a novel tetravalent dengue vaccine in healthy children in Asia: a phase 3, randomised, observer-masked, placebo-controlled trial. *Lancet*, 384, 9951, 1358–65, 2014.
25. Villar, L., Dayan, G.H., Arredondo-Garcia, J.L., Rivera, D.M., Cunha, R., Deseda, C., Reynales, H., Costa, M.S., Morales-Ramirez, J.O., Carrasquilla,

G., Rey, L.C., Dietze, R., Luz, K., Rivas, E., Miranda Montoya, M.C., Cortes Supelano, M., Zambrano, B., Langevin, E., Boaz, M., Tornieporth, N., Saville, M., Noriega, F., Group, C.Y.D.S., Efficacy of a tetravalent dengue vaccine in children in Latin America. *N. Engl. J. Med.*, 372, 2, 113–23, 2015.

26. Biswal, S., Reynales, H., Saez-Llorens, X., Lopez, P., Borja-Tabora, C., Kosalaraksa, P., Sirivichayakul, C., Watanaveeradej, V., Rivera, L., Espinoza, F., Fernando, L., Dietze, R., Luz, K., Venancio da Cunha, R., Jimeno, J., Lopez-Medina, E., Borkowski, A., Brose, M., Rauscher, M., LeFevre, I., Bizjajeva, S., Bravo, L., Wallace, D., Group, T.S., Efficacy of a Tetravalent Dengue Vaccine in Healthy Children and Adolescents. *N. Engl. J. Med.*, 381, 21, 2009–2019, 2019.
27. Logunov, D.Y., Dolzhikova, I.V., Shcheblyakov, D.V., Tukhvatulin, A.I., Zubkova, O.V., Dzharullaeva, A.S., Kovyrshina, A.V., Lubenets, N.L., Grousova, D.M., Erokhova, A.S., Botikov, A.G., Izhaeva, F.M., Popova, O., Ozharovskaya, T.A., Esmagambetov, I.B., Favorskaya, I.A., Zrelkin, D.I., Voronina, D.V., Shcherbinin, D.N., Semikhin, A.S., Simakova, Y.V., Tokarskaya, E.A., Egorova, D.A., Shmarov, M.M., Nikitenko, N.A., Gushchin, V.A., Smolyarchuk, E.A., Zyryanov, S.K., Borisevich, S.V., Naroditsky, B.S., Gintsburg, A.L., Gam, C.-V.V.T.G., Safety and efficacy of an rAd26 and rAd5 vector-based heterologous prime-boost COVID-19 vaccine: an interim analysis of a randomised controlled phase 3 trial in Russia. *Lancet*, 397, 10275, 671–681, 2021.
28. Dolzhikova, I.V., Zubkova, O.V., Tukhvatulin, A.I., Dzharullaeva, A.S., Tukhvatulina, N.M., Shcheblyakov, D.V., Shmarov, M.M., Tokarskaya, E.A., Simakova, Y.V., Egorova, D.A., Scherbinin, D.N., Tutykhina, I.L., Lysenko, A.A., Kostarnoy, A.V., Gancheva, P.G., Ozharovskaya, T.A., Belugin, B.V., Kolobukhina, L.V., Pantyukhov, V.B., Syromyatnikova, S.I., Shatokhina, I.V., Sizikova, T.V., Rumyantseva, I.G., Andrus, A.F., Boyarskaya, N.V., Voytyuk, A.N., Babira, V.F., Volchikhina, S.V., Kutaev, D.A., Bel'skih, A.N., Zhdanov, K.V., Zakharenko, S.M., Borisevich, S.V., Logunov, D.Y., Naroditsky, B.S., Gintsburg, A.L., Safety and immunogenicity of GamEvac-Combi, a heterologous VSV- and Ad5-vectored Ebola vaccine: An open phase I/II trial in healthy adults in Russia. *Hum. Vaccin. Immunother.*, 13, 3, 613–620, 2017.
29. Pollard, A.J., Launay, O., Lelievre, J.D., Lacabaratz, C., Grande, S., Goldstein, N., Robinson, C., Gaddah, A., Bockstal, V., Wiedemann, A., Leyssen, M., Luhn, K., Richert, L., Betard, C., Gibani, M.M., Clutterbuck, E.A., Snape, M.D., Levy, Y., Douoguih, M., Thiebaut, R., E.E.s. group, Safety and immunogenicity of a two-dose heterologous Ad26.ZEBOV and MVA-BN-Filo Ebola vaccine regimen in adults in Europe (EBOVAC2): a randomised, observer-blind, participant-blind, placebo-controlled, phase 2 trial. *Lancet, Infect Dis.*, 21, 4, 493–506, 2021.
30. Chavda, V.P., Apostolopoulos, V., Sah, R., Langya henipavirus outbreak. *Expert Rev. Anti Infect. Ther.*, 21, 10, 1021–1024, 2023.

31. Chavda, V.P., Patel, K., Apostolopoulos, V., Tomato flu outbreak in India. *Lancet Respir. Med.*, 11, 1, e1–e2, 2023.
32. Chavda, V.P., Vora, L.K., Apostolopoulos, V., Monkeypox: a new face of outbreak. *Expert Rev. Vaccines*, 21, 11, 1537–1540, 2022.
33. Srivastava, S., Kumar, S., Chinnam, S., Srivastava, N., Mehta, R., Mohanty, A., Sah, S., Feehan, J., de Courten, M., Apostolopoulos, V., Sah, R., Mosquito-borne ross river virus: A raising concern in Queensland. *Travel Med. Infect. Dis.*, 59, 102723, 2024.

12

Emerging Viral-Vector Technologies: Future Potential

Vasso Apostolopoulos[1]*, Pankti C. Balar[2] and Vivek P. Chavda[3]

[1]*School of Health and Biomedical Sciences, RMIT University, Bundoora, Melbourne, Australia*
[2]*Pharmacy Section, L.M. College of Pharmacy, Ahmedabad, Gujarat, India*
[3]*Department of Pharmaceutics and Pharmaceutical Technology, L.M. College of Pharmacy, Ahmedabad, Gujarat, India*

Abstract
Leveraging a variety of viral platforms, emerging viral vector–based vaccines are reshaping immunization strategies. Using vectors such as influenza, adeno-associated, HSV-1, retrovirus, Zika, alpha, and Epstein-Barr viruses, these technologies hold promise for advancing vaccine development. Approved for human use, adenovirus, vesicular stomatitis virus (VSV), poxvirus, flavivirus, and measles virus–based vaccines demonstrate efficacy and safety. Adenovirus vectors, including Ad26 and Ad5, deliver genetic material for targeted immune activation. VSV vectors show promise against Ebola and SARS-CoV-2. Poxvirus-based vaccines combat infectious diseases. Flavivirus platforms, exemplified by the dengue vaccine, offer broad protection. Measles virus vectors demonstrate versatility in delivering antigens. Viral vector–based vaccines are paving the way for a new era in preventive strategies against diseases.

***Keywords*:** Adenovirus vector, viral vectors, vaccine, delivery, Ad26, Ad5, vesicular stomatitis virus vector, poxvirus vector

**Corresponding author*: vasso.apostolopoulos@rmit.edu.au

Vivek P. Chavda and Vasso Apostolopoulos (eds.) Viral Vectors for Vaccine Delivery, (357–364)

12.1 Introduction

The emergence of new viral threats has expedited diverse vaccine development, with viral vector vaccines emerging as a significant option. With the advent of the COVID-19 pandemic, several technologies were used to develop vaccines [1–6]. Viral vector vaccines have emerged as powerful antigen delivery systems, stimulating antibody and T cell response to protect against infectious diseases using genetically engineered viruses. Among these, adenovirus vectors, particularly Ad5 and Ad26, are notable for their efficient transduction of host cells and strong immunogenicity. Clinical trials of vaccines using these vectors, such as Ad5-nCoV and Ad26.CoV2.S, have shown promising stimulation of antibody and T cell responses against COVID-19. Likewise, the Ad5 vector in the Ad5-EBOV vaccine has demonstrated efficacy against the Ebola virus. The vesicular stomatitis virus (VSV) vector is also significant due to its ability to elicit strong immune responses. Modified to carry genes from target pathogens, it promotes immunity without causing disease, as evidenced by the high effectiveness of the VSV-ZEBOV vaccine against Ebola virus disease. Likewise, yellow fever virus vectors have been successfully used in ChimeriVax-JE for Japanese encephalitis and CYD-TDV for dengue fever, showing protective efficacy in human clinical trials. Combining viral vectors can further enhance immune activation and protection. For instance, Gam-COVID-Vac and GamEvac-Combi have demonstrated notable efficacy against COVID-19 and Ebola virus, respectively [7]. Measles virus vectors have also shown promise when combined with Ad26 vectors in Ebola virus vaccines. These vaccines represent significant advancements in preventing a wide array of infectious diseases, contributing to global health security (details are presented in Chapter 13) (Figure 12.1). However, ongoing research and development are essential to fully realize the potential of viral vector vaccines in combating infectious diseases worldwide.

12.2 New Emerging Viral Vectors for Vaccines

Viral vector vaccines, using adenovirus vectors (Ad5 and Ad26), VSV, yellow fever, poxvirus, and measles virus vectors, effectively stimulate strong and effective immune responses against pathogens such as SARS-CoV-2, Ebola, and smallpox. This innovative technology is vital for advancing global vaccine development and addressing a wide range of infectious diseases [8]. As research and refinement continue, the potential applications of viral vector vaccines are vast and promising, extending to other infectious diseases, including emerging pathogens and those causing seasonal outbreaks [9–13]. In addition, viral vector–based vaccines have shown promise in other conditions, including cancer immunotherapy and genetic disorders. Engineering viruses to deliver tumor-specific antigens have shown encouraging results in human clinical trials, with some patients experiencing tumor regression and prolonged survival. As such, viral vectors, including adenovirus, adeno-associated virus, herpes simplex virus, and retrovirus, hold promise for gene therapy in cancer treatment, as summarized in [14] (Figure 12.1). Despite challenges in gene delivery, viral vectors offer efficient transduction of target cells and are currently prominent in preclinical and clinical trials. Furthermore, viral vectors can be engineered to target particular cell types or tissues, paving the way for targeted gene therapy and regenerative medicine. Adeno-associated virus vectors can deliver therapeutic genes to for genetic disorders such as hemophilia and muscular dystrophy. As our understanding of viral biology and gene delivery mechanisms progresses, the potential for viral-vectored therapies to address a range of genetic and acquired diseases will expand exponentially. Regarding vaccines, adeno-associated virus vectors show

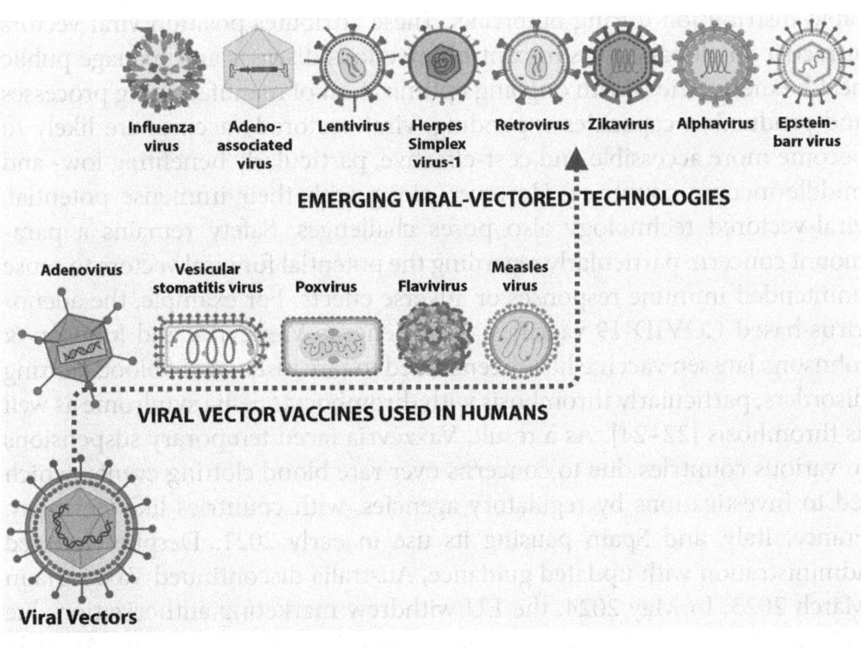

Figure 12.1 Schematic diagram of viral vectors used in vaccines in humans and emerging viral-vectored technologies.

promising features for their use in vaccines since they have low immunogenicity and efficient transduction of several cell types [15]. Such vectors have been studied in animal models and human clinical studies targeting influenza virus, HIV, and SARS-CoV-2. Their ability to stimulate immune responses shows safety in early studies, positioning adeno-associated vectors as adaptable platforms for next-generation vaccines. Other emerging viral vectors include reovirus, alphavirus, Zika virus, gamma retrovirus, Epstein-Barr virus, lentivirus [14], and influenza virus vectors [16–18] (Figure 12.1). Viral-vectored technology has applications in agriculture, where it could be used to develop vaccines for livestock diseases [19], improving animal health while protecting food security [20, 21].

12.3 Viral Vector Vaccines: What is Good and What is Not So Good

The continuous advancement of viral vectors holds promise for enhancing global health security and improving disease prevention and treatment strategies worldwide. In addition, viral-vectored vaccines provide several advantages, such as scalability, ease of production, and the capability for rapid distribution during outbreaks. These attributes position viral vectors attractive in global efforts to control infectious diseases and manage public health emergencies. With ongoing optimization of manufacturing processes and production capacities expanding, viral-vectored vaccines are likely to become more accessible and cost-effective, particularly benefiting low- and middle-income countries. However, along with their immense potential, viral-vectored technology also poses challenges. Safety remains a paramount concern, particularly regarding the potential for viral vectors to cause unintended immune responses or adverse effects. For example, the adenovirus-based COVID-19 vaccines, AstraZeneca's Vaxzevria, and Johnson & Johnson's Janssen vaccine have been linked to rare instances of blood clotting disorders, particularly thrombosis with thrombocytopenia syndrome as well as thrombosis [22–24]. As a result, Vaxzevria faced temporary suspensions in various countries due to concerns over rare blood clotting events, which led to investigations by regulatory agencies, with countries like Germany, France, Italy, and Spain pausing its use in early 2021. Despite resumed administration with updated guidance, Australia discontinued Vaxzevria in March 2023. In May 2024, the EU withdrew marketing authorization due to its association with rare thrombosis cases, including 81 deaths. As such, the risks and benefits of each viral vector platform need to be assessed thoroughly and strategies designed to mitigate potential safety concerns.

12.4 Conclusion

In conclusion, viral vector technology holds promise for revolutionizing vaccine development, as well as gene therapy, and disease prevention worldwide. While offering several advantages, safety concerns must be carefully addressed to maximize their potential in managing infectious diseases as well as other diseases and advancing public health initiatives.

References

1. Chavda, V.P., Yao, Q., Vora, L.K., Apostolopoulos, V., Patel, C.A., Bezbaruah, R., Patel, A.B., Chen, Z.S., Fast-track development of vaccines for SARS-CoV-2: The shots that saved the world. *Front. Immunol.*, 13, 961198, 2022.
2. Chavda, V.P., Kapadia, C., Soni, S., Prajapati, R., Chauhan, S.C., Yallapu, M.M., Apostolopoulos, V., A global picture: therapeutic perspectives for COVID-19. *Immunotherapy*, 14, 5, 351–371, 2022.
3. Chavda, V.P., Hossain, K.H., Beladiya, J., Apostolopoulos, V., Nucleic acid vaccines for COVID-19: a paradigm shift in the vaccine development arena. *Biologics*, 1, 3, 337–356, 2021.
4. Chavda, V.P., Ghali, E., Balar, P.C., Chauhan, S.C., Tiwari, N., Shukla, S., Athalye, M., Patravale, V., Apostolopoulos, V., Yallapu, M.M., Protein subunit vaccines: Promising frontiers against COVID-19. *J. Control. Release*, 366, 761–782, 2024.
5. Chavda, V.P. and Apostolopoulos, V., Mosaic receptor binding domain nanoparticles: towards fourth-generation vaccination. *Nanomed. (Lond)*, 18, 19, 1223–1226, 2023.
6. Chavda, V.P. and Apostolopoulos, V., COVID-19 vaccine design and vaccination strategy for emerging variants. *Expert Rev. Vaccines*, 21, 10, 1359–1361, 2022.
7. Pollard, A.J., Launay, O., Lelievre, J.D., Lacabaratz, C., Grande, S., Goldstein, N., Robinson, C., Gaddah, A., Bockstal, V., Wiedemann, A., Leyssen, M., Luhn, K., Richert, L., Betard, C., Gibani, M.M., Clutterbuck, E.A., Snape, M.D., Levy, Y., Douoguih, M., Thiebaut, R., E.E.s. group, Safety and immunogenicity of a two-dose heterologous Ad26.ZEBOV and MVA-BN-Filo Ebola vaccine regimen in adults in Europe (EBOVAC2): a randomised, observer-blind, participant-blind, placebo-controlled, phase 2 trial. *Lancet Infect. Dis.*, 21, 4, 493–506, 2021.
8. Chavda, V.P., Bezbaruah, R., Athalye, M., Parikh, P.K., Chhipa, A.S., Patel, S., Apostolopoulos, V., Replicating Viral Vector-Based Vaccines for COVID-19: Potential Avenue in Vaccination Arena. *Viruses*, 14, 4, 759–779, 2022.

9. Chavda, V., Bezbaruah, R., Kalita, T., Sarma, A., Devi, J.R., Bania, R., Apostolopoulos, V., Variant influenza: connecting the missing dots. *Expert Rev. Anti Infect. Ther.*, 20, 12, 1567–1585, 2022.
10. Chavda, V.P., Apostolopoulos, V., Sah, R., Langya henipavirus outbreak. *Expert Rev. Anti Infect Ther.*, 21, 10, 1021–1024, 2023.
11. Chavda, V.P., Patel, K., Apostolopoulos, V., Tomato flu outbreak in India. *Lancet Respir. Med.*, 11, 1, e1–e2, 2023.
12. Chavda, V.P., Vora, L.K., Apostolopoulos, V., Monkeypox: a new face of outbreak. *Expert Rev. Vaccines*, 21, 11, 1537–1540, 2022.
13. Srivastava, S., Kumar, S., Chinnam, S., Srivastava, N., Mehta, R., Mohanty, A., Sah, S., Feehan, J., de Courten, M., Apostolopoulos, V., Sah, R., Mosquito-borne ross river virus: A raising concern in Queensland. *Travel Med. Infect. Dis.*, 59, 102723, 2024.
14. Xie, L., Han, Y., Liu, Y., Zhou, Y., Yu, J., von Brunn, A., Lei, J., Viral vector-based cancer treatment and current clinical applications. *MedComm-Oncology*, 2, 4, e55, 2023.
15. Zhao, L., Yang, Z., Zheng, M., Shi, L., Gu, M., Liu, G., Miao, F., Chang, Y., Huang, F., Tang, N., Recombinant adeno-associated virus 8 vector in gene therapy: Opportunities and challenges. *Genes Dis.*, 11, 1, 283–293, 2024.
16. Mailybayeva, A., Ryskeldinova, S., Zinina, N., Zhou, E.M., Renukaradhya, G.J., Tabynov, K., Evaluation of Duration of Immunogenicity and Protective Efficacy of Improved Influenza Viral Vector-Based Brucella abortus Vaccine Against Brucella melitensis Infection in Sheep and Goats. *Front. Vet. Sci.*, 7, 58, 2020.
17. Mailybayeva, A., Yespembetov, B., Ryskeldinova, S., Zinina, N., Sansyzbay, A., Renukaradhya, G.J., Petrovsky, N., Tabynov, K., Improved influenza viral vector based Brucella abortus vaccine induces robust B and T-cell responses and protection against Brucella melitensis infection in pregnant sheep and goats. *PLoS One*, 12, 10, e0186484, 2017.
18. Tabynov, K., Influenza viral vector based Brucella abortus vaccine: a novel vaccine candidate for veterinary practice. *Expert Rev. Vaccines*, 15, 10, 1237–9, 2016.
19. Ryskeldinova, S., Zinina, N., Kydyrbayev, Z., Yespembetov, B., Kozhamkulov, Y., Inkarbekov, D., Assanzhanova, N., Mailybayeva, A., Bugybayeva, D., Sarmykova, M., Khairullin, B., Tabynov, K., Bulashev, A., Aitzhanov, B., Abeuov, K., Sansyzbay, A., Yespolov, T., Renukaradhya, G.J., Olsen, S., Onate, A., Tabynov, K., Registered Influenza Viral Vector Based Brucella abortus Vaccine for Cattle in Kazakhstan: Age-Wise Safety and Efficacy Studies. *Front. Cell. Infect. Microbiol.*, 11, 669196, 2021.
20. Brun, A., Albina, E., Barret, T., Chapman, D.A., Czub, M., Dixon, L.K., Keil, G.M., Klonjkowski, B., Le Potier, M.F., Libeau, G., Ortego, J., Richardson, J., Takamatsu, H.H., Antigen delivery systems for veterinary vaccine development. Viral-vector based delivery systems. *Vaccine*, 26, 51, 6508–28, 2008.

21. Chavda, V.P., Feehan, J., Apostolopoulos, V., A Veterinary Vaccine for SARS-CoV-2: The First COVID-19 Vaccine for Animals. *Vaccines (Basel)*, 9, 6, 631–633, 2021.
22. Al-Ansari, R.Y., Al Qahtany, F.H., Qomawi, Y., Fadoul, T., Woodman, A., Severe thrombocytopenia after Vaxzevria vaccination in a single patient: A case report. *SAGE Open Med. Case Rep.*, 10, 2050313X221091407, 2022.
23. Lane, S. and Shakir, S., Assessing Case Fatality on Cases of Thrombosis with Concurrent Thrombocytopenia Following COVID-19 Vaccine AstraZeneca (Vaxzevria) in the United Kingdom: A Review of Spontaneously Reported Data. *Drug Saf.*, 45, 9, 1003–1008, 2022.
24. Shivarev, A., Phillips, A., Brophy-Williams, S., Ford, T., Richmond, P., Effler, P., McLean-Tooke, A., Adverse event reports of anaphylaxis after Comirnaty and Vaxzevria COVID-19 vaccinations, Western Australia, 22 February to 30 June 2021. *Intern Med. J.*, 53, 2, 275–279, 2023.

Index

Printed in the USA/Agawam, MA
September 18, 2026

910661.114